Health in a
Fragile State

Africa and the Diaspora:
History, Politics, Culture

Edited by
Thomas Spear, Neil Kodesh,
Tejumola Olaniyan, Michael G. Schatzberg,
and James H. Sweet

HEALTH IN A FRAGILE STATE

Science, Sorcery, and Spirit in the Lower Congo

John M. Janzen

THE UNIVERSITY OF WISCONSIN PRESS

The University of Wisconsin Press
728 State Street, Suite 443
Madison, Wisconsin 53706
uwpress.wisc.edu

Gray's Inn House, 127 Clerkenwell Road
London ECIR 5DB, United Kingdom
eurospanbookstore.com

Printed in the United States of America
This book may be available in a digital edition.

Library of Congress Cataloging-in-Publication Data

Names: Janzen, John M., author.
Title: Health in a fragile state : science, sorcery, and spirit in the
Lower Congo / John M. Janzen.
Other titles: Africa and the diaspora.
Description: Madison, Wisconsin : The University of Wisconsin Press, [2019] |
Series: Africa and the diaspora: history, politics, culture |
Includes bibliographical references and index.
Identifiers: LCCN 2019008136 | ISBN 9780299325008 (cloth)
Subjects: LCSH: Medical care—Congo (Democratic Republic)—Luozi. | Public
health—Congo (Democratic Republic)—Luozi. | Medical anthropology—
Congo (Democratic Republic)—Luozi. | Public health—
Anthropological aspects—Congo (Democratic Republic)—Luozi.
Classification: LCC RA552.C75 J36 2019 | DDC 362.1096751—dc23
LC record available at https://lccn.loc.gov/2019008136

ISBN 9780299325046 (pbk.)

Nsi vo yitomuna beto tuna zinga, kansi vo nsi kayeti toma ko, beto i mpila mpasi mu toma zinga [If the land thrives, we will live; but, if the land doesn't thrive, we will have difficulty improving our lives].

—Mama Luezi Mbambi Jacqueline, grandmother of twenty-six, household head, Janzen intensive sample interview, 2013

CONTENTS

ILLUSTRATIONS

MAPS

TABLES

PREFACE AND
ACKNOWLEDGMENTS

A few comments on Equatorial African naming practices and conventions will assist the reader in following the references to persons and places in this book. Individual Congolese names reflect personal preferences, changing conventions due to custom, colonial impositions, and postcolonial ideologies. The result is a great deal of variation in the manner in which people use names. In this book I introduce individuals on first mention with their full titles and names, and in parentheses, the abbreviated name or names that appear throughout the book. In many cases I use the honorific prefixes *Tata* (father) and *Mama* (mother) commonly used in face-to-face conversation, especially when a junior is addressing a senior figure. *Mbuta* (elder) is also sometimes used, although its counterpart *nleke* (junior) is not so common. The campaign for authenticity, inaugurated in the late 1960s by President Mobutu Sese Seko, required the abandonment of Christian or Western names and encouraged the use of ancestral or ascending generation names. Some individuals retained the use of such additional names after the waning of the ideology of authenticity. Others reclaimed their Christian or Western names, placing them sometimes before, sometimes after, their "authentic" names.

Place-names also reflect historical convention, outside imposed wording, particular phonetic practices, and random variations. Generally European colonials and missionaries did not acknowledge the nasalized initial sound of the names of sites they created or inhabited. Thus, Nsundi, the clan name, became Sundi. Sundi Lutete, a Protestant mission in North Manianga, and Sundi Mamba, a former colonial post, are spelled as they appear on maps and textual sources, whereas references to clan and other social group names are given the phonetically more accurate Nsundi. Many other names beginning with a nasalized initial sound are similarly abbreviated in official, colonially created, sites.

Historical practices, external impositions, and conventions regarding the name Congo and Kongo are confusing to the uninitiated reader. Although all pronunciations of the word Congo are the same, popular usage and official naming have established the following conventions: Congo with a "C" refers to the Congo Basin, the Congo river (including Upper Congo and Lower Congo), the Congo Free State, the Belgian Congo, the Democratic Republic of Congo, and the Republic of Congo (Brazzaville). Kongo with a "K" refers to the historic Kongo kingdom, the BaKongo people, the KiKongo language, and the region in northern Angola, western Democratic Republic of Congo, and the Republic of Congo. A fuller explanation of these and other terms for the region and history is given elsewhere in the text.

This book, and the research project on which it is based, could not have happened without the generous assistance of many individuals—colleagues, family, friends, interested strangers, and above all the patient citizens of the Lower Congo where the research occurred. Foremost of these participants deserving mention, and acknowledgment, is Tata Professor Kimpianga Mahaniah, historian, university rector, and colleague. He agreed early on to be my "counterpart host," as required by the Institute of International Education and the Fulbright Senior Scholar Program, which funded this research. He provided logistical support and advice, lodging and support staff in Luozi, a vehicle with chauffeur, and access to his vast network of people in the region and particularly in the Centre de Vulgarisation Agricole (CVA), including the Free University of Luozi (ULL). A few individuals in the CVA and ULL are listed here, but many more are acknowledged. Diallo Lukwamusu provided intellectual reflection and logistical assistance whenever needed. Célestin Lusiama, head of Radio Ntomosono ("Radio Development"), provided ethnographic assistance and offered good conversation on many pertinent topics. Mbuta Kisolokele Thomas was my social conscience, etiquette adviser, mediator in a range of contacts, and general conversation partner. His untimely death in 2017 robbed the community of a much loved and respected elder.

Reinhild Janzen, my wife, accompanied me throughout this research adventure, including living in the CVA compound and residence in Luozi. Here, Mama Luezi Mbambi Jacqueline (henceforth Mama Jacqueline) was our household host, chef, overseer, and gatekeeper, with ready and firm guidance on every occasion; together with the staff and her granddaughters Winnie, Merveille, and Anneke, she took care of our every need. Pierre Mayimona was our genius of a chauffeur-mechanic, who not only kept the Toyota Hilux running and drove us all over, from Kinshasa to Boma, and northward to Sundi-Lutete, but was our bodyguard in those moments when one was needed, as in the Kinshasa general market; he greatly expanded our appreciation for that unique role of "boy chauffeur" upon whom Congolese road veterans depend.

I am indebted to, and here gratefully acknowledge, the many individuals who participated in one or another aspect of the intensive sample that figures importantly in this work. Professor José Dianzungu (henceforth, Professor Dian-zungu) translated the English statement of the project and letter of introduction into French and KiKongo. After we tested the questionnaire, Tata Luyobisa Luheha Jackson (henceforth Tata Luyobisa or simply Luyobisa) administered it to many of the households. Tata Luyobisa joined his wife, Mama Nsansi Bakima, to meet with us on numerous occasions to share meals, fellowship, or excursions to interesting events or places. Of special mention is the trip to Nzieta, the headquar-ters of the Church of the Holy Spirit in Africa, for a celebration of its founding. In this connection I also acknowledge with appreciation the time church president Mayangi Masamba Charles (henceforth Tata Mayangi, or Mayangi Charles) gave us to discuss the movement's origins and history. Tata Luyobisa's sudden death in 2018 robbed his family, his community, and the research effort of a true friend and ally. Mama Ndiongono kwa Nzambi Marceline stepped in to extend the questionnaire to women of eighteen to forty-five years of age, a critical cohort for understanding women and children's health and reproductive planning. I also acknowledge the survey's respondents from 105 households, who were eager to contribute to this inquiry into the status of their health and the well-being of their region.

A special thanks is due the staff at the Luozi Health Zone—Ngemba Jeanben-oit, Mansinsa Dianzenza Delvin, and Mbasani Veronique—who explained their work in detail and provided important information on the innovative nature of public health in the Congo. Chef de Cité Matondo Lufinama was of particular assistance in providing city records and relevant information to the study. I am equally grateful to the leaders and staff of the Territoire de Luozi for affording me support in my research and access to records and documents pertaining to the study. I am appreciative of the *chef de bureau* of the *territoire* for showing me the room that houses the colonial records of the region, scooped up from the storm-damaged hangar in which I found them in 1965, although they await sorting and arranging into a usable archive.

Mbuta Yoswa Kusikila kwa Kilombo (henceforth Mbuta Kusikila, or simply Kusikila) and younger brother—now also mbuta—Nkebi Kilombo Victor and his wife, Mama Bakela Nayenge Sidoni, were faces and voices from the past who gave us a special welcome on our visit to Kisiasia in Kivunda, North Manianga.

Mbuta Flaubert Batangu Mpesa (henceforth, Batangu Mpesa) welcomed us to the Congo shortly after our arrival, came to Luozi to give us a tour of his pharma-ceutical establishments, offered a fitting commentary at our Luozi farewell party (as well as a generator and light for the occasion, after a storm delayed the party for several hours), and gave us his own farewell reception in Kinshasa.

Ruth and Robert Dyabanza were welcoming neighbors in Luozi, checking on our well-being and always ready for an afternoon's cool drink in their shady house overlooking the Congo River.

I wish to acknowledge the gracious invitation from colleagues in Halle, Ger-many, for a three-month research visit in fall 2014 to participate in the Deutsche

Forschungsgemeinschaft Priority Programme 1448 "Adaptation and Creativity in Africa," under the leadership of Professor Richard Rottenburg of the University of Halle-Wittenberg. I gratefully acknowledge the program's publication of my early formulations of the perspective in this book as the working paper "Divergent Legitimations of Post-State Health Institutions in Western Equatorial Africa" (Janzen 2015b). I also welcomed the opportunity offered me by Professor Marie-Claire Foblets at the Max Planck Institute for Social Anthropology in Halle to participate in the Institute's Colloquium on Anthropology and Consultancy. I gratefully acknowledge Professor Steven Feierman's offer to take his place in these venues. The opportunity to work unencumbered in the Max Planck Institute's library in Halle is reflected in the more ample reference foundation of some of the themes in this work.

I wish to thank *African Studies Quarterly* for permission to use content and perspective in this book that were published in my article "Science and Spirit in Postcolonial North Kongo Health and Healing" (Janzen 2015a) and Indiana University Press for permission to use material and perspective published in my chapter "Science in the Moral Space of Health and Healing Paradigms in Western Equatorial Africa" in the book *African Medical Pluralism*, edited by William C. Olsen and Carolyn Sargent (2017).

Inger Anderson, antiquarian of photographic collections of the Museum of World Culture and the Museum of Ethnography, Gothenburg, Sweden went out of his way to piece together the pedigree of Josef Öhrneman's remarkable 1927 photograph of a *dumuna* moment of a Bemba *nganga* in Kolo, Republic of Congo; thank you! I also acknowledge Carlotta Image Services' permission for the use of the photo in this publication.

Among the many colleagues and scholars who have read and commented on my work, whether in seminars, conference sessions, or private conversations, I single out for special gratitude longtime Africanist scholar and friend Wyatt MacGaffey. His deep insights and high scholarly standards have been a steady influence on my own work. His review of the manuscript for the University of Wisconsin Press is gratefully acknowledged, as is that by an anonymous reader. I also acknowledge with appreciation the expert reading and editorial suggestions made by Professor Omer Galle and Zona Galle.

A special note of thanks to Professor Marike S. Janzen for helping me sift through many possible titles and identifying the one that contains the most poignant formulation of the book's complex subject with an economy of words.

A very special all-encompassing thank-you goes to my wife, friend, and scholarly companion, Reinhild Kauenhoven Janzen. She has accompanied and encouraged me at every stage of this project, from planning the proposal to critically reading the manuscript. She has encouraged and stimulated me and has provided moral support all along the way—not just of this project but of my entire career.

ABBREVIATIONS

BDK   Bundu dia Kongo (Association, church, or union of Kongo; nativist movement, political party)

CDC   Centers for Disease Control and Prevention; US government agency, Atlanta, Georgia

CEC   Communauté Evangélique du Congo (Evangelical community/church of the Congo); formerly Svenska Missions Förbundet (SMF, Swedish Mission Society); Église Evangélique de Manianga et Matadi (EEMM, Evangelical Church of the Manianga and Matadi)

CRPL   Centre de Recherche Pharmaceutique de Luozi (Pharmaceutical Research Center of Luozi)

CSEA   Communauté du Saint Esprit en Afrique (Community, Church of the Holy Spirit in Africa); formerly Dibundu dia Mpeve a Nlongo en Afrika (DMNA)

CVA   Centre de Vulgarisation Agricole (Agricultural Extension Center)

DMNA   Dibundu dia Mpeve a Nlongo en Afrika (Church of the Holy Spirit in Africa)

DOM   Département des Oeuvres Médicales (Medical Department of the CEC)

DRC   Democratic Republic of the Congo

ECC   Église du Christ au Congo (Evangelical Church(es) of Congo); postcolonial national Protestant council in DRC

EJCSK	Église de Jésus Christ sur la terre par le prophète Simon Kimbangu (Church of Jesus Christ on Earth by the Prophet Simon Kimbangu)
FOREAMI	Fonds Reine Elisabeth pour l'Assistance Médicale aux Indigènes du Congo Belge (Queen Elisabeth Foundation for the Medical Assistance of Indigenous Peoples of the Belgian Congo)
GAVI	Global Alliance for Vaccines and Immunization
HAV	Homme Adult et Valable (Viable Male Adult); Belgian Congo census category of one adult male worker
IME	Institut Médical Evangélique (Evangelical Medical Institute); Kimpese, Lower Congo
MAF	Mission Aviation Fellowship
MAP	Medical Assistance Program International
NGO	nongovernmental organization
PHC	primary health care
RDC	Republique Democratique du Congo (Democratic Republic of the Congo)
REGIDESO	Régie des Eaux (Water Works Parastatal Organization)
SMF	Svenska Missions Förbundet (Swedish Mission Society)
SANRU	Santé Rurale du Congo (Rural Health of the Congo)
ULL	Université Libre de Luozi (Free University of Luozi)
UNDP	United Nations Development Programme
UNICEF	United Nations International Children's Emergency Fund
USAID	United States Agency for International Development
USOFDA	United States Office of Foreign Disaster Assistance
WHO	World Health Organization

Health in a Fragile State

INTRODUCTION

This book examines the legitimation of power and knowledge in public health and health care in the wake of the collapse of the Zairian/Congolese state in the 1980s and 1990s. Of special interest are the institutions and services that emerged in the wake of this collapse and how they came to terms with the challenge of endemic diseases. The diseases they confronted were the common tropical scourges of malaria, severe respiratory infection, severe childhood diarrhea, bilharzia, occasional outbreaks of trypanosomiasis, infant protein deficiency, tuberculosis, HIV/AIDS, typhoid, and seasonal flu. The institutions and the knowledge they used included churches, universities and institutes that train medical practitioners, nongovernmental organizations (NGOs) both national and international, local and regional ad hoc alliances and actors, and local government. The book illuminates the paradox of the persistence of these well-understood diseases in the context of reasonably well-stocked medicine supplies, an array of knowledgeable experts, and relative peace in the region. As the book's title suggests, a fragile state produces fragile health, whereas legitimate institutions with authority empower those who work in them to achieve improvements all around.

The research site is the three health zones in the Luozi Territory, also known as the Manianga, in the Lower Congo—north of the Congo river, between the capitals of Kinshasa and Brazzaville to the east, and to the west the Mayombe and Cabinda regions at the Atlantic Ocean (map I.1). This region has a turbulent health history tied to the caravan routes that carried global trade, including the slave trade, from the seventeenth century through the late nineteenth century, then became the site of entry for King Leopold's Congo Free State. How this historical backdrop lives on in structures, population distributions, and memory is an important dimension of the postcolonial story of health and health care.

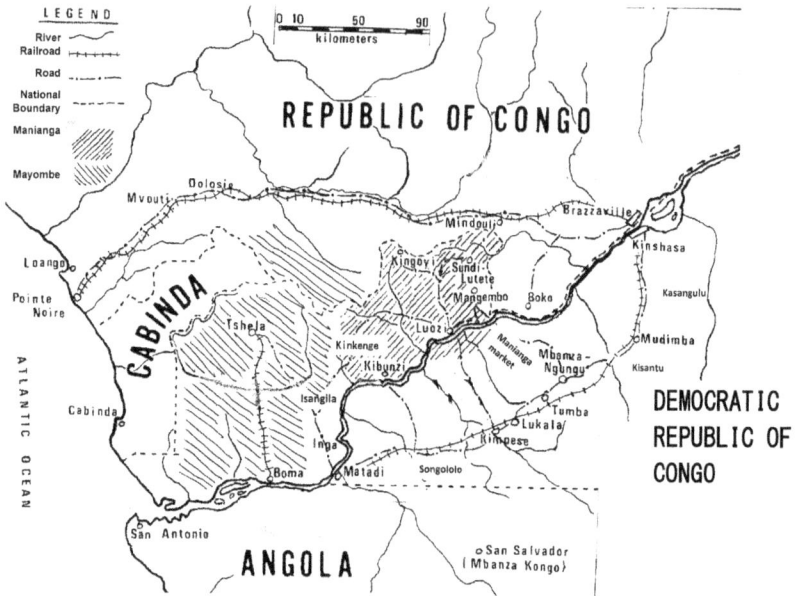

MAP I.I. Manianga region in the Lower Congo. The name Manianga, or Manyanga, derives from the historic market along the main caravan route from Mpumbu market at Malebo Pool (today's Kinshasa) to the Atlantic and Congo river ports at Boma and Vivi (near today's Matadi), and Atlantic ports of Malemba, Kakongo, and Loango. These routes were especially heavily frequented during the eighteenth and nineteenth centuries, the heyday of the Atlantic slave trade. Map by author.

With this historical backdrop in mind, within the setting of three adjacent health zones north of the Congo river in Lower Congo, the book analyzes the manner in which these institutions that carry the load of medical expertise in public health and health care establish their legitimacy: that is, how they promote knowledge, how they generate support from the populace and from national and global affiliations, and how they wield institutional and professional power. Fuller discussion of the concept of legitimacy and its use in institutional analysis occurs throughout the text. In a society where the state is conspicuous in its fragility, to be effective these institutions must not only coordinate routine tasks of inoculation campaigns, emergency care, and day-to-day medical work; they must also offset the considerable fear of illicit power, suspicion of authority, all kinds of popular rumors, and the occasional antisorcery movements that threaten individuals and public figures. These institutions have become power brokers, surrogates of the state.

The work's analysis suggests that these nonstate players in public health and health care are likely to be effective in addressing disease and promoting health to the extent that they enjoy full legitimation. A detailed analysis of institutions in relation to particular diseases or groups of diseases demonstrates where and how effective interventions and care are at work. For example, annual city inspections of household latrines to avert sewage-borne diseases demonstrates the legitimacy of local government as an institution involved in public health, and WHO-directed measures of trypanosomiasis outbreaks show the legitimacy and efficacy of very fragile health zone networks established in the 1980s, despite the collapse of the National Ministry of Health. Other cases, such as high levels of malaria infection and the rising incidence of seasonal flu, demonstrate the limits of efficacy resulting from limited institutional legitimacy.

The study's significance is evident in this and other societies where the state is weak or where global neoliberal policies have eroded state-sponsored institutions and services, and where alternative initiatives and agencies have been created to fill the void. The appropriateness of this analysis in the Lower Congo is evident where several centuries of institutional disruption due to the global commerce, slavery, colonialism, and postcolonial upheaval have eroded public trust and impeded the development of centers of expertise in an important realm such as health and healing. An analysis of legitimation also illuminates widespread fears of illicit power and recourse to rituals of protection and cleansing deemed necessary for well-being.

CRISIS AND CREATIVITY: STATE COLLAPSE AND THE RECONFIGURATION OF INSTITUTIONS

As often as commentary on the Congo has been phrased in terms of crisis and creativity, the reader of these lines may well ask "Which crisis?" and "Whose creativity?" Authors on events of the late nineteenth and early twentieth centuries have used "death of a tradition" (Vansina 1990), the "breakdown of a moral order" (Vos 2015), outright "catastrophe" (Ekholm 1991), or the KiKongo *kimongi* ("plague"; Kusikila 1966) to describe the negatively transformative impact of change on the Lower Congo and its people. Without minimizing those events, this work focuses on a very recent round of crisis and creativity that reached its climax with the 1998 name change of the country from Zaire back to the Democratic Republic of the Congo following the overthrow of longtime dictator Mobutu Sese Seko. The crisis continued into the era of Joseph Kabila Kabange, who did not seek reelection in late 2018 (the president as of June 2019 is Félix Antoine Tshisekedi Tshilombo). The main driver for the crisis of the 1980s and 1990s and beyond was the crisis of state. It is necessary to give this phenomenon momentary focused attention in order to understand its pervasive impact on health, and the distinctive contours of the creative response taken in dealing with the crisis.

The collapse of the Zairian/Congolese state did not occur all at once; nor was it ever total. The phenomenon of state collapse must be seen here, and in other cases, as occurring sector by sector, region by region, and in particular time periods. The crisis in centralized, state-sponsored health care and public health of the 1980s and 1990s was forecast by the collapse of a number of other state institutions due to mismanagement, loss of financing, or both. Entire sectors of government-run life came to a standstill. Some were simply abandoned, and life went on without them. This was the case with the postal system. By 1990, and continuing into the 2010s, buildings that once housed postal clerks selling colorful postage stamps with pictures of tropical flowers and wildlife stood empty. Other sectors were replaced by alternative structures. This was the case with the Université National du Zaire (UNAZA), with campuses in Kinshasa, Lubumbashi, and Kisangani, each featuring a specialized focus, and research and training institutes to match. In the 1970s this structure operated effectively, with ample national funding. When funding dried up, its unitary model gave way to thirty or more smaller universities financed and administered by local leaders, churches, and private groups, sometimes with the support of international NGOs. The Free University of Luozi is an example of this type of institution.

The Manianga region of the Lower Congo, which is the focus of this study, was never in the fifty postcolonial years the scene of civil war; nor was it ever occupied by a rebel army. It is situated relatively close to the capital, Kinshasa, and the major national port of Matadi, and thus enjoys relatively easy access to the economic and political hubs of urban national life. Throughout the postcolonial period, local levels of government have been filled by officials carrying on the daily tasks of administration. State collapse here has meant very slim or missing tax revenues; fiscal crisis that rendered currency worthless; and nonpayment of staff, obliging them to make their living another way. As in many other regions of Zaire/Congo, local or regional militias or mobs have arisen to take things into their own hands, with belated national military action that has killed a number of "resisters" and terrified the populace. Yet the north bank of the Lower Congo has been a relatively peaceful setting by Central African standards. As elsewhere, events of the 1980s and 1990s forced regional elites and health care practitioners to create alternative structures to administer hospitals and clinics and to find funding for their operations.

The crisis of the Zairian state was reflected in the diminished role of the Ministry of Health. It was also reflected in negligible income from public funds (0.9 percent) for public health and health care, at a rate of 3.7 percent of gross national product (GNP). Thus 99.1 percent of all funding for public health and health care was from private or other nongovernmental sources (World Health Organization 2012). This contrasted dramatically with Botswana's 61 percent governmental expenditure for public health and health care (4.2 percent of GNP), the highest for any African country. Botswana's proportion of health spending coming from the government was higher than that of the United States, at 44.1 percent (13.7 percent of GNP), and just below Germany's 77.5 percent (10.5 percent of GNP; WHO 2012). In sum, the DRC's public expenditures for public health and health care were almost nonexistent, necessitating private financing or simply causing an increasing health disparity between those with means and those without.

Many scholars have weighed in on the collapse of the state in Zaire/Congo and other state settings. Only the general outlines of this literature can be reviewed here, insofar as it is relevant to grasping the unfolding picture of public health and health care infrastructure in the Manianga, the Lower Congo, and beyond. In their exhaustive study of the "rise and decline" of the Zairian state, published before the paralyzing riots of the early 1990s, Crawford Young and Thomas Turner (1985, 8–12) define the state as a series of historical characteristics common among nations in the post-nineteenth-century world. States claim exclusive authority over a bounded territory and sovereignty among nations. They usually attach to the state a nation, which is the identity as a people. And they possess institutions of rule, an organizational expression of hegemony, a framework for governance, a legal system (that is, predictable rules), and an idea or ideology that grants the state authority by consensus of the governed. The authors review the ways in which the Zairian state under Mobutu faltered on most of these criteria, especially by the mid-1980s. But paradoxically, the Zairian state was not carved up by invading neighbors; it has survived at least nominally for fifty postcolonial years. Young and Turner (1985, 45–46) offer this assessment of the Zairian/Congolese state, which holds true twenty years later: "The [Congolese] state persists as an important concept in the social imagination; the image of a powerful, efficient, and rational state serves as a normative counterpoint to the derelict 'empirical state.' Thus the moral entitlement of the state to hegemony is not challenged, even while its regulations are widely ignored. The possibility of a resurrection around the normative image remains present."

James Ferguson's phrase the "shadow state" (2006) captures an important dimension of state weakness. The shadow state is a structure of bureaucratic and political roles, yet it lacks the economic strength to achieve the services and level of presence expected of states. He relates this shadowness to the neoliberal economic pressures that open service sectors to global commoditization, with governance by large global corporations.

Fiscal tightening imposed on African and other states by the structural adjustment programs of the World Bank and the International Monetary Fund have been seen as particularly crippling for the health and health care sector. Increases in chronic diseases, the rise of malnutrition in children, and the general immiseration of the poor have been traced in study after study to such fiscal belt-tightening at the national level (Pfeiffer and Chapman 2010). Other, more indirect effects on public well-being include the imposition of fees for health care services where once public financing carried such services; cuts to public-sector services such as education, agriculture, water, and public works; unemployment caused by layoffs of public-sector workers and income declines resulting from wage cuts for those remaining; privatization of state industries that often leads to layoffs; removal of state subsidies for food transport and food price supports; currency devaluation; and general increases in inequality (Pfeiffer and Chapman 2010, 152). Critics of structural adjustment emphasize that health is not a commodity that can be economized for greater profit and economic development; it is a right, or at least a basic human need that is compromised if health care infrastructure is short-changed.

All the adjectives used by scholars writing about failed states apply to the DRC, a state that is variously called "shadowy" (Ferguson 2006), "fragile" (Fund for Peace 2012), "hollow" (Rusca and Schwartz 2012), or "crumbling" (Dizolele and Kambale 2012). In the DRC the post-2011 presidential election paralysis brought charges of gutting the electoral process with parliamentary manipulation, ballot rigging, lost ballots, and hasty certification by an apparently bought-off electoral commission.

The particular reasons for the state's failure go well beyond the outside-imposed fiscal tightening of the 1970s and 1980s. Mobutu's Zaire was a classic case of a patrimonial state, in which the elite helped themselves to the basic resources of the land and doled out favors to their friends and dependents in exchange for loyalty, some services, and support, rather than investing in systematic development of essential services such as education, health care, communications, urban development, and roads. The patrimonial state, in this kind of scenario, is a structure of personalized patron-client relations. Under such circumstances, some analysts claim, development does not take place. The productive resources of the land are drained off for personal ends and deposited in Swiss banks. This is the standard understanding of corruption.

A different understanding of the patrimonial patronage state is proposed by Patrick Chabal and Jean-Pascal Daloz (1999). According to them, the very chaos that ensues from structural adjustment or other types of disorder becomes a resource that may be managed as patronage. This is not the kind of development that development experts intend, but it is nevertheless a political system that seems to thrive. Elites translate social disorder into patronage resources that shore up the loyalty of their client networks, as they help their friends and others who are loyal to them. Western-style development does not undermine the viability of "neo-patrimonialism" (Gerhart 1999). Although this kind of patronage is anti-thetical to the public interest, it works as a system of maintaining power.

The DRC was not the only state to experience such a decline. Many states across Africa and elsewhere felt the transforming winds of loss of confidence in their ability to serve the needs of their citizens. There was a major shift in the 1970s and 1980s away from attempted state-sponsored health programs to other kinds of arrangements that were sometimes called public-private partnerships or outright privatization. Privatization of major sectors of the economy and social services was usually accompanied by the rise of project-specific nongovernmental agencies and the outsourcing of services, including health care (Rusca and Schwartz 2012). These moves were usually accompanied by the rise of neoliberal economic regimes and "global health" (Geissler, Rottenburg, and Zenker 2012, 8–9). Thus, the weakening of states in the decades of the 1970s to the 1990s was usually accompanied by an ideological shift on the part of international donors from working through state structures to working directly with NGOs with project-specific goals that ignored or bypassed local and national jurisdictions. In this regard the DRC was not exceptional but supertypical.

A comparative perspective on state failure or collapse is helpful in situating the DRC among nations, and the Territory of Luozi within the DRC. The Fund for Peace keeps a score sheet on state resilience and fragility, with the following main indicators: a nation's cohesion, that is, the orderliness of its overall governance structure and institutions; its economic status, whether it is productive, maintains trade and internal flow of resources, and has a stable currency; the legitimacy of the state and human rights, as reflected in the well-being of minorities and of the effectiveness of judicial institutions to protect their rights; and last, the state's social and demographic trends, including whether its citizens are fleeing as refugees or are internally displaced in significant numbers (Fund for Peace 2018). From 2012 through 2018—that is, in the period of the current project and analysis—the DRC ranked between the second and sixth most fragile state globally, after Somalia, Central African Republic, South Sudan, and now Syria and Yemen on the Failed State Index.

And yet during these same years several African states succeeded in wielding strong state structures to enhance public health and health care programs. Botswana, where 61 percent of overall health and health care expenditures were state-originated, was the first African state to offer free AZT medications to HIV-positive sufferers. In Uganda, where strong state-sponsored initiatives had brought HIV/ AIDS infection rates down from 35 percent to 5 percent of the populace, similar coordination of national public priorities led to the rapid containment of an Ebola outbreak in Gulu in 2000. Through coordinated national public health measures, international agency intervention, the tracking of suspected carriers, laboratory testing, and close national monitoring of the isolation of infected individuals, the outbreak, which had produced 425 infections and 225 deaths, was contained within four months.[1] Rwanda represents a third instance of significant state coordination in public health and health care, as in other service realms. With the use of systematic digital record keeping, Rwanda has launched an initiative to track child health in local centers, and to monitor the results of other health improvement campaigns. One of the dramatic goals in this initiative is to eliminate chronic malaria.[2]

Scholarly awareness of strong states and the analysis of areas of effective governance in Africa has been recently supported by work such as Thomas Biershenk and Jean-Pierre Olivier de Sardan's focus on effective bureaucracies and projects in Africa (2014). It is important to keep in mind this range of state capacities as we explore further details of the health and health care institutions that emerged in the post-collapse era of the Zairian/Congolese state.

PRIMARY HEALTH CARE AND HEALTH ZONES AS THE PHOENIX RISING FROM THE ASHES

The impact of the collapse of the Zairian state on public health and health care services featured the simultaneous shrinking of centralized supply lines, and the loss of effective coordination of programs, while the new primary health care structure promoted by the World Health Organization (WHO) introduced the health zone as the framework for services. (The prototypes of the health zone in the DRC that preceded the WHO program will be detailed in chapter 4.) Primary health care and the health zone format was the phoenix rising from the ashes of and replacing the centralized Zairian national health system. The phoenix is a mythical bird in ancient Greek legend that is able to spread its wings and take flight after being burned to ashes in a fire. A symbol of miraculous renewal or revival after death, it is one of a number of symbols of resurrection used by early Christians and appears on tombs of martyrs in the catacombs in Rome.

Following the spirit of the 1978 Alma-Ata Declaration of "Health for All by the Year 2000," Zaire adopted the basic primary health program for health zones across the country; the Territory of Luozi constituted three of the country's three hundred initial health zones, which ultimately became over five hundred (map I.2). In the course of the 1980s, the zones were organized from the ground up. Basic care in the form of the services of a trained nurse with essential drugs was to be accessible to all. No one was to have to walk farther than 15 kilometers for this care. Each health zone was organized into local primary health posts, regional midlevel centers, and a central regional hospital. In the local centers nurses carried out basic care and public health initiatives such as children's inoculations and care for basic illnesses. Ideally they were to refer the most serious cases up to hospital centers. Medicines and other resources were to be distributed from central stocks to the local centers.

The entire Zaire program was coordinated under a national directorate headed by Martin Ngwete, who holds a PhD in public health, and his staff of Congolese and expatriate consultants.[3] By 2000, about half of the clinics were administered jointly by the state and faith-based organizations—that is, mission or independent church entities. In some ways the Zairian public health program was ahead of WHO's primary health care program. As will be described in more detail in chapter 4, pilot health zones had been developed at several hospitals across the country. Thus when WHO launched its international program, Zaire already had a working

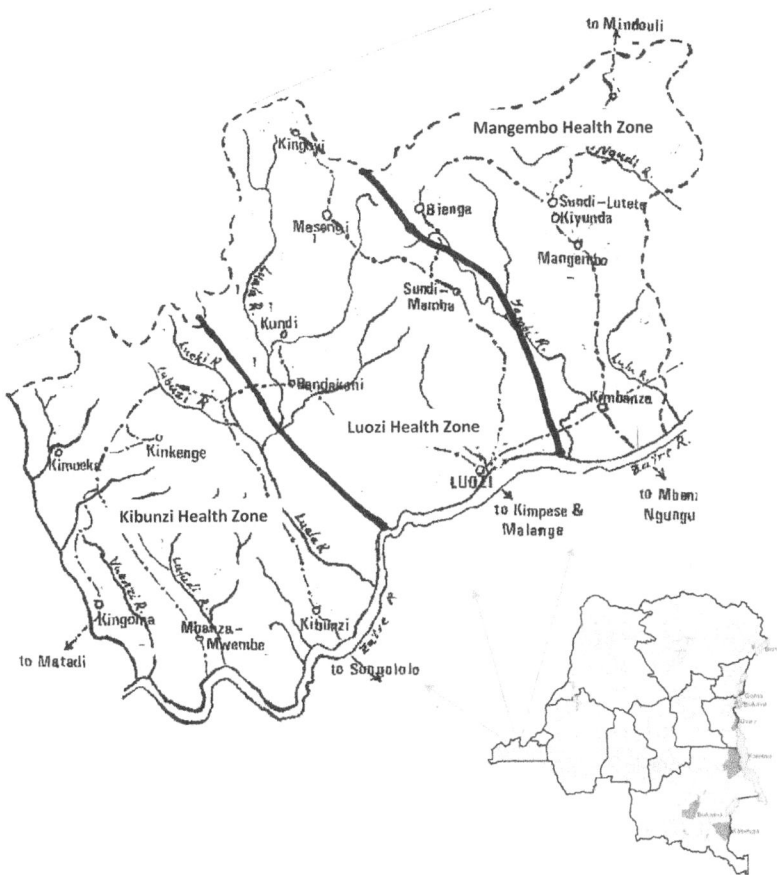

MAP I.2. Health zones of Kibunzi, Luozi, and Mangembo within the territory of Luozi (the Manianga), province of Bas-Congo, Democratic Republic of Congo. Detail at right, the 500 health zones in the DRC. Arrows identify the three health zones in the Luozi Territory. Map by author.

model of the health zone that became a foundation on which to build a national program with international funding (Baer 2007).

Because of the unreliable availability of state medical supplies, the primary health care system in Zaire was purposefully created in such a way that multiple, redundant supply networks would operate parallel to the government sources (Janzen 2002, 255–57).[4] These arrangements allowed hospitals and health zones to negotiate separate supply arrangements with international or private sources. The wisdom of such multiple structures was seen amid the turbulence of the wars and governmental changes of the 1990s.

By the late 1980s, the Zairian government's role in the primary health care system, as in every other service sector, had deteriorated. Inflation soared to 1,000 percent per year. In one two-month period, there were five Ministers of Health.[5] The entire national budget became unreliable. At this point the government exited the public health and health care business entirely. The Ministry of Health became nonfunctional, as did other ministries of the Zairian government. Observers began to speak of the collapse of the state. The 1991 riots in Kinshasa by Zairian soldiers and the destruction of many private enterprises brought the country into a state of deep moral and economic crisis. Along with infrastructure such as the postal system, roads, and ferries, now too the primary health care zones were threatened because governmental workers were no longer paid, or if paid, their salaries were as worthless as the hyperinflated currency. After the riots in 1991 foreign partners like the United States Agency for International Development (USAID) and Canadian International Development, Belgian assistance, and organizations like OXFAM and UNESCO withdrew because it became impossible to conduct their affairs. In 1993, the primary health care directorate in Kinshasa was pillaged by soldiers, medicine stocks were stolen, vehicles were taken, and personnel abandoned their posts.[6]

Local supervision by motivated and interested individuals became everything in new efforts at public health. In this sector, as in education and food production and distribution, private initiatives and faith-based organizations were all that was left. Where village nurses understood the issues, local clinics survived. The same was true of hospitals and clinics. But many hospitals and clinics now of necessity became fee-for-service operations, dependent on their local constituency, students, or patients, all the while searching for support from outside agencies of the church, the United Nations, or other private sources. In Zaire and elsewhere in Africa, the NGO became the structural wherewithal of health care delivery. "Zairian crisis" became a way of life.

The medical sector had been largely nationalized by the Zairian state under Mobutu. Former mission- or church-operated institutions, as well as independent ventures, were incorporated into this national structure. The collapse of these state-sponsored structures and supply lines in the late 1980s and 1990s obliged health workers and policy leaders to radically reform the institutional framework through which such services were organized, if there were to be any services at all. An array of alternative institutions—lower-level governmental entities, churches, international and local NGOs, private enterprises, and ad hoc coalitions—picked up the pieces to try to provide continuing public health and clinical health care.

There is an ironic aspect to this story: social and political crisis provided the fertile ground for creative solutions, for innovation. Whether out of desperation or opportunism, the loss of legitimacy of one set of institutions called forth efforts by individuals and groups to create alternatives to carry out a much-needed and desired service. The challenge of endemic diseases and the desire to promote health have brought into being a series of creative initiatives, social movements, institutional innovations, and entrepreneurial ventures.

The cultural seed of this process of creative relegitimation from within society, at least in the Lower Congo, is the deeply rooted Kongo notion that the chaos of failed authority is perceived as a sickness to be healed by the re-creation of authority, order, and justice.[7] Rituals such as the *dumuna*, which accomplished this historically and continues to do so in certain settings today, will be portrayed at greater length in chapter 6. Although Kongo thinking prescribes a transcendent anchoring of such renewals of authority, in the contemporary world of businesspeople, brokers, academics, clerics, diplomats, and politicians, the process of creative renewal may take surprising turns that are only later recognized as enduring institutional re-creation. The history of Kongo is dotted with such renewals and visions of dilemmas resolved (Janzen 1977; 1982, 323–26).

The fragmentary condition of institutions and initiatives handling public health and health care in the Lower Congo has deeper roots than the economic, political, and ideological crises of the postcolonial era. Such fragmentation also reflects a historical condition of past institutions and regimes. Kingdoms and chiefships arose and declined in the face of precolonial coastal mercantile trade. *Minkisi*, the units of knowledge and technique of the past, were invented, served for a while, and then were discarded, to be supplanted by other *minkisi* or Western colonial knowledge or scientific ideas.

The story of health, healing, and problem solving is couched in a crazy quilt of social forms and institutions. These include the landed estate (*nsi*), which has continued right up to the present from the dawn of cultivation; the village (*vata*), of the same ancestry; the house, or community (*nzo*); the local kin group (*dikanda*); the unilineal clan (*mvila*); and various emanations of chiefship, precolonial (the *kimfumu nsi*, or *kimfumu mpu*), colonial (the *mpalata*, morphed into the *secteur*), and postcolonial (again *secteur*) via the *commune*. Alongside all these deep social forms are those created by postcolonial initiatives, including local, regional, and national governments; the churches—Catholic, Protestant, Kimbanguist, Prophetic—as corporate institutions, with their varied programs in education, development, and health care; and businesses and enterprises, both individual and larger corporate affairs. All are nominally expected to be licensed, registered, or recognized by the state. Yet the collapse or extreme fragility of the state calls into question the very legitimacy of these institutions and social formations, and represents a hindrance to their effective operation.

The question therefore becomes, How do we understand the alternative, hybrid institutions that claim power under the shadow of a weak state? This work illuminates the creativity in play when the state fails and others who care ramp up alternative structures and initiatives to maintain and improve health. This inquiry will also reveal the limits of what can be done within a weak state in a neoliberal global economy.

Luozi and the Manianga, the Setting of the Study

The town of Luozi is named after the Luozi River, which flows into the mighty Congo River about 150 kilometers downstream from Kinshasa. This location is halfway between the old market of Manianga, atop a high hill just downstream from a series of rapids, and Isangila, at the beginning of rapids farther downstream, in the middle of a 63-kilometer stretch of relatively slowly running water, where the Congo River is two kilometers wide. Luozi is the capital of the Territory of Luozi, colloquially known as "the Manianga," which is bordered on the east and north by Congo-Brazzaville, on the west by the Mayombe, and on the south by the Congo River (map I.1).

Luozi's commercial center near the ferry I had known in the 1960s was still there, but in the ensuing five decades the town has spread throughout the valley

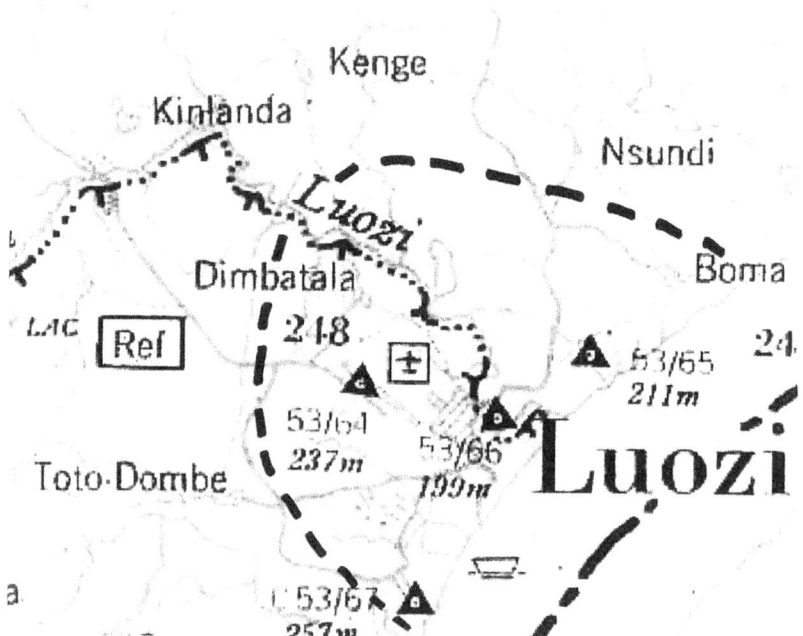

Map I.3. Luozi in 1958 (hatched pattern to left of the *L* of *Luozi*) and 2013 (inside the dotted line); surrounding villages are being annexed to the town with urban laws and land registries. Map by author. Source: Detail of Map of Territory of Luozi, Geographical Society of Congo, 1960.

and hills. Seven surrounding villages—Ntoto Ndombe, Dimbatala, Kinlanda, Kenge, Nsundi, Boma and Kibusi—are being annexed to Luozi, in recognition of their de facto engulfment by the town and the residents' desire to be part of the larger community. Sprawling new settlements have grown in all directions from the commercial center and these villages (map I.3)

The iconic Congo River beach, where the ferry departs and arrives four times per day, provides Luozi's main contact to the national corridor of cities beyond for people living north of the river in the Manianga district—the Territory of Luozi. At this beach trucks, buses, cars, motorcycles, bicyclists, and pedestrians gather to cross the majestic river. Impromptu market stalls sell meals, snacks, smoked fish, *chikwanga*, bread, coffee, beer, soft drinks, bottled water, cigarettes, dry goods, cell phone time units, and tire repair materials to this waiting crowd. A modern five-story hotel is nearing completion on the Luozi side of the river for visitors, tourists, merchants and others needing lodging at the waterfront. Facing Luozi on the southeast bank of the river is Kibemba, a small settlement of makeshift stalls, with vendors of food, dry goods, and cell phone time units. For the unfortunate traveler who arrives after the last ferry of the afternoon has returned to Luozi, there is also a hotel of modest proportions alongside the residential houses of fishers who

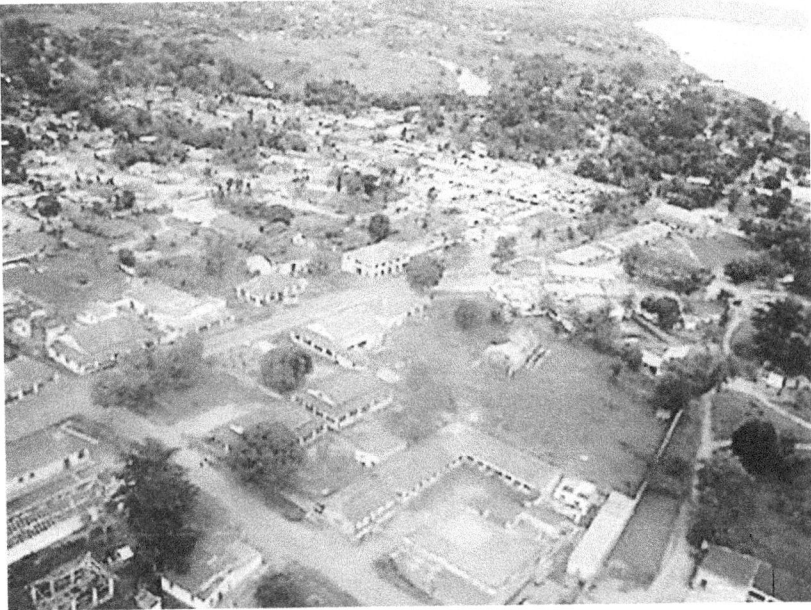

Figure I.1. Aerial view of Luozi commercial district. Luozi River visible upper center; Congo River upper right; sprawling residential areas visible below horizon. Source: Missionary Aviation Fellowship pilot, posted to internet, ca 2010.

in their dugout canoes make their living on the river, providing the fish that are readily sold in the ferry-side eateries and in town.

Several major roads—wide red lines on international and internet maps— converge in Luozi: the RN (Route Nationale) 12 from Matadi to Congo Brazzaville, which runs parallel to the Congo River, and the RP (Route Provinciale) 111 from Kimpese across the ferry northward, joining the RP 112 to the Luala Valley and on to Kingoyi in the northwest. Although these roads are all dirt, they are occasionally maintained by workers with hoes and shovels and intermittently by a heavy-duty crew that builds and repairs bridges. The roads, as rutted and rough as they may be, provide avenues of travel for cargo trucks, cars, motorcycles, and pedestrians, and for the very occasional world tourist who tests the elements, logistics, and infrastructure to drive across Africa following the wide red lines in their touring atlas. Although there is weekly bus service between Luozi and Kinshasa, most of the transportation is done on trucks that combine cargo with passengers. These trucks can be seen unloading and loading on Luozi's Commerce Avenue in front of the main market.

Every morning of the week there is much noisy activity at the central market at the lower end of Avenue du Commerce and around the corner and on the main commercial streets: selling, buying, and trucks and buses arriving from or leaving to distant places, packed high with luggage; sacks of manioc, onions, and bananas; bags of charcoal and other products, and people and small animals on top of that. Civic authorities have opened two other markets. Despite this attempt to localize selling and buying in markets, petty commerce occurs wherever people congregate or move, especially alongside thoroughfares and or at main intersections. On the margins of and surrounding the central market are the stores of merchants, money transfer houses (mainly Amis Fideles Yokasan), money changers, pharmacies, hardware stores, general stores, beauty salons, restaurants, and bars (figures I.2–I.4). So far Luozi lacks banks of any kind. There are many pharmacies in Luozi, bearing such names as La Benediction de Dieu or Pharmacie la Main Sainte, selling imported drugs, locally manufactured medicines (in particular the trademarked Manalaria and Manadiar, produced by the Centre de Recherche Pharmaceutique de Luozi [CRPL]), and in the market, traditional medicinal ingredients. Beauty shops are festooned with paintings of fashionable hair styles and smooth skin, luring the customer with such slogans as "Maison Elikia: Ici sécrèt des méches" (here the secret of the hair extensions) and "Beauty is not born, it is made."

Several thousand of Luozi's approximately 15,000 inhabitants are school children, who stand out on the streets in their white shirts, dark blue trousers and skirts, and—for the girls—required modest hairdos, walking to or from their schools in the early morning, at noon, and again in the late afternoon. Luozi is highly regarded as a place to raise children and youth, for several reasons. It is a safe place; children are seen running around on their own, riding bicycles, playing soccer,

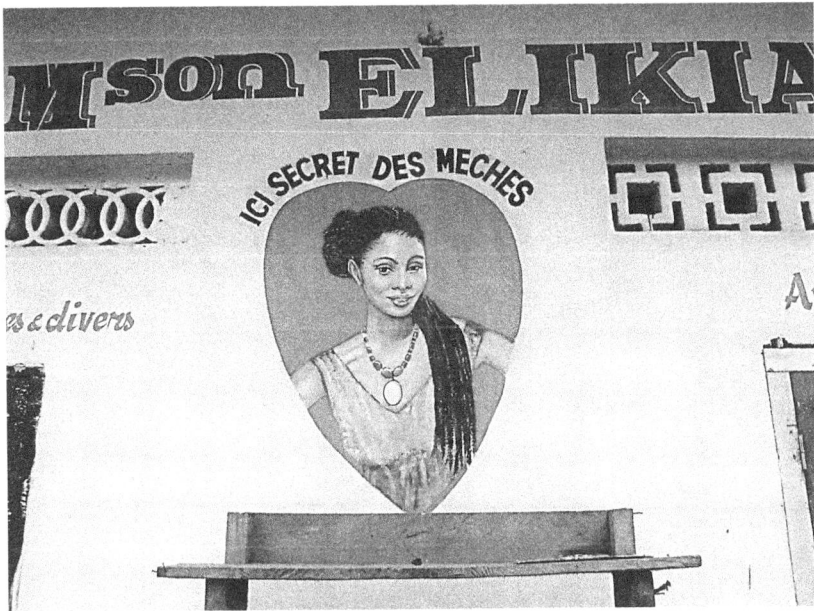

FIGURE I.2. Sécrèt des mèches—the faux hair lock. Artist Emmanuel Mvibidulu's portrayal for a Luozi hair stylist of the latest fashion. Photo: Reinhild Janzen, February 2013.

walking the streets in groups, attending soccer games in the stadium, fetching goats from their day's grazing, and running errands for parents, whether to stores, to markets, or around the neighborhood. Another reason Luozi is a child- and youth-friendly place is the sheer variety and number of schools: eleven primary schools, twelve secondary schools, four institutes of higher education, two universities, and four maternity schools (Mahaniah 2009, 41). Indeed, it would seem that the major industry in Luozi is education, the production of educated youth and young adults.

The school uniforms of the weekdays are exchanged on Sunday for clothes as fancy and colorful as possible. The streets are filled with brightly dressed women, men, and children often shaded by bright umbrellas in the morning's tropical sun on their way to Luozi's fifteen churches. Two churches are of the mainstream Communauté Evangélique du Congo, derived from the Swedish Covenant Church mission; there is also the Catholic church, Notre Dame du Perpétuel Sécours, opposite the central market. Half a dozen churches are independent African churches deriving from the Kongo prophetic tradition's early twentieth-century movements, including the Kimbanguist church. Other religious communities include the Salvation Army; the Seventh-Day Adventists; the Pentecostal church; a Bahá'í congregation, The Way; and a small Islamic community and mosque.

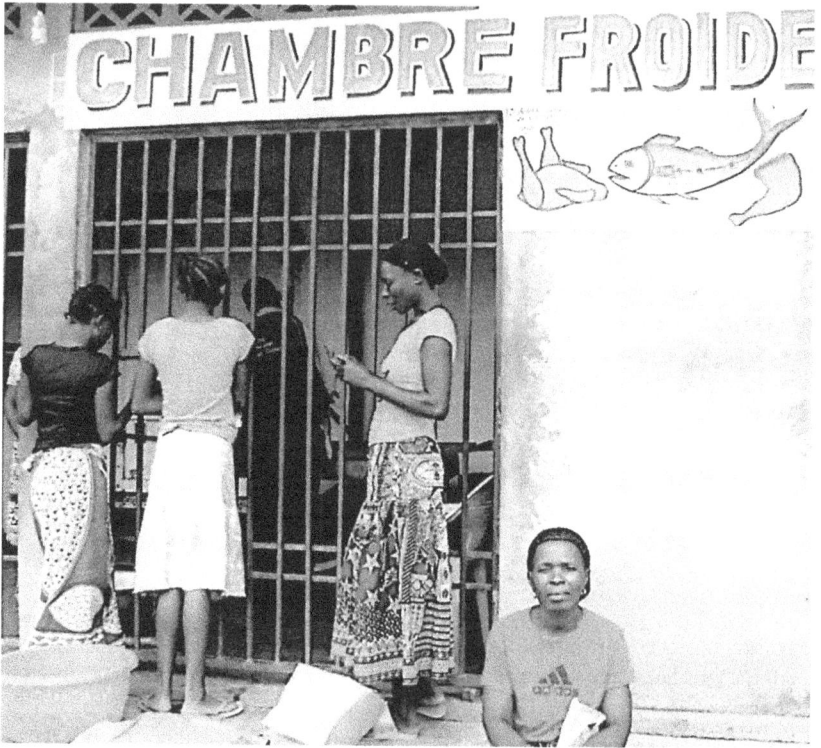

FIGURE I.3. Women shopping for fish at a cold storage shop while checking cell phones. Photo: John M. Janzen, 2013.

The bright colors of worshipers on their way to their gatherings corresponds to the energetic sounds of singing and especially the rhythm of the instruments that always accompany group singing: the double-membrane *bandi*, long single-membrane *ngoma*, and *ngulu-ngulu* friction drums; iron double gongs; tin and gourd rattles; and horns, whistles, and other sources of rhythm that inspire worship. The people of Luozi and the Manianga are spirited in their religious devotion, and tolerant. Often one finds adherents of different affiliations within the same clan, family, or even couple. This religious diversity and intensity reflects a century of mission work by Western churches and several centuries of Christian influence in the wider Kongo area, deriving from the sixteenth-century Christianity of the Kongo kingdom, and from the eighteenth-century Kongo prophetic tradition.

From late afternoon to dusk women are seen returning from their fields with loads of firewood on their heads or the evening's food in their *mpidi* baskets on their backs. At the same time children collect the goats that have been picketed on

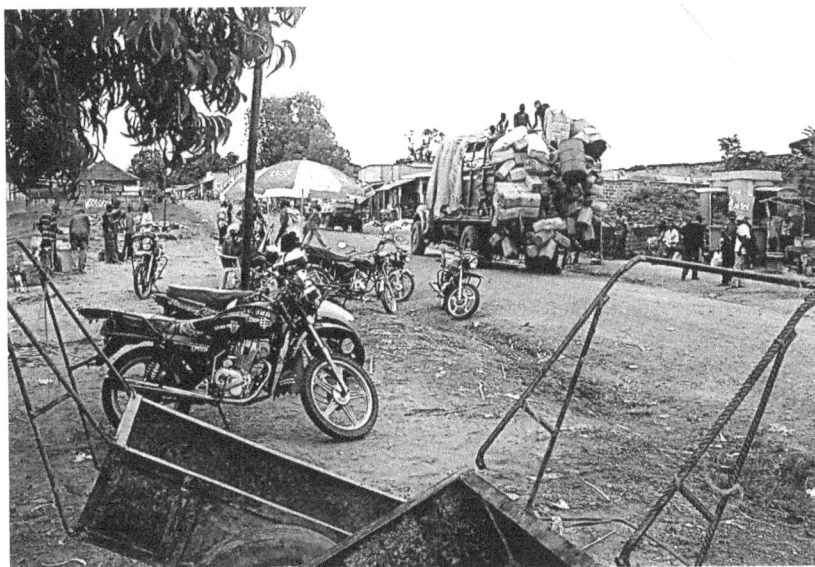

FIGURE I.4. Avenue du Commerce, Luozi, on market day. Truck being loaded for transport; carts and taxi-cycles parked at street side. Photo: John M. Janzen, April 2013.

grassy corners for the day and are now bleating as if to plead with their owners to come fetch them. The same scene before sundown includes motorcycles, their headlights breaking the growing darkness, carrying a young family home, with father driving, mother and children hanging on. Sunset comes early—around 6:00 p.m.—this close to the equator, and whatever evening life will happen will occur in the family gathering at home to a meal, often harvested or earned that very day at a field, a market, or a job. This scene, showing Luozi as a rural subsistence village-like town, demonstrates how close to the nub life is in this part of the Congo for most people. A few bars near the market keep after-dark hours, especially those with generators and television sets, suggestive of a more urban life.

But there are also scenes that feature the wider connections of travel and communication, linking this town on the Congo River to the wider world. Most Wednesdays around noon the air is shattered by the overhead sound of an airplane buzzing the city to announce its presence before landing at Luozi's airfield alongside the intersection of Commerce Avenue and the road north past the university—at the crocodile monument. Air service that was once provided by Air Brousse has been taken over by Mission Aviation Fellowship (MAF) to carry mail and any passengers who can pay the $100 fare from Kinshasa, or to evacuate medical cases to Kimpese or Kinshasa. But far more widely used than air travel are messages on cell phones and the internet, which have been available to Luozians since about 2005, when three companies—Tigo, Airtel, and Vodacom—installed their towers at the higher elevations and hills of Kilemba and beyond the university. Encouraged by the government, which saw the usefulness of digital communication for security purposes, these companies took advantage of the burgeoning market for cell phones worldwide. Shops and vendors of time cards sprang up around town to accommodate the ubiquitous use of phones, and more limited email use. Previously the only airwaves in Luozi had been the three radio stations: Radio Yenge (Joy) of Batangu Mpesa; the radio of the Protestant Church; and Radio Ntomosono ("Development"), owned and operated by the Congolese NGO Centre de Vulgarisation Agricole (Agricultural Extension Center).

The town of Luozi is organized into four residential quarters: Bidimio (with forty-nine streets, including the top administrator's residences at Kilemba, overlooking the river), Luvwezo (twenty-six streets, including the police camp near the river and the prison), Mbandu (with twenty streets, including the central market), and Nzadi (twenty-six streets, including some large residences near the river). These streets are not marked with street signs, so the inquisitive stranger will be quite lost; even some residents do not know the name of their street. However, the *chef de cité* assured me that the streets were indeed known, and only a shortage of funds hindered putting up street signs. The streets were the basis in 2012 of a city-wide census that identified men, women, boys, and girls. A not-to-scale map was drawn up by the *chef* himself for the benefit of census workers. This, and the old cadastre maps that were shown me reluctantly, are the only maps I could find of Luozi; no published map exists of the town in its present, or even recent, elaboration—just as there were no maps of Kinshasa commercially available in 2013.

Luozi, in Congolese legal terms, is a *cité* rather than a *ville* (100,000 inhabitants or more). As a cité Luozi has no tax-levying authority; no *décret-loi* has established its independent legal existence. Its budget is determined and paid by the provincial government, just as its chief executive, the *chef de cité*, is appointed by the provincial governor (figure I.5). Other public entities or levels of organization with which the city shares responsibility include (1) the territorial government with headquarters in Luozi, including the chief territorial agent and his assistants, the adjoint chief, and a variety of staff who occupy the offices near the football stadium and the territorial court; (2) the seven villages (map I.3) that predate Luozi but are now being incorporated into Luozi; (3) the sectors (in this case Mbanza Ngoyo to the north and Mbanza Mona to the west); (4) the health zone structure, which administers hospitals, health centers, and local health posts, as well as public health services such as vaccinations, and reports to the government on matters of population and disease epidemiology; (5) the city water system, administered by a local branch of the national parastatal Régie des Eaux (REGIDESO), now being privatized by decision of the national parliament; (6) eleven mutual aid societies representing

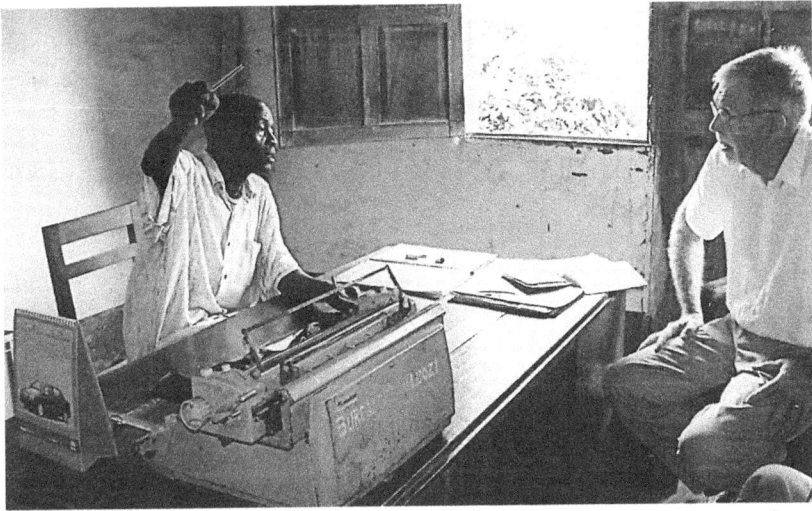

FIGURE I.5. Chef de Cité Matondo Lufinama explains the work of Luozi city government to anthropologist John M. Janzen. Vintage Royal typewriter and carbon copies provide necessary office technology. Photo: Reinhild Janzen, January 26, 2013.

Luozi residents from the ten sectors of the Manianga (Territory of Luozi), plus one for residents from elsewhere in Congo and foreigners, especially in matters pertaining to burials in Luozi's three cemeteries.

Despite this apparent lack of autonomous authority, the cité has substantial administrative responsibility, as Chef de Cité Matondo Lufinama explained to me. He oversees a staff that includes a police force, secretaries and assistants for the registration of civil affairs such as marriages, and a cadastre service to approve building applications and landholding permits. The cité is also responsible for cleaning the streets (hiring push carts or trucks to haul away refuse piles created by residents and market-stall keepers), and for annual inspection of Luozi's 2,600-some residential households for adherence to the pit toilet ordinance.[8]

Luozi is blessed with an abundance of health care institutions and specialists, thanks to a history of planners who chose the territorial capital for their main hospitals, to the 1984 adoption of WHO's program of primary health care, with health posts, health centers, and general referral hospitals in each health zone. One of three health zones in the Manianga, the Luozi Health Zone, uses the old state hospital (built in 1949 along the road up to Kilemba administrators' residences) as one of three referral hospitals in the Territory. The Catholic hospital (Hopital des Soeurs Catholique) across Commerce Avenue from the market, and part of the Catholic diocese complex, is in the health zone a health center. Yet it functions much like the hospital it was created to be in the 1950s. Luozi thus effectively has two hospitals. Multiple health centers and private clinics are scattered throughout the town. In Kinsemi, ten kilometers west of Luozi, a well-supplied health center has been created in his home community by Dr. Joseph Kapita-Bila, well-known in Kinshasa for his pioneering work in HIV/AIDS research. Luozi also has many pharmacies with usually well-stocked shelves. The innovative CRPL, founded and headed by Batangu, produces malaria prophylaxis and cures from herbs grown in valleys above Luozi and in the wild. These medicines are exported to Kinshasa for far wider distribution. Luozi is also home to healers (*banganga*) and herbalists.

Although these establishments are visible in buildings, signs, and advertising images, other—mostly unresolved and less visible—issues abound. People said that they hoped someone—government, an international NGO, they themselves applying their own intelligence—would alleviate the national economic crisis that affected them personally, making it difficult to pay for health care and tuition for their children's schooling. The vivid evidence of this economic crisis comes in the form of reference to occupations or sources of livelihood of most households. Some households are self-identified as cultivateur/cultivatrice. But many of those in which at least one adult member practices a profession, such as teacher, administrator, medical doctor, nurse, lab technician, or merchant, the other spouse, usually the wife, is identified as cultivatrice. Sometimes individuals with a profession will have a second identity as cultivateur. This focus on food production is reflected in the layout of the town, with loosely neighboring large yards with vegetable gardens and room for a few chickens, pigs, or goats. Many Luozians also have private fields outside of town, or in their ancestral villages, if these are within a day's walk or short drive. This is evidence of the fact that professions and trades do not pay well, and that there are few opportunities for professional advancement. The study's intensive sample reveals that 16 percent of Luozi's residents are adult children living with and being supported by their parents.

The urban allure of an education followed by a salaried job is a chimera for many. Luozi is, on the one hand, a territorial capital with institutions of government, higher education, health care, and religion, and it is a commercial hub at the convergence of roads to the interior and to the ferry, which connects with bigger urban centers. On the other hand, Luozi has the visage of a rural town, with every household growing its own food. But this is a deceptive visage that reflects the structural bind imposed by a specific kind of economy without many public services, that requires the people to pay for everything, where global commodities are cheaper than what is locally made, but where people are obligated to grow their own food to survive. Yet Luozi is not a village with clan-based settlement patterns, land tenure, and community decision-making. The layout of residences is very decidedly based on surveyed, registered lots purchased by individual residents or developers from preexisting clan land chiefs or other individual owners (Kalusebolo Mattlola 2013).[9] Resident households are mostly variations of nuclear families or single-parent families. According to Thomas Kisolokele, however, many people substitute regional associations for clan adherence.[10] The associations are most important as burial mutuals, with several new cemeteries emerging as the expression of nonvillage, nonclan sodalities.

Even after four months' residence, and memory of the town forty years before, Luozi remained challenging to visualize and therefore to conceptualize as an urban place and community. Despite Luozi's high number of educational institutions, government offices, and health care institutions, it had the feel of an agricultural village. Formerly whitewashed old colonial buildings had a generally run-down appearance, with rusting metal roofs, but the women and men walking the streets alongside these buildings were very fashionably dressed. Despite the presence of numerous medical centers and hospitals, and a thriving public health network in Luozi and the territory, malaria, a disease with known cause and cure, affected many people and killed numerous children every year. Most people owned and used cell phones, yet the postal system was completely defunct. Much attention was paid to development, but the roads were very bad, there was little public budget for improvements, and not a single bank in town could offer loans. The money transfer houses around the market (such as Amis Fideles Yokasan) represent a unique adaptation to the weakness of the local currency alongside the regular legal use of international currencies, such as the US dollar and the Euro. There are numerous examples of thriving individual businesses, but also high unemployment among the young.

High youth unemployment and the high percentage of young adults living with their parents hints at deeper contradictions of national Congolese political life lurking just beneath the surface of the apparently peaceful, bucolic town of Luozi. Unmentioned thus far in this profile of the town and its hinterland region is the garrison of the Congolese National Army's special forces about a mile west of town and within sight of the territorial agents and staff residences at Kilemba Heights, where the transmission towers of the cell phone companies rise into the sky. Five years earlier (in 2008) the forces were called in by the territorial agent when youth and antagonists loyal to Muanda Nsemi's nativist Bundu dia Kongo mobbed several local offices and carried out violent actions against property and persons.[11]

In a showdown in Luozi between Nsemi's followers and the military, at least twenty-five of the partisans were killed. Nsemi's political party was outlawed, although he continues to be a member of the national assembly. However, Nsemi's pamphlets proclaiming independence for the BaKongo and a return to pre-Christian ancestral religion and customs can be seen in the hands of groups of youth on Luozi's streets. Several observers said that although there is calm in the streets, the issues have not gone away and the youth, particularly those without education and without work, are more frustrated than ever.

To what extent do these local sentiments reflect structural absences due to a collapsed or fragile state in the midst of a neoliberal global economy. The sketch of the setting of this research into postcolonial and twenty-first-century health and health care following the collapse of the state must go beyond Luozi and the Manianga to the national, even global economic context. An entry I wrote in my field journal upon arrival in Kinshasa in January 2013 captures the features of this wider neoliberal context that is the Democratic Republic of the Congo.

Neoliberal global economy has never been clearer to me than in recent days in Kinshasa. The literature I've read refers to global transfers of resources, information, people, and capital, with power residing somewhere in the hands of those who control or take advantage of these flows, those who control the nexuses of networks. The overwhelming evidence of this economy is everywhere, showing clearly the differentiation between the big players and the struggling, marginalized pawns. Government—here the RDC—may be a facilitator, but probably not the main driving force in shaping things. Current RDC policy seems to support open flows of currency—dollars, euros, francs—in the form of investments of all kinds in exchange for resource concessions. This is the "liberal" aspect. The Chinese build and pave roads (e.g., the airport road, Blvd 30 Juin, the Kin-Matadi road) in exchange for concessions of precious metals and minerals. Food importers of all kinds (e.g., Seaboard, of the flour mills) have a ready market that can undercut local food producers. A Japanese lumber and construction conglomerate is exporting huge logs from Congo's rainforest. They are floated downstream from Kisangani, loaded onto log trucks that daily haul several dozen loads through clogged Kinshasa streets and down the newly paved highway to the Matadi port, where they are shipped to their destination to become veneers and fiberboards for the global construction industry. Information technology, in the form of telecommunications companies—Vodacom (S. African), Airtel (Indian), Tigo (African, headquarters in Kigali)—are doing a booming business at every corner in cell phones, time cards, subscriptions, and cash transfers. The cell phone has revolutionized the ways and extent to which people can be in touch, locally, regionally, globally. And rates are really cheap, ca. $38 for one Samsung phone plus time. Fewer people use internet and email, but the means exists with the three companies mentioned. Our Tigo modem cost $30; a top-use 4 GB monthly subscription, plus initial hookup, $50. Small shops with solar panels, small generators, a laptop, and time cards for sale, plus food and drink, constitutes an internet or "cyber-café." In this structure of open flows of everything, anything can be commoditized. That is, it has a price and can be bought and sold, in infinitely reducible units. So, at intersections or traffic stops, a young man is selling single time cards for cell phones; another street side vendor was hawking singly or in handfuls: funnels, coat hangers, food bits, plastic tubes of water, items of clothing, even used passports! The ubiquitous taxibuses move masses of people across the megalopolis of Kinshasa—100 sq. kms, 13 million estimated inhabitants—because there is no public transportation. Even the buses of yore are long gone.

Neoliberalism is antithetical to, or simply ignoring of, public investment in infrastructure or welfare, social services/health care programs, pensions, unions, any kind of reinvestment of resources into redistributive public programs. The painters of *l'art populaire* depict the realities noted here—e.g., minerals being carried off, masses being squeezed, environment trashed, the future compromised.

RESEARCHING HEALTH ANTHROPOLOGICALLY

Health, as an object of research, is framed by philosophical abstractions regarding themes that guide or reflect domains of action in a society (such as adaptation, stability, security, and well-being). It is also rendered accessible through statistical indicators—above all, birth rates, death rates, and the incidence of disease—that are usually seen in publications of health organizations such as WHO, the Centers for Disease Control in the United States, and the health zones in Congo. Health as an object of research is also evidenced in the realm of sentiments, signs and symbols, expressions of poetry, and embodiment; it is interiorized in the body and organs, and exteriorized in words and various perspectives projected toward others as health or sickness, suffering or joy. Thus health is for anthropology a topic that is equally fitting for qualitative and quantitative study, for reflections of a theoretical or philosophical nature as well as of contemporary or historical ethnography.

The present research was designed to integrate all of these perspectives to determine the current status of health in a region of western Central Africa, and to assess the extent of progress made in recent years toward overcoming some of the disease challenges that defined an earlier era. The central focus of the project was to understand the institutions that ensured the continued investment in levels of health gained, and advantages achieved, during the crisis years of the 1980s and 1990s and beyond.

The research project was more open-ended than I had anticipated, full of surprises and discoveries. The ripple effect of the collapse of state structures and the concurrent introduction of public health zones rearranged institutions in unforeseen ways. But in other respects I found connections that looped back to the earlier work of my *Quest for Therapy in Lower Zaire* (1978) and *Lemba 1650–1930: A Drum of Affliction in Africa and the New World* (1982a). Although the prominence of healers had diminished since the 1960s, complex cases of illness and the search for social causes still produced quests for appropriate therapy. Evidence of the historical impact of the precolonial coastal trade, including the slave trade, emerged frequently in surprising ways, having to do with memories and fears of hidden illicit powers, loss, or death.

Identifying Inspirations, Collaborations, and Facilitators

Vana kiese—"to give joy"—was the drink of choice at the large reception hosted for my wife, Reinhild, and me at Batangu's elaborate Kinshasa house/laboratory/ production facility in late April 2013. This liqueur was a joint product of Batangu's pharmaceutical processing company and his brother's agricultural products processing plant, both in Luozi. In addition to imported and local beers, the menu on the lavishly set table included several kinds of meats, including *muamba nguba* (groundnut stewed chicken), *chikwanga* manioc bread, a pasta salad, and fried caterpillars. The thirty guests represented Batangu's friends and acquaintances from the world of education (including the rector of the new Université Kongo in Mbanza Ngungu, whose board of trustees he chaired), local government officials, professors and graduate students of other Kinshasa institutions of higher education, his pharmacy colleagues, and Manianga elites. Such lavish hospitality within warm relations is an important ingredient of the successful research enterprise in Congo. Establishing and maintaining contacts with the public, with government, and with professionals, is critical to carrying out anthropological research on a topic as sensitive and volatile as health and healing. Therefore featuring the personalities and projects on which anthropological attention is focused is an important dimension of this research.

Here I wish to go beyond the lines of credit already enumerated in the acknowledgments section to recognize the intellectual, as well as social, contributions that individuals have made my research career and to this particular project, both of which have built on enduring relationships. Whereas fifty years ago I was welcomed into Kongo society as a foreign student, a stranger, now I was received and hosted as Professor Janzen by other professors, directors, businesspersons, and medical doctors. Whereas previously people who endured my questions and presence politely seemed to be pleased that I wished to study their language and customs, now these peers wanted to know what my research project entailed, what my hypothesis was, and how my career in anthropology was shaping up. Several of these individuals will be introduced here, and their contributions to my understanding of Kongo life and thought made explicit.

Batangu, pharmacist, entrepreneur, national deputy, and educator, is a continuous thread connecting earlier scholarship with the present project in Lower Congo. This son of the far northwest region of the Manianga—Kingoyi—is the founder and director of the CRPL, a research and manufacturing company that is today widely known for marketing Manalaria, an antimalarial prophylactic, and Manadiar, a malaria treatment that calms the fever and diarrheal effects of the disease. Because of his successful bid for national parliament in the 1990s, Batangu may, in elite circles of Kinshasa, be addressed by the title "Honorable," but he does not insist.

Batangu has often told his story of his earliest acquaintance with the project I conducted with William Arkinstall in the 1960s how it decisively altered the course of his career. He repeated this story at our farewell party in Luozi and again at the already-mentioned reception in Kinshasa some days later. While he was a student in pharmacy at the University of Montreal in the 1970s, he received a research paper that originated in the seminar Arkinstall and I led with Don Bates at McGill University. The herbarium of medicinal plants Arkinstall assembled in work with healers in the Manianga was of particular interest to Batangu. Inspired by such an affirmation that Manianga was a resource for medicinal plants, he determined to launch a research and development institute on his return home. This he did, without any outside help, creating the CRPL.

Later in the 1970s, Batangu, by then a national deputy, traveled to the United States with a sampling of medicinal plants that he had determined had potential for curative purposes. He visited me at the University of Kansas, where I introduced him to the director of the Department of Pharmaceutical Chemistry, which has an extensive botanical herbarium. This lab identified Batangu's plants and affirmed their medicinal potential. Unfortunately, in the wake of Congo's descent into chaos and corruption, the collaboration we had hoped to develop did not materialize. But in 1982, in connection with a large-scale comparative study of healing ritual networks in Kinshasa, Dar es Salaam, Swaziland, and Cape Town (Janzen 1992), I was able to visit Batangu in Kinshasa and to renew acquaintances to see his urban pharmacy where he sold the products coming from the fields, forests, and research labs of Luozi, as well as commercial drugs.

When we arrived in Congo on January 2, 2013, and word of our presence spread through the grapevine, Batangu called to welcome us. When Arkinstall, his wife, Karin, and daughter, Rhylin, visited Luozi in late April, Batangu came to join us. He gave us an extensive tour of the plantation of medicinal plants, the residence he had established in a new section of Luozi near the plantation, his research facility, his radio station, the entire complex. Throughout this tour Batangu's videographer filmed us. At our Luozi farewell dinner, with about fifty persons present, Batangu and I related this history of mutual inspiration dating back to the early 1970s. This too was filmed and became a part of an edited DVD titled "Rencontre Scientifique Luozi Avril 2013."

In Kinshasa a few days later, at his own reception for us, Batangu introduced us—the Janzens—by relating the same history of encounters and mutual enrichments in Montreal and Kansas, and now Luozi and Kinshasa. Batangu then turned the floor over to me with instructions to explain how I became interested in the Congo initially. "What inspired you to come here, study our history, culture, health, and healing, and to return again forty-five years later?" I began my response in KiKongo but quickly switched to French because I was on complicated identity terrain. Also, the hour was getting late, and I surmised that despite my audience's love of speeches they would want a brief three- to five-minute response. The temperature and humidity in the room were both at ninety-five. In abbreviated form, here is what I said.

As a nineteen-year-old conscientious objector to military service, I responded to the opportunity to go to the Congo under the Pax voluntary service program of the Mennonite Central Committee. My brother-in-law had gone into this program before me, and we all admired him. So for two years, from 1957 to 1959, in what is now Bandundu Province on the southern savanna, I worked in construction and education, and did a bit of medical work, mainly bush ambulance driving. During my final six months I was overseer of a crew of about twenty-five carpenters and masons who were building a hospital at Mukedi mission station near Kilembe, in the heart of western Pende country. To this gathered group of Congolese postcolonial elites, I recalled the impact of the Léopoldville riots of January 1959 on the mood of my workers, and on me, just eighteen months before the independence of the Congo. The workers were often sullen and angry, not with me personally—I visited their homes, ate meals with them, and had many conversations—but rather with the colonial system that had taken their land and shortchanged their freedom and prosperity. A short four years later the beautiful new hospital would be torched by the militants of Pierre Mulele, although later it was restored and is again in use.

When I returned to the United States to finish college, I chose to continue my studies in anthropology and African Studies because I had many questions about what I had seen and experienced. I found that there was a great need in the United States and the Western world for experts who could interpret to students and the general public what was happening in Africa, especially the new countries facing their independent national development. When I received grant funding to conduct my doctoral research, I chose the Kongo region of Lower Congo because it had been much more deeply affected by contact with the Western world than the southern savanna region where I had served in the Pax program (the impact there was more subtle but also quite significant). I chose the north bank of the Congo region, the Manianga, because it had been less extensively studied, apparently, than other regions.

I landed in Kivunda because of my acquaintance with Carroll Yoder, an American who was teaching at Sundi Lutete secondary school under the Teachers Abroad Program (TAP). Meanwhile, I learned that another anthropology student, Wyatt MacGaffey, would be conducting research on the south bank at the same time. Over the years our friendship and research collegiality has been a great inspiration to me. Kisiasia village is where communal mayor Mbuta Kusikila offered me lodging in his house in 1964. Years later he would confess to me that he had done this for two reasons: because he was genuinely interested in what I had come to study and for surveillance purposes.

I had wanted to return to the Manianga to see what had transpired in the realm of health, healing, and health care in the years since my earlier research. The audience of about thirty guests in Batangu's spacious reception/meeting/dining room vigorously applauded my speech and would have had many further questions had I not excused myself to return to our hotel through dense Kinshasa traffic to prepare for our departure the next day. Several weeks later Batangu would assume the rectorship of the Université Kongo at Mbanza Ngungu, where he could promote scholarship and the teaching of science for the development of his national community.

My first encounter with the people and culture of the Manianga was in my dissertation research in 1964–66. A postdoctoral project with Arkinstall followed in the same region in 1969 and led directly to the publication of the book *The Quest for Therapy in Lower Zaire* (Janzen 1978), following the two seminars at McGill University in which Arkinstall and I, together with medical historian Bates, studied quests for healing in Lower Congo and Quebec.[12] A 1982 return to Kinshasa and several short assignments in Central and Southern Africa in connection with the books *Lemba* (Janzen 1982a) and *Ngoma* (Janzen 1992) permitted some engagement with Manianga people near their home.

The present book builds on that earlier work and contributes to the body of Western Equatorial African—Kongo—scholarship. During the 1960s and 1970s African studies was a booming field that sought to document and understand the emergence of new societies from colonialism. Anthropology and other social sciences were at the center of this scholarship. In the 1970s the Joint Africa Committee of the Social Science Research Council and the American Council of Learned Societies launched a research planning project on health and healing in Africa. Historian Steven Feierman and I were invited to serve as cochairs of this project, and we ultimately published much of the research in the volume *The Social Basis of Health and Healing in Africa* (Feierman and Janzen 1992).

Together, and with the help of other scholars, we organized a series of workshops, conferences, and publications to shape new research and policy on critical questions of health, public health, culture, and the direction of health care, and the collaborative relationship of African medicine to cosmopolitan medicine. Particularly the June 1980 conference at Emmanuel College, University of Cambridge, titled "African Medical and Health Systems as Systems of Thought, Causality, and Taxonomy" (Janzen and Prins 1981) became instrumental in shaping research projects. The conference involved scholars and health care practitioners from Africa, Europe, and North America who were conducting their own work and training students. Several Congolese scholars participated in this conference, and their work would shape all studies on Lower Congo health and healing in subsequent years. Jean Masamba ma Mpolo, theologian and psychotherapist, spoke on the issue of witchcraft in health and healing, hypothesizing that bewitchment represents an unconscious effort at personality integration vis-à-vis a social "group ego." In his pastoral and clinical counseling Masamba sought to help the patient realize fuller self-actualization and self-confidence (Masamba ma Mpolo 1981). Kimpianga Mahaniah, historian, had written about religious history of the Manianga. He presented an overview of the diversity of healing modes and traditions in the growing metropolis of Kinshasa, at a population of 2 million in 1980 (Mahaniah 1981). Also Congolese philosopher V. Y. Mudimbe sketched a perspective from Western philosophy, especially the work of Michel Foucault, in the analysis of African healing around harmony, emulation, analogy, and sympathy, the four universal categories of resemblance (Mudimbe 1981).

Masamba ma Mpolo's work would influence a generation of Congolese and international theologians, pastoral counselors, anthropologists, and scholars of religion concerning the difficult issue of witchcraft suspicions in personal mental health and morality, and in sketching a course of contemporary thinking that does not simply dismiss as false belief this common dimension of African thought. After a season serving with the World Council of Churches in Geneva, Switzerland, he returned to Congo and taught at the Protestant seminary in Kimpese, Lower Congo, until his death in 2000.

Mahaniah took a similar trajectory to that of Masamba, serving for a decade with the World Council of Churches in Geneva as head of the African Development department. Following a decade in Geneva he returned to the Congo, where he taught African history and development in several institutions in Kinshasa and the Lower Congo. Then in the 1980s he founded an independent development NGO in the Manianga, the Centre de Vulgarisation Agricole (CVA). This modest sounding outreach center began as a publishing initiative for Congolese writings on issues of economic development and cultural renaissance. In due course the CVA, with its headquarters in Luozi and Kinshasa, would found the Free University of Luozi, which has become a major institution of higher education in the Lower Congo and especially the Manianga.

Mudimbe's writing on philosophy in Africa and generally on critical scholarship in and on Africa became well known. He was forced to flee the Congo in the 1980s when President Mobutu tried to co-opt him into his political elite. He received political asylum in the United States, where he taught at Haverford College and Stanford and Duke universities.

When I returned in early 2013 to do a follow-up study of health, healing, and health care, I wondered how many people I would find whom I had known from my earlier visits. Throughout the four-month stay Reinhild and I met individuals who had been seminal facilitators and informants during my early fieldwork. There was Mbuta Kusikila, former teacher and mayor of Kivunda commune (now again called a *secteur*), who in 1964 received me in his office, listened to my explanation of my project, and then promptly invited me to live in his village house, with his younger brother, in the Nsundi clan section of Kisiasia. Reinhild joined me for part of this stay in Kisiasia.

Now we visited Mbuta Kusikila in his retirement house in Tadi, the commercial center at Kivunda, where he spends his time cultivating his garden of vegetables and special plants for medicinal applications. He proudly brought out of his library cabinet the copy of my dissertation I had shipped him in 1967, although he had not been able to read the English. He was intent on showing me the nutritional-medicinal substances he had invented from plants in his garden or the wild, work inspired by our early research. I gave him a French copy of my book *The Quest for Therapy in Lower Zaire* (1978), which had been researched in his commune, and showed him the passage where I describe his assistance in the project. He had transferred his village house to his younger brother, Nkebi Victor, who with his wife Sidoni still lived there. Another day they received us on the same veranda where we had often stood, overlooking the main village street. They invited us to come inside, and we sat in the same solid wooden armchairs as in 1965. Nkebi had become the head of the local Nsundi clan section, and in his responsibility for allocating land to all his dependents he asked me for the local maps I had drawn in my earliest research in the 1960s.

Many of the people with whom we had special relations—hosts, friends, informants—had died, as we learned from their descendants, friends, and neighbors. Pierre Nzuzi, once head of a section of the Kimbanga clan at Kisiasia, who had been very helpful in reconstructing the Kimbanga genealogy and the settlement and political history of his group, had died, as I learned from his son Kukelana, who contacted me several years ago from his residence in Spain. But then there was the accidental meeting with Nzuzi's cousin Nsimba Jacques, who with his wife greeted me in the Sundi-Lutete hospital, where he was recuperating from surgery. When I appeared at the door of his hospital room during a tour of the facility, he looked up with surprise on his face, came forward to look at me up close, and exclaimed, "John, c'est vous?" (Is it really you?) After the surprise of a face-to-face encounter after forty-five years, he assured me that the Kimbanga clan genealogy I had left with his cousin Nzuzi was now safely kept in his house.

Launching the Study

The Fulbright Senior Research Fellowship that funded this study requires a solid relationship to a host in the country where the research is conducted. I am deeply indebted to Professor Kimpianga Mahaniah for offering to serve as a counterpart, host, and interested partner in this research. When I wrote him in 2011 about my interest in returning to the Manianga for a research project, he offered endorsement and a generous package of infrastructural supports in Luozi—lodging, caretaking staff, a vehicle, and a circle of handlers who not only looked after us but introduced us to a range of contacts in government, health care, education, and the community. I could not have hoped for better research assistance.

I used several anthropological methods. The most common was that hallmark of anthropological fieldwork, participant observation—just hanging around, watching others, and being part of the action if possible. Each activity may render visible ideas, values, or cultural conceptions, seen or formulated in a particular context. I observed medical institutions, particular cases of illness, and trajectories in the pursuit of health care. These all serve as testimonies to structures of thought and action.

I also developed a questionnaire that was used in formal interviews of households. The results became a compendium I call the intensive sample. Anthropologists use inquiry by questionnaire to achieve a more balanced understanding of specific areas of behavior, knowledge, values, and opinions. The questionnaire, titled "The Social Reproduction of Health / La réproduction sociale de la santé / *Mtombuka a zungu mu mavimpi*," was administered in either French or KiKongo, depending on the preference of the interviewee. The following six topics were covered: (1) Household composition / La composition du ménage / *Bonso buena mbutuka*; (2) Occupation / *Kisalu* / *kisalanga konso muntu* (*Bakala 1, Nkento 2*) *kia kedika*; (3) Illness episodes experienced in past year, treatment, result / Episodes de maladie, traitement, resultat (dans l'année dernière) / *Tandu kia bimbevo ye ndiakusunu (mu mvu yi viokele)*; (4) Around the house / Autour de la maison / *Kinzungidila kia nzo*; (5) Meaning of health / Sens de la santé / *Mavimpi*; (6) Family planning / La planification familliale—*Nkubukulu a mbutulu*.

This part of the study yielded returns from 105 households in Luozi and in the North Manianga region of Kivunda and Sundi Lutete. The selection process produced what anthropologists call an opportunistic sample, including individuals or households intentionally selected for their likely differences in health and disease manifestations. In Luozi this included middle-class—professional—and other households that benefited from the city's pure water system; households of merchants, government administrators, and teachers; and members of churches that practice healing rituals. Included intentionally were households of cultivators who lived beyond the city water system, and of fishers on the river. During a trip north to the Kivunda region, we interviewed a similar cross-section of cultivators, educators, and craftspeople. From all these groups we sought to include approximately equal numbers of women in different age cohorts: 50–70, 40–49, 30–39, and 18–29 (tables I.1 and I.2). Interview respondents in the intensive sample were told explicitly at the beginning of an interview that their participation was voluntary. They were also asked if they wished to have their names remain anonymous or were willing to be identified with the results. The large majority wished to be identified. However, with the exception of a few credits of quotations at the beginnings of chapters, respondents are only identified by social, demographic, or occupational category.

TABLE I.I. Household heads in intensive sample, by occupation and gender

	male	female	total
Administration / bureaucrat	4	1	5
Artiste-Peintre / artist-painter	1		1
Bibliothecaire / librarian		1	1
Chauffeur, mecanicien / chauffeur, mechanic	5		5
Commercant / merchant	4	2	6
Cultivateur, cultivatrice / farmer	39	80	119
Cusinier, domestique, ménagère / cook, domestic, household manager		5	5
Electricien / electrician	1		1
Enseignant / teacher, professor	8	3	11
Etudiant / student		2	2
Exécutif (CVA, etc)/ executive	2		2
Forgeron / blacksmith	2		2
Guerisseur / healer	1		1
Industrie, travailleur / worker	1		1
Infirmier / nurse	2	1	3
Juge / judge	1		1
Macon / mason	2		2
Maitress d'ecole / headmistress		2	2
Menuisier-charpentier / carpenter	5		5
Pasteur, aumonier /pastor, chaplain	3		3
Pecheur / fisher	11		11
Photographe / photographer	1		1
Tailleur, couturier / tailor	2	3	5
Technicien de laboratoire / laboratory technician	1	1	2
Total household heads			197

SOURCE: Janzen intensive sample.

Important information for the wider study was available in public records of the city and territory, in church offices, and in publications available in libraries and individual holdings. Particular attention was paid to the health zone office, where public health initiatives have been created and records kept since 1984. Territorial offices were a source of statistics and information in the annual reports. City records were a further source of statistical and anecdotal information on health and population.

TABLE I.2. Respondents by age, gender, and household composition

Ages of heads	Head and Spouse		Grown children (appearing in mother's age group)		Children under 18 (appearing in mother's age group)		Total households and individuals (appearing in mother's age group)	
	M	F	M	F	M	F	Households	Individuals
70s	2	1	1	1	0	0	1	5
60s	9	5	5	6	3	7	5	35
50s	24	14	20	17	11	14	14	100
40s	21	24	24	19	42	38	24	168
30s	31	35	0	0	57	61	36	184
20s	11	25	0	0	27	24	25	87
Total	98	104	50	43	140	144	105	579

SOURCE: Janzen intensive sample.

OUTLINE OF CHAPTERS

The book is organized into three parts. Part I, "A History of Population and Disease in the Lower Congo," provides an overview of the main trends of population and disease in precolonial, colonial, and postcolonial eras. Part II, "The Social Reproduction of Health," investigates the nature and capacity of domestic and public institutions in the social and economic determination of health, including the configuration of public health and health care institutions that prevailed during and after the crisis of the 1980s and 1990s. Part III, "The Legitimation of Power and Knowledge," examines the condition of those institutions in terms of their acceptance by the public, the professions, and the wider world; the strength of their organization; and the efficacy of their work.

Chapter 1, "Population Decline and Rise," is premised on the assumption that a full understanding of contemporary disease and of the way some diseases are remembered requires historical background. The chapter tracks a regional demographic and epidemiological history during precolonial mercantilism, including slavery (until ca. 1870), and the transition to the colonialism of the Congo Free State (1877-1908) and the Belgian Congo (1908–60). After establishing a baseline of credible population and disease numbers in the 1930s, the chapter reviews evidence for and an explanation of the massive population decline through 1900, which was followed by a gradual rise in population after 1930 and throughout the colonial era until 1960. Chapter 2, "Postcolonial Population and Disease Trends," reviews the extent of population growth, the advent of family planning, and the broad outlines of disease epidemiology. A discussion of the principal diseases of the Manianga gives an overview of diseases from 2003 to 2012 as recorded by the

Luozi Health Zone, a profile of their causes and manifestations, and a description of how they are dealt with by the community and by health care institutions. This profile of diseases is also compared to findings from the study's intensive sample.

Chapters 3, 4, and 5 portray the social reproduction of health as seen in the productive and organizational support of public health practices, health care practitioners and institutions, and popular ideas and images of health. Chapter 3, "Health in Household, Family, and Clan," applies the concept to North Kongo social and economic organization, reviews Kongo domestic social organization, and features the household within a bifurcating pattern of access to land, the essential resource sought by the majority of the population, through clan membership on the one hand, and through civil land titles on the other. Both models produce and reproduce health as each provides the essential resources for households and families to care for basic and emergency needs. The chapter includes a case study of household production and reproduction in relation to health care and educational costs. It also sketches the health care costs and patterns of use in representative examples drawn from the study's intensive sample.

Chapter 4, "Public Health and Health Care Institutions, Reconfigured," continues this line of presentation and analysis, and includes a portrayal of Congo's neoliberal political-economic environment. A discussion of local government and health portrays the chiefship/sector/commune in colonial and postcolonial eras, and the critical role local government has played in clean water provisioning and sewage containment, as well as the public health dimensions of dispute settlement and the maintenance of public order. The chapter records the 1984 launch of the health zones, first as prototypes, then under WHO auspices, and discusses the system's transformation in the 1990s. The chapter also describes the resurrection of earlier church medical services, now under Congolese Protestant and Catholic leadership. A discussion of Luozi's waterworks tells the remarkable story of the design and installation of a pure water system in Luozi in the early 1990s, on the eve of the collapse of the state, and the role of the regional elite in this project. The section also includes a brief account of rural pure water and sanitation installations and their upkeep, or lack thereof.

Chapter 5, "Rejoicing in Our Bodies: Popular Meanings of Health," situates popular understandings of health gleaned from the survey question "What is health to you?" alongside definitions of health employed in global health organizations and biomedicine. Distinctive themes that emerge in popular ideas of health are quality of life, including children's education; "force in our bodies," or ability to work; purity or cleanliness of body, house, and yard; sanctity, peace, and benediction; "rejoicing in our bodies" and having hope; physical, mental, and social well-being; and agency to make right decisions. The chapter also sketches health-related concerns respondents voiced in the same breath as their vivid depictions of how they understand health.

Chapters 6, 7, and 8 explore the legitimation of institutional power and knowledge, with a culminating assessment of how such legitimation affects the efficacy of disease control, in particular of the nine current principal diseases. Chapter 6, "*Dumuna*: Creating Authority from Below," examines social legitimation in light of both classical Western theories and Central African ideas of power and legitimacy, including the view that loss of control is sickness, and that social healing, or restoration of authority, brings about physical health. The classical academic theories, rooted in statecraft, need to be supplemented with theories that define the nature of legitimation in entities outside the state, or under the shadow of a fragile or failed state. Central African ideas of legitimacy of power and knowledge importantly recognize the threat of illegitimate power outside of instituted authority. Of particular importance in this study is an appreciation of governmentality beyond the state, formulated usefully for present purposes as "divergent legitimations." The chapter elaborates on the multiple constellations and applications signaled by the North Kongo ritual *dumuna*: in confirming healers' interventions in patients' lives, in family blessing, as a reflection of the importance of sound alliances as building blocks in long-term societal stability, and in inaugurating chiefs. Creating chiefships is a form of social healing, and prophetic appropriations of *dumuna* include faith healing and inauguration of prophetic healers.

Chapter 7, "Science, Sorcery, and Spirit," examines the integration of science into popular and elite thought, alongside other modes of knowledge. The opening section reviews the scholarship on science, culture, and distinctive African ideas. A discussion of the salience of evolutionary biology for malaria and sickle cell anemia examines how these issues are understood by both medical and scientific figures in Kongo society, and the impact of medical knowledge, especially modern genetics, on the people and families who have to contend with the sickling syndrome. The subsequent section presents the debate over whether to examine kinship at the time of a misfortune or sickness; this reflects the existence of a moral universe in which the perception of misfortune prompts the desire to know who and what are behind the matter—forces ranging from crocodiles, fish, carrion-eating birds, humans, nature spirits, and energy transfers. The examples considered bring out both positive advantages and the negative potential of *mfiedulu*, the examination of kinship and other relationships. The chapter traces the distinctive features of the contours of personhood, the source of much of the concern over misfortune and health in Kongo thought. The chapter closes with a close-up portrait of a young professional who, as a newly minted MD, seamlessly joins medical science with faith healing, becoming a fully qualified healer in a prophet church in order to address the "whole person."

Chapter 8, "Legitimation and Disease Control," revisits the principal diseases of the Manianga in terms of their clusters of features, the way they are handled, and the institutions that handle them. The work's hypothesis about institutional legitimacy and efficacy in treatment is repeated here so it can be applied to each of the "divergent legitimations and diverse diseases." Sewage-born diseases and the regulation of sources of water are largely handled by local government. Diseases affecting maternal and child health are largely handled by the health zones and local clinics, centers, and hospitals, with the collaboration of national and international NGOs. Dangerous diseases—that is, those that are regarded as international hazards—are addressed by the same NGOs working with the health zones. Steady-state diseases, such as malaria and bilharzia along rivers, are treated on an individual basis and not as social conditions. New diseases, such as diabetes and diseases with increasing incidence, such as the global flu, are hardly spoken about, and little is done about them. The chapter's analysis thus recognizes where institutional legitimacy and efficacy gives way to spotty or even no attention. The most serious of these diseases is the global seasonal flu, which is not considered within the orbit of anyone's responsibility. The same is true of the public aspects of treating malaria. A number of respondents lamented the missing authority of the state, which they wish would address the shortcomings in public health and health care delivery to achieve the pictures of health they imagine.

The book's conclusion offers ideas on wider relevance of the study. The interplay of knowledge and power is pivotal for effective control of disease and enhancement of health in the Manianga region of the Lower Congo, and in many similar regions across the globe. This work has focused particularly on the way in which multiple kinds of knowledge have been developed to heal the conditions that affect many people in the region, and on the social and institutional structures in which this knowledge has been couched. Of particular concern has been the process by which such structures acquire and maintain their legitimacy in the face of the historical rise and decline of specific instances of public order. The evisceration of public authority—whether by global trade, colonial conquest, or corruption and destitution under postcolonial despots—results in a paralysis of public institutions, including health care institutions, leading to the lingering incidence of well-understood diseases and conditions of ill-health. This situation, chronic in the region, justifies scholarly analysis into the nature of social legitimacy: what it is and how it is lost, re-created, maintained, and engaged.

PART I

A History of Population and Disease in the Lower Congo

I

Population Decline and Rise

There was a war between the people (*bisi-nsi*) and the government white man from Mpioka on the Congo river. This was before there was a station at Kikenda, by which time the people had accepted the foreign government. The white man arrived with his soldiers to Kimbedi, but the people ran. Mbemba, of a Kimbanga clan, who may have been land chief there, was killed by a ball from his gun. They then cut off his arm. He traveled on a litter (*kipovy*). Only white man Si-Si-Si travelled on horse (*punda, cavalo*).

—Kimbanga elders, Kisiasia village, to J. M. Janzen, April 1969

Workers on the railroad Matadi to Ango-Ango fled to their villages to escape the grippe that was spreading from Matadi, and needed be forced to return to work. In addition to the grippe, epidemics of dysentery, malaria, and sleeping sickness are reported.

—*Régistre des Rapports sur l'Administration Générale*, Congo Belge, 1916,
    Luozi Territorial Archives

Although this work is largely a study of twenty-first-century health and health care in the Lower Congo region of Western Equatorial Africa, the historical record of birth and death rates provides important clues for many contemporary conditions, modes of adaptation, and cultural attitudes toward particular diseases. The centerpiece of this historical demographic backdrop (table 1.1) is the dramatic fluctuation of total population numbers during the past three centuries: falling population from 1700 to 1930, by as much as 50 percent according to some sources (Sautter 1966), with other sources concentrating much of this decline in the years of the Congo Free State—1880s to 1907 (Hochschild 1998). Then the population rose from about 1930 until the end of colonialism in 1960 (Trolli and Dupuy 1934; Nicolai 1961; Feierman and Janzen 1992, 25–37). In the postcolonial period, total population nearly tripled, and in the twenty-first century we see the emergence of family planning in some regions, a direct indication of the self-conscious effort

TABLE 1.1. Timeline of political history and population trends, Lower Congo, 1800–2010

Timeline	Key Events	Luozi Territory pop.	Pop. decline/ growth/yr	Birth rate/ 1000/yr	Death rate/ 1000/yr	Infant mortality rate/1000/yr
1800	Peak of slave trade; 15,000 deportees/yr at Congo Coast ports	50,000 estimate				
1865	End of Atlantic slave trade					
1881	Stanley opens Manianga station					
1885	Berlin Conference founds Congo Free State		–2% estimate			
1898	Matadi to Kinshasa RR completed		–5% estimate			
1908	Congo Free State ends; Belgian Congo begins		–5% estimate			
1921	Upsurge of prophetic movements		–2% estimate			
1935*	Judicial reforms create local government courts	70,000	1%	29	16	300
1960**	Independence of DRC	88,000				
1984	WHO introduces Primary Health Care–Health Zones	150,000	3%			
1991	Département de Médecine created; Luozi waterworks					
2000***	All-Africa War, DRC fragmented; Bundu dia Kongo active	160,000	2%	18	5	80
2010****	National & regional elections	180,000	2%			66

SOURCES: *Trolli & Dupuy 1934; Svenska Missionsförbundet 1939; **Soret 1959, 6; ***Territoire de Luozi, Rapport Annuel, 1987; ****Luozi Health Zone records; other local, national, and WHO sources given in chapter.

on the part of couples, especially young women, to take control of their lives by limiting the number of their offspring.

Although population numbers by themselves do not translate easily into healthy or unhealthy conditions, they do provide a backdrop that can illuminate the overall health conditions of the populations concerned. Rising or declining birth rates clearly indicate the conditions of reproduction and of women's and infants' health. Similarly, rising or declining death rates, especially by population age and gender cohorts, offer clear pictures of the relative health of these groups and of the entire population in question.

Following this chapter's presentation of the demographic backdrop to the health story of the Manianga and the wider region of the Lower Congo, chapter 2 introduces the principal diseases of the Manianga that were monitored by the health zones in the decade from 2003 to 2013. It discusses how these diseases are regarded by the populace, and how they are dealt with by the medical and public health community. Some of these diseases are the same ones that ravaged the population in earlier times when they were not as well understood.

A number of related topics are necessarily included in the present chapter: slavery and precolonial commerce and how they transformed society; colonial domination of Western Equatorial Africa, which further transformed society; the connection between forced labor, population displacement, and the outbreak of contagious killer diseases like malaria and sleeping sickness; and the colonial labor policy that sought adult male workers and, back in the villages, fertile women to produce future workers. In many cases these policies dictated the types of records that were kept, and that would be available to later generations, including researchers.

Understanding the historical dimensions of health in an anthropology of contemporary health such as this is advantageous for grasping the long-term impact of the juxtaposition of today's local economy of food production and relational exchange with the commoditized global economy. This complex set of factors is of long standing, dating back at least to the seventeenth century. Precolonial commerce and the colonial extractive economy were the precursors of today's globalization. Population and health issues that arose from this background are thus still with us today. Fernand Braudel's "longue durée" is uniquely suited for conceptualizing not just the background of social structures but also the nature of memory.[1] People of the Lower Congo do speak of their ancestors, of the conditions they experienced, and of change. But as importantly, memory may be unconscious, instilling moods and related behaviors created by those ancestral conditions. The paranoid fear of someone else taking your or your kinsperson's vital essence—the core metaphor in sorcery (*kindoki*)—may be rooted in the collective memory of the thousands who disappeared into slavery, of the population diminishing, and of entire clans being decimated by disease.[2]

Establishing a Demographic Base Line

The earliest systematic population figures for Western Equatorial Africa—the Lower Congo in general and the Manianga in particular—are from the 1920s and 1930s, well within the era of Belgian colonialism. We will need to examine the sources, especially with regard to the allegation by numerous scholars and popular writers that a "50 percent decline" in the population of the coastal region and river corridor occurred from the seventeenth to the early twentieth centuries (Sautter 1966; Sanderson 2000), or during the period of the Congo Free State (1885–1908) in particular (Hochschild 1998). These, and other sources from Belgian colonial demographers Giovanni Trolli and Lucien Louis Dupuy (1934) and from Swedish medical doctors (Svenska Missionsförbundet 1939), attest to the then-very recent return of population growth following either localized areas of negative population trends or evidence of recovery from significant epidemic diseases.

Going backward in time, the evidence for birth and death rates becomes ever more vague, although historians use ships' records to establish the numbers of Africans removed from the continent by gender, age, and ports of departure, and occasionally by societies and regions of origin. These figures are then associated anecdotally with the sources of such population in the interior of the continent. Moving forward in time, population numbers become more frequent and reliable, with colonial and postcolonial annual government reports that include basic demographic information. Since the 1984 public health reforms in the Democratic Republic of the Congo (DRC), as in many countries of the world, the health zones of the primary health care structure have tracked population and epidemiological developments.

One demographic baseline for the Territoire de Luozi, the Manianga, as provided by colonial demographers Trolli and Dupuy (1934, 43), is 70,093 inhabitants in 1933, out of a total number of "Bakongo" in the district of Bas-Congo of 588,148. Within the Luozi Territory the totals are, for men over fifteen, 14,672; for women over fifteen, 19,699; for boys up to fifteen, 18,178; and for girls up to fifteen, 17,544. Infant mortality for 1933 was 322 in the first year after birth, or 33 percent of live births (1934, 74). The overall birth rate was 39.4/thousand, the mortality rate was 16.39/thousand, and the growth rate per annum was 23.11/thousand (1934, 78), or 2.3 percent, a highly suspect figure, as will be explained shortly.

Trolli and Dupuy's records reflect the colonial regime's intention to show off in a most favorable light the impact of the Fonds Reine Elisabeth pour l'Assistance Médicale aux Indigènes du Congo Belge (FOREAMI), focused on the BaKongo region of Lower Congo and the Nsele just upriver from Kinshasa. The effect of the record, bristling with seemingly scientific statistics, is to display an overall healthy population growing by several percentage points annually, with only pockets of disfunctionality. The book also demonstrates the adult male labor potential that a healthy population can provide. Yet it displays at least two distorting features that call into question the validity of its conclusions. First, the figures for numbers of adult males (15–45) and for elderly males (45 up) are misleadingly high, as they represent de jure customary population of men who originate from home villages as opposed to those who are actually present. Second, there is no historical backdrop showing conditions prior to this ostensibly improved health situation.

Only in an appendix can the discerning reader discover that 44 of 236 chiefdoms in the Lower Congo—around one-fifth of all local administrations led by the colonially appointed medallioned (*mpalata*) chiefs—manifest a death rate equal to or greater than the birth rate (1934, 80–81). Not surprisingly, the largest number of these chiefdoms is located where the population has experienced the longest and most intensive interaction with the colonial state and commercial activity: Mayumbe and Bas-Fleuve at the coast; Seke-Banza north of Boma; and Matadi, near Isangila rapids and the Manianga market, close to where Congolese laborers dug out roads in the hills around the rapids and pulled Henry Stanley's high, iron-wheeled vehicles carrying the boat and the steam engine to the next flat water on the Congo River. A close reading of the appendix of this work reveals that seven "disappearing chiefdoms" were in Basse-Sele near Kinshasa/Léopoldville.

Trolli and Dupuy reject the idea that labor recruitment was a contributor to the negative growth rate in these areas, in spite of the fact that half the men were absent from their homes. This figure may be grossly underreported, due to the way that Belgian colonial demographers categorized populations as living in *milieu coutumier* ("customary milieu") or *milieu extra-coutumier*. Seasonal or oscillating laborers, even if they were absent for years, were counted as belonging to their *milieu coutumier*. This practice continued several years into the postcolonial period.

The authors also reject disease as a factor in negative population statistics, although they enunciate the then-current Belgian colonial policy of not recruiting workers from chiefdoms where women's infertility is a serious concern. Explanations for these "disappearing chiefdoms" are contained in policy recommendations that chiefs be provided with greater authority so they would be able to impose food crop assignments on the population to ensure that there would be two harvests per year instead of just one, and would be able to limit the movement of women and girls to avoid "prostitution" as a means of livelihood contributing to the "moral degeneration" of the society (1934, 74–80). Today one would infer that high infertility of women, possibly due to disease or malnutrition, was a cause of the low birth rate, which, together with the high infant mortality rate, led to the disappearance or at least the shrinkage of these communities. Early colonial administrators, embarrassed by the high death rates and shrinking populations, sought to remedy the situation by controlling local populations, minimizing travel or migration out, and increasing food production.

A second source for a population and disease baseline in the 1930s are the records kept by the Svenska Missionsförbundet (SMF) under the Service Auxiliare de l'Assistance Médicale aux Indigénes—a pre-FOREAMI program—to carry out surveillance of five chiefdoms in the area of the SMF's hospital at Kibunzi in the southwestern corner of the Manianga. The SMF survey, combined with records of public health interventions, reveals a more disastrous population profile, directly due to colonial labor and resettlement policies. Tracking of actual resident population, rather than the colonial government's *population coutumier*, reveals that the population categories for old men (age forty-five and up) and adult males (fifteen to forty-five) had about 6,000 fewer individuals than their female counterparts, out of a population total of 18,000 (which would have been 24,000 had the missing men been included). In other words, a quarter of the population was absent: away at work projects, off trading to earn money for taxes and purchases, or deceased. In the category of the elderly, 602 resident men compare to 3,606 women; in the fifteen to forty-five age group, 1,007 resident males compare to 4,103 females (table 1.2). This offers a clear picture of prior living conditions under the Congo Free State. Elderly men, who were now largely missing, would have been prime labor prospects during the Congo Free State era of thirty to forty years earlier.

The SMF medical effort, under Gustav Palmaer from 1911 to 1926, developed methods to fight against sleeping sickness with a focus on the same five chiefdoms in the southwest region of the Manianga. Field surveys and treatments begun in 1920, in addition to hospital treatment at Kibunzi and infant feeding programs begun in 1924, were the main thrusts of the SMF public health interventions. By 1926, 30,000 people had been examined, and 1,024 cases of sleeping sickness treated; in 1924, the year it was opened, Kibunzi hospital treated 1,217 sleeping sickness cases out of a total of 14,791 patients. This tireless field and hospital effort achieved a reduction of sleeping sickness infection rates to 3 percent of the population by 1930, from the 5 percent of several years earlier, and to near disappearance by 1938. Projecting a 5 percent infection rate for sleeping sickness back several decades would provide a picture of falling overall growth rates from this disease alone, which had a near total mortality rate for those infected, not to mention malaria, diarrhea, dysentery, typhoid fever, seasonal flu, and other severe diseases. Table 1.3 shows a population with considerably lower infant mortality rates than are shown by Trolli and Dupuy, but with an annual growth rate of only 1.31 percent.[3] We can therefore conclude that the Trolli and Dupuy population growth estimate, based on customary membership in a descent community, is inflated by at least a percentage point.

The state's interests were well served by special concentration on sleeping sickness, since eliminating it as a health crisis improved the survival of potential labor and yielded a dynamic population that reproduced itself. But diseases and infestations such as bilharzia and other waterborne diseases that could not be treated in hospitals were of concern, at least to the missions. From 1927 until 1932 an annual

TABLE 1.2. Population in five southwest Manianga chiefdoms, 1938

			Age and gender							
			45–up		15–45		3–15		0–3	
Chiefdom	# villages	Pop.	M	F	M	F	M	F	M	F
Kibunzi	22	2,574	93	504	158	557	447	451	154	180
Bamba	27	3,977	147	753	241	861	813	732	220	210
Kinkungu	16	2,088	92	404	141	462	351	385	129	124
Bulu	18	2,173	64	432	143	457	396	396	141	144
Kinkenge	81	7,402	206	1513	324	1,766	1,384	1,299	452	456
Total		18,214	602	3,606	1,007	4,103	3,421	3,263	1,096	1,114

SOURCE: Svenska Missionsförbundet 1938.

TABLE 1.3. Births and deaths in five southwest Manianga chiefdoms, 1938

Villages	Pop.	Births		Deaths		Deaths 0–1		Deaths 1–3		Infant mortality rate (%)
		M	F	M	F	M	F	M	F	
Kibunzi	2,574	48	81	21	28	9	3	2	8	9.30
Bamba	3,977	55	50	10	20	1	3	7	14	3.81
Kinkungu	2,088	42	48	23	20	3	3	7	5	6.67
Bulu	2,173	35	39	25	23	8	3	4	5	14.86
Kinkenge	7,402	64	69	62	60	3	3	34	30	4.51
Total	18,214	244	287	141	151	24	15	54	62	7.34

SOURCE: Svenska Missionsförbundet 1938.

health survey was carried out in sixty-four villages in five districts or colonial chief-doms, first by Palmaer and then by his successors and colleagues of the SMF.[4] Until 1938 the Swedish mission carried the major load for public health in the entire region around Kibunzi. Hygiene maps were kept of villages, indicating loca-tion (whether in a tsetse-infested valley or on a hilltop) and showing water sources, bathing places (whether infested with bilharzia or not), paths, number and types of houses (grass, mud, brick), number and types of toilets, and the overall hygienic condition of village (e.g., "assez propre").[5] Also listed are the names of clans and nearby abandoned village sites, reflecting the impact of labor recruitment, resis-tance wars, or moves for health reasons.

Projecting back in time all contagious and therefore potentially fatal diseases, as well as diseases that restrict fertility in women, heavy labor recruitment of adult males, and infant mortality rates of up to one-third of births, as seen in both the Swedish mission medical research and Trolli and Dupuy's data from the 1930s, we have plenty of evidence for the factors contributing to a declining popula-tion. In the Manianga, the highest mortality rates were in two chiefships along the river: Mbu, near the old Manianga market and Stanley's Manianga station; and Bulu, west of Luozi near the rapids that required massive labor to move Stanley's boat and wagons overland. Both are along the old caravan route north of the river that ran from Mpumbu at Malebo Pool to the port towns of Vili, Matadi, Boma, and Banana on the Congo River and Cabinda and Loango on the Atlantic Ocean coast.

GLOBAL PENETRATION OF WESTERN EQUATORIAL AFRICA (1650–1884)

As we project our base population data back into the Congo Free State and the mercantile trading period before that, we face a more formidable challenge in sort-ing out salient causes of high mortality rates and low birth rates—main factors in a declining population. One of the main sources of evidence of a population decline at some point in the past in the Congo River Valley and in the western lowlands of the Luala River Valley is a much lower population density there—as low as fewer than eight per square kilometer, compared to thirty-five per square kilometer in the northern regions of the Manianga, in the border areas between the two Congos (Nicolai 1961, 8) (map 1.1).

The Congo River, from its mouth at the Atlantic Ocean, is navigable for about one hundred miles to the port city of Matadi. Just east of this point the river rises through a series of rapids until it reaches another level stretch, at Isangila, and widens to two kilometers across at places such as the Luozi crossing. This stretch is navigable eastward to the site of the old Manianga market, which used to provi-sion caravans. The river rises through another series of rapids until it broadens out in the Malebo Pool between Kinshasa on the south bank and Brazzaville on the

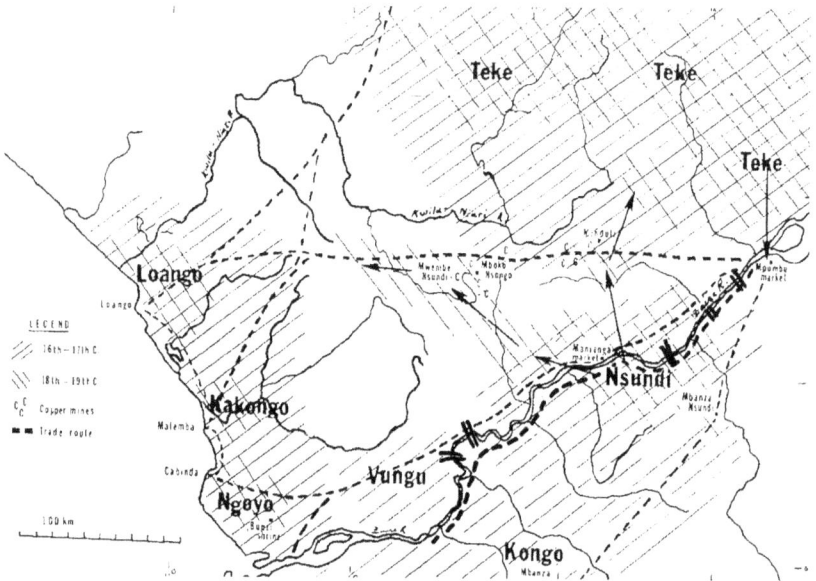

MAP 1.1. Precolonial trade caravan routes from Mpumbu Market (at today's Kinshasa) to the Atlantic coast ports, via Manianga market on the Congo River. Rapids on the Congo River below Kinshasa, to east of Manianga market, then again downstream at Isangila and Inga, made river travel impossible. Ocean vessels could reach Matadi or Vivi; upstream, Isangila to Manianga was navigable; further upstream, Malebo Pool to Stanleyville/Kisangani was navigable. Map by author. Sources: Vansina, *Tio Kingdom of Middle Congo 1880–1892*, 1973; Mahaniah, *Carte postale du Territoire de Luozi*, 2009.

north. From there it is the sluggish, broad river whose main arteries and tributaries drain the entire Congo Basin, the heart of the African continent.

The Lower Congo has been the gateway to Equatorial Africa over much of the past five centuries and is of special interest regarding the health of its inhabitants. From the seventeenth century until the 1890s (Bontinck 1983), Central Africa was in contact with the rest of the world via footpaths that were trodden by travelers walking or being carried on tipoyi-litters, or porters carrying loads on their heads, from Mpumbu market at Malebo Pool to coastal ports in Angola at Ambriz, Ngoyo, Boma, Kakongo (Cabinda), or Loango. The main route from Mpumbu to Manianga passed south of the Congo River through Mbanza Nsundi (near today's Inkisi), and crossed the river just below the rapids of Manianga, where the river is quite narrow (today's Mpioka). From there, one route continued on the south side of the river to Ngoyo. On the north side of the river, another route continued toward Boma, with a fork off toward Loango through the Luala Valley. Large canoes plied the river a thousand miles upstream in the entire Congo Basin, and downstream between the rapids from Manianga to Isangila in the Lower Congo, and beyond Vivi out to the Atlantic Ocean.

The riverain and overland caravan routes were heavily traveled. This early commerce was at once lucrative and devastating to communities along the trade routes. By the eighteenth century up to 15,000 slaves were being brought overland to the coastal ports of Congo every year, many coming from the deep interior via the Mpumbu market at Malebo Pool, others from Lower Congo. The sale of slaves, ivory, copper, and dye in exchange for guns, trade goods, cloth, liquor, and other European luxury goods directly provided a vigorous economy for those involved in it, and indirectly for their communities. Local food production was stimulated by the passage of many slaves and traders through the area. As Célestin Lusiama remarked in driving past the distant hilltop Manianga market site in 2013, today's popular collective memory of Manianga market is that a variety of local people, such as criminals, antagonists in feuds, debt pawns, and junior clan members of the merchants were likely to end up in the middle passage to the Americas.[6] In this same tradition, Stanley (1885) wrote that one of his Zanzibari helpers was kidnapped at Manianga in 1881.

Local stories of Manianga market offer several versions of its origin. Congolese historian Kimpianga Mahaniah (2008, 44–46) places its beginnings in the seventeenth and eighteenth centuries. Local sources tie the market to Nkenge day of the traditional Kongo four-day week, thus its one appellation Nkenge-Manianga. Another source suggests that it was founded by a chief from the Nsundi stronghold (a province of the Kongo kingdom) to the south of the river. The market and ties to the trading network gave the rulers of nearby Kimbanza, which paid tribute to the *ntotila* king of Nsundi, a connection to larger political systems of the region (Pirenne 1959).

How did this global trading system, which included massive slave trade, affect the local population of the Lower Congo? Historian Jan Vansina, who has reviewed the sources and literature of European mercantile penetration of Equatorial Africa and its effect on population numbers (1990, 218–20), considers the differential impact of the extraction of productive adult males versus females, the introduction of venereal diseases that can affect reproduction, and the destabilizing raids. Slave numbers by year, ages, and genders are known; only a third were women of childbearing age. According to Vansina, slavery alone would not have changed birth rates and death rates enough to result in a negative population trend. The population imbalance of women over men that was seen in our baseline statistics appears to have existed even before colonialism. In fact, the accumulation of wealth in people—*bantu mbongo*—was a well-known strategy of traders, clan heads, and men in general in Kongo society. The majority of adults in a typical precolonial Kongo village might have been slave women married to free men, producing children for them for economic purposes: "Our ancestors' money," noted Lusiama, regarding the return of former slaves to their former masters' settlements in the northern Manianga.[7]

The only circumstance in which Vansina allows that precolonial slave trading would have taken the population into a negative trend would be during peak levels of raiding and extraction, with destabilization, flight, and serious and widespread diseases that caused infertility in reproductive-age women. Scholars have long postulated an "infertility zone" along Western Equatorial Africa's Atlantic coast, extending into the southern savanna (Larson 2003; Hunt 2011). This is confirmed by the widespread proliferation of healing cults and medicines with fertility enhancement as their main focus in the region. On the north bank of the Congo River, the Lemba association (Janzen 1982a) provided a ritual-economic pattern of exchange to redistribute some of participants' earnings within their own kin communities, thereby "sealing them off from the capricious effects of global mercantile capitalism" (Miller 1988, 201–2). But Lemba, along with other *minkisi*, highlighted the reproductive importance of couples, households, and individual women. This suggests that there may well have been widespread infertility, or concerns for the reproductive effectiveness of women, families, clans, and communities, although we cannot establish even the approximate rates of reproduction of the period before 1880.

ROCK BREAKER AND THE
CONGO FREE STATE (1885–1908)

In the 2012 annual report of the Territoire de Luozi, as in previous annual reports, the date of the origin of the administrative region is given as 1881, when Stanley established the Manianga post.[8] This was during Stanley's five-year employment with the Société Anonyme Belge pour le Commerce du Haut-Congo, which morphed into the Congo Free State after the Berlin Conference of 1885. Stanley spearheaded the establishment of base camps on the north bank of the Congo River from its uppermost reach by ocean vessel, at Vivi (just above today's Matadi) and Isangila (above a series of rapids), and sixty-three kilometers higher upriver at Manianga, where there were again rapids partway to Kinshasa at Malebo Pool. Stanley and later the Free State acquired the nickname of Rock Breaker—*bula matadi, bula matari*—for the heavy work of clearing boulders and digging roads around the rapids of Vivi to Isangila, and from Manianga to near Kinshasa (Stanley 1885). The boats were used on the sixty-three-kilometer stretch from Isangila to Manianga, past today's Luozi, and were again assembled at Kinshasa for use upriver. The Société Anonyme, through Stanley, recruited local laborers to dig roads and to pull the boats and steam engines on huge iron wagons around the rapids.

Stanley's writings about these efforts to create posts, connecting roads, and a network of chiefs who could deliver workers conveys the spirit of heroic courage in laying the groundwork for civilization and trade, fighting against the odds of raw nature and "whimsical, cunning" natives (1885, 170). Locally Stanley is known for the whip that he apparently used on workers and for the big iron wheels used to portage his steamboat in two sections on roads hewn out of rocky hills around the rapids of Isangila and Manianga (figure 1.1). The wheels survive in various monuments (figure 1.2).

His chapter on the Manianga region is mainly about his week-long near-fatal bout with malaria (figure 1.3). Given his determination to create the exploration and trading network of posts and connecting river passages, he appears not to have devoted much of his reportorial energy to understanding or describing the local customs. Nor does he offer much in the way of accounts of health, disease, and his own and the Société's impact on the population. We are interested in the likely connection between the activity of Stanley and his associates and the empty and low population areas along the river, in the western lowlands of Manianga,

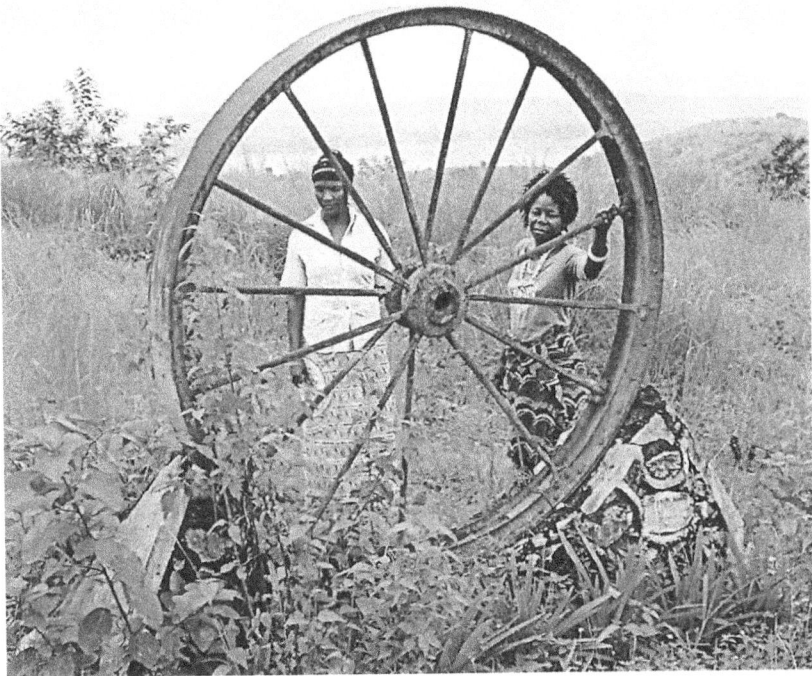

FIGURE 1.1. Henriette Kalusebolo Mattlola (*left*), clerk of civic affairs of the city hall of Luozi, and Charlotte Matondo Nlandu, librarian, posing behind one of Stanley's wheels mounted by colonial agents atop Kilemba Heights, residence of territorial administrators, overlooking the Congo River at Luozi. Photo: John M. Janzen, 2013.

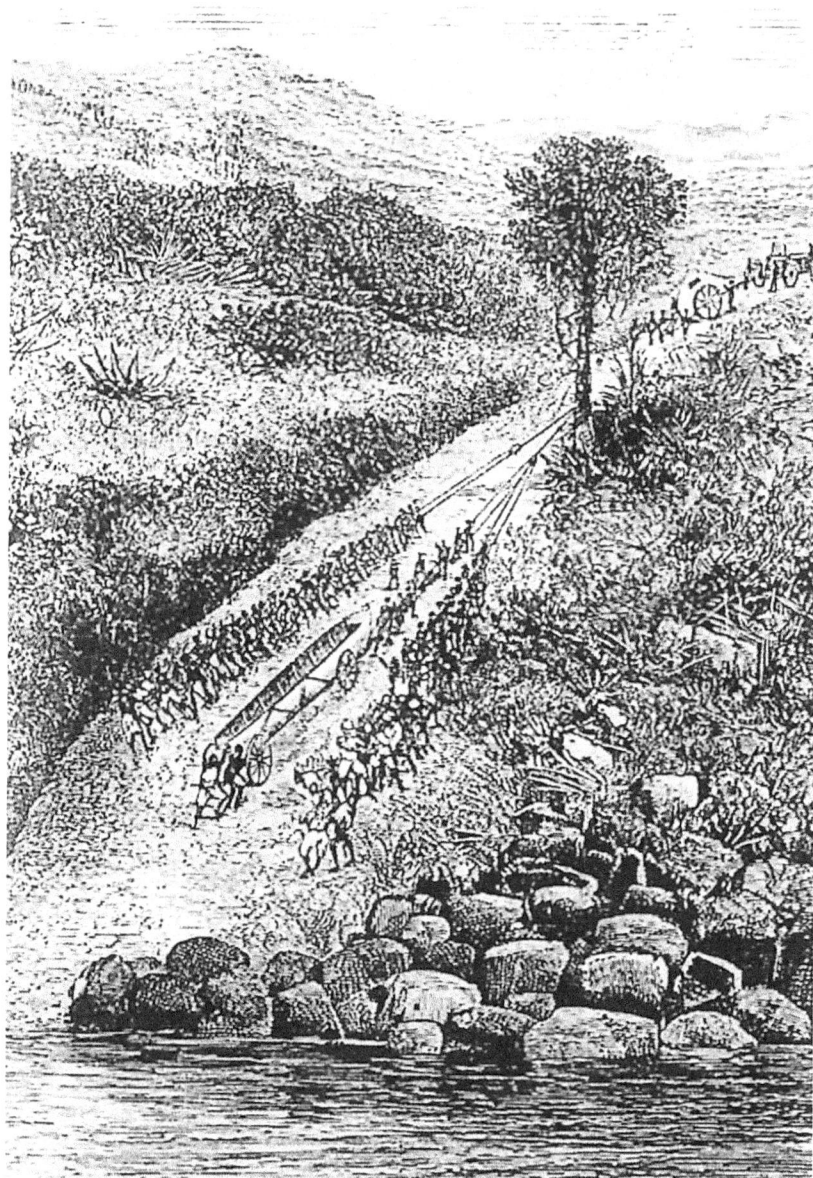

FIGURE 1.2. Congolese workers dragging Henry Stanley's steamboat and steam engine on huge wheels over steep roads dug out of rock around rapids on the Congo River. For this and other rock-breaking work, Stanley, the Congo Free State, and the Belgian Congo, gained the name *bula matadi* ("break rock"). Stanley's twelve iron wheels are scattered around Manianga as monuments. Source: H. M. Stanley, "Ascending the Nyongena Hill," in *The Congo and the Founding of Its Free State*, vol. 1 (1885), 229.

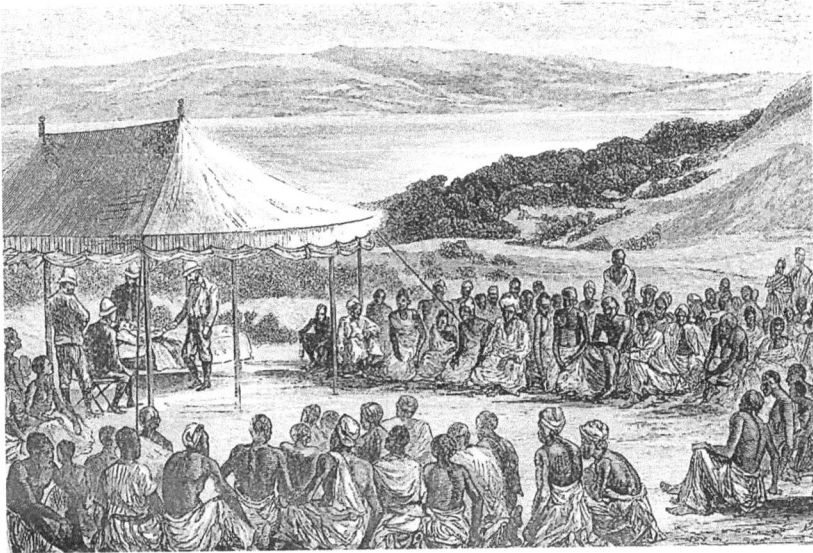

FIGURE 1.3. Stanley on malaria sickbed at Manianga Station overlooking the Congo River. Stanley, believing himself to be near death from malaria, summoned his expedition and local observers to instruct them about carrying on. He survived. Source: H. M. Stanley, *The Congo and the Founding of Its Free State*, vol. 1 (1885), 274.

and south of the river. Local oral tradition and scholarly research help us piece together a more accurate picture of this connection.

Interviews with several lifelong residents of Luozi—Kitoko, Muanda Mbamba Albert, and Bavedila Mboti Nkala—whose elders would have been eyewitnesses to the events of the late nineteenth and early twentieth centuries, suggest initial curiosity about the strange whites, later interaction with them, then resistance due to their heavy-handed and exploitative ways. One account by the son of a fisher on the Congo River describes Stanley arriving by boat, traveling upriver to the rapids of Manianga, turning back, and slowly exploring the coastline. Another account describes an elder who could speak English conversing with the strangers, who they thought might be albinos. Another thread of narrative has to do with the way the whites seized terrain, particularly the heights of Kilemba, which provoked the river's water spirits, who are thought to have destroyed a bridge the whites had built to cross the stream to get to Kilemba.

One of Stanley's men was nicknamed Mpakasa, buffalo, for his physique and his brusque ways. It was he who occupied Kilemba by force. But following the flood that washed away the bridge, and a bad dream, he was forced to negotiate with local landowners for the purchase of the site. Buffalo was always in charge, and he taught his people to deceive the public and to seize people to gain access to them for work projects. His labor recruiter they called Mabienga Mbanzi—"He who produces pain in the side."[9] He tried to recruit people to build the roads and to carry loads, including carrying the whites on *tipoyi* hammocks. A tax was also imposed, but many people resisted. This led the new authorities to build a prison with guards for those who didn't work or pay. Many others fled.

It appears, however, that the heaviest labor recruiting came a few years later when the river route was abandoned as a colonial shipping option by the Matadi-to-Kinshasa railroad. Up to eight thousand workers were needed each year for this project. From 1881 until the railroad was completed in 1898, the burden on the local population was heaviest, with workers needed in the Lower Congo corridor as porters to carry the cargo caravans, recruitment for railroad construction, and taxes for everyone. The Free State did not have enough agents to do this through population censuses, so they simply recruited wherever they could, by whatever method, as many workers as possible.

GROWING RESISTANCE AND HEALTH IN THE HEART OF DARKNESS

Joseph Conrad's brooding *Heart of Darkness* recounts his journey in 1890 with agents of the Free State along the caravan trail south of the river, a trek from Matadi to Kinshasa with sixty porters, and from there on a riverboat up the Congo, in the employ of the concessionary company the Société Anonyme Belge pour le Commerce du Haut-Congo. Conrad describes the sickly porters, the abandoned villages, and the "horror of it all" (1965, 14–16). Of a Matadi construction site, he wrote:

> A slight clinking behind me made me turn my head. Six black men advanced in a file, toiling up the path. They walked erect and slow, balancing small baskets full of earth on their heads, and the clink kept time with their footsteps. Black rags were wound round their loins, and the short ends behind waggled to and fro like tails. I could see every rib, the joints of their limbs were like knots in a rope; each had an iron collar on his neck, and all were connected together with a chain whose bights swung between them, rhythmically clinking. . . . All their meager breasts panted together, the violently dilated nostrils quivered, the eyes stared stonily up-hill. They passed me within six inches, without a glance with that complete deathlike indifference. (12)

And of the caravan trek from Matadi to Kinshasa, he wrote:

> Next day I left . . . with a caravan of sixty men, for a two-hundred-mile tramp. No use telling you much about that. Paths, paths, everywhere; a stamped-in network of paths spreading over the empty land, through long grass, through burnt grass, through

thickets, down and up chilly ravines, up and down stony hills ablaze with heat; and a solitude, a solitude, nobody, not a hut. The population had cleared out a long time ago. Well, if a lot of mysterious niggers armed with all kinds of fearful weapons suddenly took to traveling on the road between Deal and Gravesend, catching the yokels right and left to carry heavy loads for them, fancy every farm and cottage thereabouts would get empty very soon. Only here the dwellings were gone, too. Still I passed through several abandoned villages. There's something pathetically childish in the ruins of grass walls.

Day after day, with the stamp and shuffle of sixty pair of bare feet behind me, each pair under a sixty-pound load. Camp, cook, sleep, strike camp, march. Now and then a carrier dead in harness, at rest in the long grass near the path, with an empty water-gourd and his long staff lying by his side. A great silence around and above. (15–16)

The railroad project from Matadi to Kinshasa decimated the countryside further, as people were rounded up to work and others fled. Up to eight thousand workers per year were drawn from villages in the region, of whom often less than half returned. Entire communities fled northward to the hilly border region between the Belgian and French Congo to escape the recruiters.

For a time a virtual state of war existed between some of the African communities in the middle Lower Congo and the Free State government (Cornet 1947). Colonial writers portrayed the construction of this railroad as a heroic battle in which 132 Europeans, named on a plaque overlooking a precarious gorge east of Matadi, gave their lives. The estimated, and surely underreported, 1,800 Africans who died are also mentioned but remain anonymous. There is no mention of the contingent of Chinese workers brought in to complete the work because it had become increasingly difficult to recruit local labor.

Records of the Swedish missionaries permit a glimpse of the resistance that was waged over taxation and forced labor recruitment. In 1893 Swedish missionary Carl Borrisson wrote that Free State agent Eugene Rommel set up a station south of the Congo River at Kasi to recruit labor for the railroad project. His technique to force men to work was to capture their wives and children and hold them hostage. The savagery of this tactic provoked an armed attack by the local community, in which Rommel and of some of his helpers were killed (Axelson 1970). The leader of the rebellion, Chief Nzansu, notified the missionaries that they were not in danger. Of course, reprisals by the state followed. Another recruitment post was set up north of the river at Nganda, near the Swedish mission. There too, under the leadership of one Mbonza, a state agent was killed, which led to reprisals, further attacks, and the burning of villages and destruction of fields. Entire regions became empty of villages; some relocated to within close range of the missions out of a sense of greater safety from the depredations of the Free State (Axelson 1970, 264).

Carving out the railroad through the Crystal Mountains east of Matadi, and later through mountains near Thysville, was particularly treacherous for workers, who were forced to work long hours removing stone under adverse conditions. Dysentery, malaria, and sleeping sickness, exacerbated by hunger, took their toll.

Postcolonial geographer Henri Nicolai offers the most plausible scenario of how this "opening up for civilization" relates to the empty or low-population zones in the western and southern reaches of the Manianga (1961, 42–52). Having thoroughly analyzed soil type, agricultural techniques, and ethnicity, and having found no possible difference between the regions with low and high population density, he turned to history for an explanation. Although he did not have population records from the Free State period, he does cite several colonial reports that acknowledge excessive labor recruitment, the abandonment of entire villages, and later, regions where economic developers encountered fertile lands in the Luala Valley that had no apparent landowners. That is, the claimants to these lands had simply vanished. However, in the course of inviting in settlers from elsewhere in the Manianga, who then began to cultivate these lands, neighboring landowners gradually were able to reconstruct clan identities and land claims for the empty lands. Nicolai postulates that the lands colonized for the Kundi paysanat scheme had been unworked for sixty years—that is, since the heyday of massive Free State labor recruitment from 1890 to 1900.[10]

But it was not just labor recruitment that killed off entire villages. Rather, the villagers whose men were forcibly recruited to the Free State projects, especially the railroad, fled into lowland forest shelters. These lowland forests, which may have seemed a safe refuge, or were the only refuge available, were infested with trypanosome-carrying tsetse flies, which infected large numbers of people with a disease for which there was no effective cure. Starvation finished off many of the children.[11]

In any event, reports of atrocities in the Congo by independent observers (Lagergren 1970) had by 1908 so embarrassed the Belgian king in the international arena that the Belgian parliament confiscated the territory of the Congo from Leopold II. Some concessionary companies found their activities curtailed, but others continued as before. Some agents were asked to leave, but others continued, as was the case with agent G. Bolant, who had been *chef de poste* at Luozi on the Congo River between Isangila and Manianga.

Belgian Colonialism, Public Health, and Population (1908–1960)

In 1909 Belgian officer Bolant returned to Luozi to find that his headquarters had been completely pillaged by the local Africans. Doors and hinges had been removed from all the buildings. Furniture, tools, tables, chairs, hoes, machetes, and storage chests had all vanished. His inventory of what remained included long saws, a dozen metal sheets from a boat, the drill for making rivet holes, and other metalworking instruments used in boat making. The smith's bellows, shovels, and oil barrels were gone. A boat that had been put in the protection of inhabitants of the local village of Lemba could still be used. Bolant wrote in his report that he would live in a remaining mess hall initially, and his African troops could live in grass thatch houses (Luozi State Archives, 1909–15).[12] Now working for the Belgian colonial government instead of the Congo Free State, Bolant began to make trips into the interior to establish a census base for taxation, to try to connect up with the prior Congo Free State medallioned *mpalata* chiefs. But these chiefs, the main connection of the colonial administration to the African population, were now being threatened physically by their own people. Several villages along the northern border had moved into French Congo to escape Free State and Belgian colonialism. Many *mpalata*, called by messenger to report to Luozi, did not bother to show up to bring their tax revenues. Others, on trying to round up their people from the forests where they were hiding, were met with gunfire from their own people.

The agents' reports from 1909 on offer a picture of the state of the health and well-being of the region prior to the effective imposition of the second colonial government. Although the paths were well-kept, except parallel to rivers, where people used canoes to travel, and although streams were traversed by bridges, many villages were unswept or even overgrown with tall grass, giving the inhabitants the chance to flee when the agent did his tours of inspection. The women were at work in the fields and the men away in Matadi or French Congo selling their animals to have money for the tax.

In 1911, Bolant reported that the *mpalata* of the northern region, where local political structure had been decidedly acephalous, had very little authority over the inhabitants. The people still fled their villages when he arrived; the *mpalata* would go into the forest to look for the people, but they would shoot their guns at him. A chief working closely with the colonial government was assassinated. One messenger recruiting workers for the port project at Boma was threatened with death. For several years an entire region in the Manianga highlands kept such messengers and tax collectors at bay through force of arms. Following an ambush of the colonial finance officer Driesen, who was registering the population and collecting taxes, the state launched a "punitive expedition" in the region where people were hiding themselves in the tall grass and forest, and opened another state post in the midst of the recalcitrant area. Several additional colonial officers came to help out, and for a time around 1912 they maintained a kind of military occupation.

By 1913 the officer reported that the hostilities had abated. After this initial repression of the population, the local administration began, in 1916, to keep a political report of "l'etat d'esprit" of the population and of the major activities of government (Belgian Colonial Government 1916).[13] The trade economy continued much as before, with caravans of porters providing the major means of transport. In 1917 the government recruited four hundred porters for the Mayombe region, and there were still no European merchants in the entire Territoire de Luozi. The population resisted imposition of quotas of cash crops—in this case Aleas fiber, a kind of sisal—and food crops in certain areas.

Epidemics of flu, dysentery, and malaria, in addition to endemic sleeping sickness, raged in the area. Workers on the railroad project northward from Matadi to Ango-Ango in the Mayombe forests fled to their villages to escape the flu pandemic of 1918, in the process spreading it further. The colonial response was to round them up and force them to return. Careful field research by this author in the north Manianga established that in the early decades of this century villages had taken to living in dense forest near streams and rivers, instead of the typical open-air hilltop sites they preferred. Such residence in the habitat of mosquitoes and tsetse flies undoubtedly contributed to the rising rate of these diseases.

These adversities were followed by widespread antiwitchcraft and messianic movements among the Bakongo in 1921. Chiefs sometimes had their own prophets, *bangunza*, which prompted further military expeditions through the area to remind the natives of who was boss. Such was the public administration of the early Belgian colonial government.

Only by 1930 had population begun to increase in the areas of the caravan trails and the regions that served as the source of labor for the railroad project (Trolli and Dupuy 1934). This increase was reflected mainly in the northern Manianga region. Well into the 1960s regions on either side of the stretch on the Congo River between Matadi and Kinshasa, alongside the still wide portion of the river between the two cataracts, there was an eerie emptiness. Only occasional hilltop villages could be seen. Along the lowland rivers in the western Manianga, there remained almost totally deserted areas (Nicolai 1961).

The Belgian colonial government struggled to gain control over health issues in its vast territories, but this came only with a massive and continuing repression that the subjects, or victims, resented. The FOREAMI "franchised" campaign, limited to the Lower Congo, was an effort to coordinate public health initiatives and the treatment of major epidemic diseases. It utilized the energies and the infrastructure established by the missions, in particular the SMF.

The colonial struggle against hamlet dispersion was perhaps the baldest instance of health policy serving the purpose of political control. In a 1932 declaration on "Hygiene des villages" (FOREAMI 1933), the health branch of the colonial government recommended stricter control of hamlet dispersion to facilitate health and administration. The Belgian colonial government used the Lower Congo and Upper Nsele regions as test areas to enact forced hamlet relocation into larger, administratively compact settlements. The declaration indicated that the dispersion of settlements should be strictly forbidden "because that makes the work of our sanitary agents and doctors physically impossible." It recommended that in the case of African chiefs who did not or could not control dispersion, the colonial government was to intervene directly to deal with the problems. Enforced public health in the form of huge projects to cut grass, demolish unused buildings, drain marshes, and even impose a village relocation or other mass public works would induce a spirit of cooperation, the author recommended. Hygiene and public works became the punishment for recalcitrance in the face of colonial authority (Janzen 1978, 41–44).

Belgian public health in the Congo was as paternalistic and repressive as its overall colonial regime. Its primary aim was to build a healthy workforce of docile natives. The ideology of the defective or distinctive *mentalité indigène* justified a special approach to Africans' access to open and free care, and restricted their participation in the upper-level medical professions: physician and public health officer.

A further indicator of Belgian colonial authorities' control of the population was an accurate accounting of who lived where, what the local organization was, who were the chiefs, judges, and clan members, and what kind of labor force could be identified. The first censuses available in the Territoire de Luozi are from 1920. They include quite detailed inventories of villages, houses (or households), and numbers of adults (over fifteen) and children (under fifteen, determining reproduction rates). Whatever Congo Free State records there may have been were destroyed by partisans in 1907.

The 1920s census of Masangi sector in the north of the Manianga provides a slice-in-time view of a population and administrative unit that was considered a successful example. The first medallioned chief, Madiongo, had died of dysentery on June 7, 1921. According to agent Leon Cartiaux, territorial administrator, a qualified successor was found in the person of Kiodi, whose long rule was still remembered in the 1960s when I lived in the region. The census covered village inhabitants, the number of households in each village, as well as village head (*duki*), clans (*luvila*), clan sections (*belo*), and judges operating to resolve conflicts. This was a long decade prior to the judicial reforms of the 1930s that created the sector tribunals. The seventeen villages of Masangi sector (or chiefdom) offer a glimpse into population structure early in the Belgian colonial period (table 1.4), which may be compared with the very late colonial and early postcolonial population structures (table 1.5).

The 1920 Masangi census reveals a fairly low occupation rate per house: barely two individuals per unit. Also, it shows the low ratio of resident men to women that we have encountered in the Trolli and Dupuy demographic study. It is impossible to decipher the infant mortality rate or the population growth or decline rate from this census, but the ratio of 581 women to 494 children (birth–15) suggests a high child mortality rate as well as high infertility in women, resulting quite possibly in a population that is in decline due to endemic or epidemic disease.

TABLE 1.4. Census of villages of Masangi Sector, 1920

Village	Household heads	Men	Women	Boys	Girls	Total individuals
Banza-Sungu	21	11	14	11	12	48
Kibangu	18	11	14	5	7	37
Kimbaku	54	39	40	18	19	116
Kimbanga	36	17	27	13	17	74
Kimbuala	42	25	34	14	15	88
Kimpondo *	31	27	24	14	9	74
Kingila *	52	49	34	20	19	122
Kinkungu	29	20	21	11	10	62
Kintadi	81	63	70	27	23	183
Kisiasia	46	33	36	14	16	99
Kumbi	24	17	19	11	14	61
Masangi	36	22	29	16	14	81
Miami	11	6	7	3	4	20
Minsenga	14	10	12	6	7	35
Nianga-Ngoyo	39	25	33	12	14	84
Nkaka	27	16	22	11	12	61
Sundi-Lutete	160	99	145	34	42	320
Total	721	490	581	240	254	1,565

SOURCE: Census by Territorial Agent, Luozi Territorial Archives, 1920.
*More men than women.

Just who are the people of these villages, and how are they related to each other? The figures do not reveal the residential dynamics of North Kongo society, in a community situated on a landed estate at the center of which is a matrilineal cemetery forest, the *makulu*, an ancient village site. Men living in the village customarily move from their childhood residence with their father to their matrilineal village at about age fifteen, where they take their places behind their maternal uncles. Women, who grow up in their father's home, move at marriage to reside with their husbands. If and when they are widowed and do not remarry a sibling of their husband, or are divorced, they would move to their own matrilineal clan home, where they would be given a space to build a house and a field to cultivate. On death, they would be buried in their matrilineal *makulu*.

A sizeable number of the inhabitants of these villages would have been slave clan remnants who were bound to their masters, women usually marrying their masters and producing children who would remain in their masters' possession, and would be buried in the master's *makulu*. The numbers of a colonial census are more fluid in their significance than they seem at first sight. They are, however, an accurate depiction of the numbers of individuals who are making a living off the land in a particular place. This geographical-environmental motif is a significant factor in overall health and well-being in the Manianga region.

TABLE 1.5. Census of villages of earlier Masangi Sector, 1964, having become part of Kivunda Commune (present and absent individuals listed)

Villages	Population (present/absent)				
	Men	Women	Boys	Girls	Total
Banza-Sungu *					
Kibangu *					
Kimbaku	63/111	112/74	124/46	98/52	397/283
Kimbanga	52/79	92/66	108/35	96/29	348/209
Kimbuala	40/69	69/59	72/44	65/30	246/194
Kimpondo	44/79	84/54	90/44	124/90	347/267
Kingila	62/123	110/78	80/54	89/94	341/137
Kinkungu	43/44	55/36	49/22	58/21	205/123
Kintadi	123/189	180/136	191/103	177/66	671/494
Kisiasia	49/91	88/55	76/41	64/37	277/224
Kumbi	20/45	41/35	48/34	35/27	138/142
Masangi	35/61	61/48	52/40	50/28	189/198
Miami *					
Minsenga *					
Nianga-Ngoyo	54/52	84/35	76/16	90/15	304/118
Nkaka	26/36	44/25	19/29	35/11	124/101
Sundi-Lutete	127/183	214/128	226/87	208/57	775/473
Total	1,117/1,162	1,234/781	1,159/595	1,129/557	4,639/3,095

SOURCES: Kivunda Communal Census, 1965. A detailed census by the author of Kisiasia village in 1964 showed a near doubling of households from 46 in 1920 (table 1.4) to 71 in 1964 (table 1.5).
*Consolidated or moved to another sector.

From early on the Belgian colonial population record keepers and planners tracked the adult male who was tellingly identified as an *homme, adult et valable* (HAV)—one man, adult, and viable (for work, thus one labor unit). The official age of the HAV was fifteen to forty-five years. Boys below fifteen and men over forty-five were recorded separately. Because the sites of colonially imposed labor or wage-earning opportunities were often at a distance from the home village, population records also needed to track the number of those present and those absent, presumably away at work. A policy of annually oscillating labor migration came into being, as is reflected in colonial population statistics through the 1908–60 era, and even after that for a few years into independence.

At first it was mostly adult men who were away, but in the course of time, particularly after World War II, women increasingly joined their husbands at these away places, and entire families begin to exist away. Yet throughout the colonial period and into the postcolonial era, the jural concept was that all Congolese have a natal village where they are officially at home. For many years Congolese people seem to have lived with this conceit. Many village houses were built by those whose adult lives had been spent in cities or at work sites elsewhere. The village and its resident population were identified as *population milieu coutumier*, and all others identified with that origin were put into the category *population hors milieu coutumier*. In table 1.5 these are shown as the "present" and "absent" population. Tables 1.4 and 1.5 contain figures from the 1920 census of Masangi and the records of the same villages from 1964 Kivunda communal records, respectively. Masangi devolved into a *groupement* in 1950s reforms that created a more inclusive sector, Kivunda, which then became a commune at independence. In the post-Mobutu era in Congo, Kivunda has been renamed a *secteur* and Masangi again a *groupement*. Four of the villages were consolidated with neighboring communities or dissolved.

The present/absent categories in table 1.5 reveal that in all cases but two, women far outnumber men, sometimes two to one. In other words, these villages are communities where more than half the men are away working in cities or overseas, leaving their women behind to deliver and raise children and practice subsistence agriculture to feed them. Only in two settings—Kinkungu and Nianga-Ngoyo—are there about as many men present as absent. These are communities that enjoy sizeable forests, allowing for lucrative cultivation of food and cash crops. In the postcolonial setting the numbers of resident men indicate the carrying capacity of forest and savanna agriculture. Absent men, women, and children also indicate the extent of urbanization in this Western Equatorial African region. The population of mostly absent men and subsistence cultivator-child bearing and rearing women also grew dramatically. The resident population doubled in forty-four years; the total de jure population quadrupled in that period.

CONCLUSION

This chapter deals with the ups and downs of a number of contagious diseases that endure in the Lower Congo region and in much of Equatorial Africa, the forces and conditions that have aggravated them, their consequences for the human community, and the ways in which they have been handled. An effort has been made to detail population figures and trends in connection with these disease histories. Accurate population figures are available only from the twentieth century (during the Belgian colonial era), but projections back in time allow for insights into the era before such figures were available (under the Congo Free State and during the earlier years of mercantile trade). In the Manianga region evidence points to Stanley's actions during the early Congo Free State as a time of serious population displacement, flight, and exposure to the conditions of disease. A bit later even more serious disease outbreaks and population decimation occurred in connection with the construction of the Matadi to Kinshasa railroad.

2

Postcolonial Population
and Disease Trends

Why would we want to limit births by family planning if there was such a significant decline in population in our history? Isn't population growth a good thing?

> —Elderly gentleman's question to J. M. Janzen following a lecture at the Free University of Luozi, April 2013

Bulenda kana kuandi mu kubika zi mbutulu za munzo evo makanda meno?
Do you practice family planning in your house or your clan?
Inga. Yes.
If Yes, would you explain your reasons.
Kidi nzo eto ya kala ya mbote ye tunga bana beto bua mbote. So that our house will be well, and to be able to raise our children well.
How many children do you want to have?
Batatu. Three.

> —Wife and mother of two, age thirty-nine, with nine years of schooling (intensive study sample)

Health, the Demographic Transition, Population Records

Postcolonial administrators and their record keepers continued meticulously recording population figures for a few years. However, in the course of time they became unable or unwilling to keep extracting the kinds of information that a heavy-handed colonial government had demanded of the people. Kivunda communal records of 1962 show an attempt to render population figures transparent by making explicit the various locations of the men, no doubt with much effort spent on interviewing.

The entire 1962 population of Kivunda was 14,264. It included 2,401 men, 4,201 women, 3,845 boys, and 3,817 girls. Of the men, 1,809 were under-forty-five-year-old "HAVs" (*homme, adult et valable*); 592 were "retired," or over 45. Of this base population, 608 men and women were "*populations flotantes*," or residents at non-village settlements like government posts, mission/hospital/school complexes, industrial sites, and the like. The category of adult men was further differentiated into "men in villages" (296), "men in the territory" (374), and men "outside the territory less than four years"—thus short-term labor migrants (605). This left 385 men unaccounted for, presumably long-term residents outside of the territory or men who were deceased. This detailed elaboration of the whereabouts of men relating to their economic endeavors was never repeated in subsequent years. But it confirmed the dramatic population increase both in the villages and in the non-village population living and working elsewhere, and the growing out-migration. These records do not indicate whether the rise in population was due to rising birth rate or to a falling mortality rate, especially among children. This latter was the case, as further trends and records demonstrate.

The last year for which the distinction milieu coutumier versus milieu hors (or extra-) coutumier was used by territorial (as well as provincial and perhaps national) record keepers was 1987.[1] In the Territory of Luozi the customary setting (basically village inhabitants) accounted for 120,000 persons, in contrast to 30,000 in the extra-customary setting, thus a total of 150,000 persons. Continuing the earlier gender distribution, women outnumbered men in the villages by 26,000, whereas the numbers of women and men were about equal in the nonvillage settings. Numbers of children as compared to adults rose substantially over what they had been in early twentieth-century colonial reports (for example, in Kivunda in 1920, the ratio was 1:1)—to 2:1 in the village setting and nearly 3:1 in the extra-village setting. The birth rate in the entire population was 1.81 percent on average (varying between 1.69 percent and 2.64 percent), while the crude death rate was 0.52 percent on average (varying between 0.24 percent and 0.98 percent), representing a population growth rate of 1.29 percent per annum. More children were surviving than were decades earlier, and population was increasing. A comparison of these birth and death rates with those from one of the most reliable early twentieth-century sources, the Swedish Medical Mission at Kibunzi, reveal a significantly declining birth rate in the fifty years from 1938 to 1987, as well as a declining mortality rate, although the overall growth rate remained about the same.

A note of caution about the validity of these figures is in order. The old colonially created distinction between the village and nonvillage setting was obsolete and basically arbitrary, impossible to track. Other realities were imposing themselves on the entire attempt to record annual population figures. Many Maniangans were by this time dividing their lives between village and city, keeping two homes, one in each location. Schoolchildren were often away at school when the censuses were taken, and it was arbitrary whether they would be counted in their ostensible matrilineal village community or at the extra-customary school location. Then too, social unrest, war, and difficult economic conditions in the cities of Kinshasa and Brazzaville resulted in the 1980s and 1990s in fairly massive temporary displaced populations occupying the villages of the Manianga; they had either returned to their natal or clan locations or simply found a safe place for a few years. Administrators told me also that a lack of personnel to cover the necessary work of record keeping during the 1980s and 1990s resulted in erroneous or intentionally distorted numbers. In perusing several years of population numbers in the territory's annual reports, I found some wildly fluctuating figures. Although the Congolese Civil War of 1998–2005 did not physically reach the Manianga—it was the only territory of the Lower Congo not invaded by rebel troops—the economic crisis of the war had an overall negative impact on local government and infrastructure, demographic record keeping included.

Perhaps because of the tumult of the war and collapse of state funding, a new style of population record keeping emerged in the mid-1990s and 2000s that was more realistic and also served political and public health needs. As the anticipation of more honest national elections grew in the post-Mobutu era, officials sought to establish a realistic understanding of their population base, as opposed to the often inflated or fabricated one before that time. The revised territorial population records began to focus on actual residence, including residence in villages, schools, medical and church posts, industrial or business centers, and emerging towns, including the territorial "capital" of Luozi. The premise of matrilineal clan adherence of all residents was abandoned for an annual accounting of who resided in a given locale when the census was taken.

Then too the 1984 creation of the health zone, a national public health or primary health administrative structure under the rubric of the World Health Organization's "Health for all by the year 2000," introduced a new independent population and epidemiological tracking framework. I was able to compare the results of these two sets of figures, although the health zone I could track, one of three in the territory, was like apples compared to the oranges of the territorial reports that were generated from the ten sector records. Eventually health zone records began to appear in the territory's annual report, in particular the occurrence of reported epidemics, numbers of persons affected, and related deaths. Health zone figures, kept independently, tended to focus on maternal and infant health, births, and childhood vaccinations. These records were generated by local primary health posts, the more centralized health centers, and the central referral hospitals. I suspected that deaths of elderly individuals were often not entered in the health zone records where such individuals died at home and were buried without a visit to a health post, health center, or referral hospital.

All indications from these population statistics, however flawed, point to a doubling of the population in the postcolonial period (1960–2012), due mainly to a decline in mortality rates—including infant mortality, which had already begun a significant decline in the second half of the colonial period (post-World War II).

A reliable total population figure for the Manianga at the year 2000 would be 160,000, against the backdrop of growth rates for the entire Democratic Republic of the Congo (DRC) of 2.7 percent per annum (World Health Organization 2000a). The exact size of the émigré population remains difficult to track, but it may be close to 1.4 percent/annum, the difference between the national Congolese growth rate and the recurring figure of 1.3 percent for the Manianga (Territoire de Luozi 2000, 2002, 2010, 2011).[2] But the modest Manianga resident population growth figure also needs to take into account the emerging popularity of fertility limitation, or family planning, which is evident in the global population figures and from anecdotal findings gleaned from the intensive sample.

NATALITY DECLINE IN THE SECOND PHASE OF THE DEMOGRAPHIC TRANSITION

The demographic background of this first picture of health in the Manianga has shown a twofold and possibly threefold increase in population over the past seventy to eighty years, due to a decline in mortality from about 1930 on, rather than an increase in natality, or the birth rate. In fact, there is a hint, in the latter phase of this period, of a decline in natality. It is not clear when this decline in birth rate from 1938 to 1987 begins (table 2.1). However, a sampling of reproductive-age women in Luozi and in the Sundi Lutete region in 2013 revealed a very deliberate effort on the part of couples to limit the numbers of their children (table 2.2). Whereas women in the fifty-to-seventy age group had given birth to an average of eight children, with five surviving, those in their forties had given birth to an average of five children, with 4.9 surviving. Women in their thirties said their ideal number of children was from one to three, half or fewer than the number of offspring of their mothers and grandmothers. This is an enormous contrast. Most of these women had entertained using or were using some form of birth control. The women we interviewed revealed the values that such wishes embody in the reasons they gave for engaging in family planning.

TABLE 2.1. Birth, death, and growth rates, Kibunzi and Southwest Manianga (1938) and Luozi (1987)

	Kibunzi and Southwest Manianga, 1938	*Luozi Territory, 1987*
Birth rate (%)	2.9	1.8
Death rate (%)	1.6	0.5
Growth rate (%)	1.3	1.3

SOURCES: Svenska Missionsförbundet 1939; Territoire de Luozi, *Rapport Annuel*, 1987.
NOTE: According to these sources, both death and birth rates have fallen as population growth has remained constant at 1.3 percent per annum. This is half the rate noted by the World Health Organization for the DRC at large, suggesting that the Lower Congo, or the Manianga, may not be typical for the entire country.

- *Kidi luzingu lua bana luakala lua tomakobama*—so that the life of our children will be better
- *Kidi nzo eto yakala mbote ye bana beto buambote*—so that our home and our children will be well
- *Mu diambu dia nsi yeto yo yikidi kuandi mpasi*—because our country has problems
- *Pour bien scolariser nos enfants et la conjuncture de notre pays n'est pas bon*—to be able to educate our children, and because the economy of our country is not good
- *Pour bien scolariser nos enfants et invester*—to be able to educate our children well, and to be able to invest

These explanations, a sampling of the total, emphasize the education of children and quality of life as the path to well-being in the face of a troubled national economy. They reflect the powerful forces of widespread girls' education against a backdrop of generally improving public health conditions. However, they are sentiments and behaviors pitted against entrenched, especially male, voices in Lower Congo society.

"Why would we want to limit births by family planning if there was such a significant decline in population in our history? Isn't population growth a good thing?" These were the words of an elderly gentleman in the audience of my lecture at the Free University of Luozi in April 2013, near the end of my research visit. In my lecture I presented a profile of historic Lower Congo population, identifying some of the likely causes of the 50 percent population decline during the mercantile and slave-trading era and during the Congo Free State era. I then pointed out, in a somewhat ironic perspective, the apparent growing popularity of family planning. I shared preliminary data on desired limits to family size among young married women based on my research. Although there were numerous

TABLE 2.2. Childbearing patterns and preferences in Luozi, by age of woman in 2013

	Ages of women			
	50s to 70s	*40s*	*30s*	*20s*
Births per woman (ave.)	8	5.5	4.4	2.1
Surviving children (ave.)	6.5	4.9	3.9	1.9
Children deceased	25%	9%	12%	8%
Years of schooling (ave./range)	6.5 (2–15)	7.1 (4–15)	7.9 (4–15)	7.3 (2–12)
Ideal, anticipated number of children, as expressed by woman (average)	N/A	4 to 6	1 to 3	1 to 3

SOURCE: Janzen intensive sample, 2013.

women in the audience, including some who had participated in the survey, none chose to rise to answer the gentleman's question. The topic of family planning—population control and limitation of offspring—remains a delicate one.

Vanished and Vanishing Diseases

The declining mortality rate of the late colonial era (until 1960) continued into the postcolonial period. Although enhanced maternal and child care, clean water sources, and sewage facilities like pit toilets were important factors in this trend, other factors included the vanquishing of particular diseases, including leprosy, smallpox, polio, and trypanosomiasis, or sleeping sickness. The first three of these are transmitted person-to-person and thus can be dealt with by tracking relations of contact and attempting quarantine, as well as treatment with medicine or prophylaxes, and by vaccination in the case of smallpox. The last one, sleeping sickness, involves insect and mammalian vectors that are much more difficult to control. Still, advancing medical research, knowledge of the diseases, and the availability of medicine had rendered all four either fully or nearly eradicated by the time of our 2013 research project.

Leprosy

Nearly fifty years ago, on April 8, 1969, I accompanied Dr. William Arkinstall and Kibunzi nurses Tata Nsinga and Tata Lelo to the Kimpevolo Leprosy Colony, which had been founded in 1932 by Swedish mission medical personnel. Arkinstall, a recent former medical director of the Kibunzi hospital and at the time an independent researcher with me on the *Quest for Therapy* project, retained his authority as a visiting doctor to carry out this public health detail. He was to determine which of the ten or so remaining inhabitants of the colony were to be sent home or given other accommodations. In any case, his main mission was to provide the medical-scientific judgment that would close the leprosarium. In addition to the relatively low degree of contagion that leprosy reflected, by 1969 medicines and treatment methods had progressed to where outpatient care was the commonly recommended treatment for the disease.

Kimpevolo, like many leper colonies in the Belgian Congo, as elsewhere in Africa, was a small society unto itself created by the medical policy of isolation, reinforced by colonial administrative muscle, and lived out by reluctant subjects who accommodated themselves to life in an alternative society. With up to seventy residents at its most populous, Kimpevolo had refashioned itself into a semblance of a Kongo village. A chief emerged; a hunter was appointed. Residents were given land to cultivate in the immediate vicinity and in neighboring clan lands, an arrangement enforced by colonial authorities. Although the legal codes and recommended practices of those registered as lepers allowed short visits home, it did not permit nonleper spouses to cohabit at Kimpevolo. Often such couples separated or formally divorced. Common-law families emerged within the leper community. Kimpevolo's recent history had seen two such families, one with three children, the other with one. But without the glue of normative social structure, interactions between individuals were often chaotic. As soon as we entered Kimpevolo, several individuals complained about the antisocial behavior of one man.

Leprosy had long been an iconic disease of otherness and stigma in the Western world. The predisposition of Western Christian missions to take up the cause of lepers, and of the colonial government to enforce the special identity-shaping status of these subjects, meant that careful records were kept of leprosy in the Lower Congo early on. In the FOREAMI report of 1932, nine hundred lepers were identified by region. The medical conditions of the progression of the disease are detailed; the indigenous terms are noted. Despite this rigorous organizing and categorizing of lepers, the stigmatizing and identity-transforming character that Westerners projected onto the disease only partially penetrated Kongo social norms. The near total disappearance of the condition from the public health checklists echoed what happened at independence in many African countries. In Mali, for example, Silla has documented the dissolution of leper colonies and the engagement of former leprosy patients in a campaign for full human rights as national citizens (1998). Only by their admission to mainstream society as full citizens with rights could the lingering stigma of the disease be dispelled. In the Manianga, apparently, the continuing availability of funds for leprosy work from the international Leprosy Mission (figure 2.1) means that the image of leprosy as a special disease is being perpetuated from outside the community, even though the incidence of the disease is miniscule and the contagion rate very minimal.

Smallpox

Smallpox was a common contagious disease in early postcolonial Lower Congo, with epidemics breaking out occasionally, although a vaccine was known. Although smallpox was much more dangerous than leprosy, there was ironically no history of quarantine of those infected or exposed, either in Kongo society or in Western medical institutions. The last outbreak reported by medical authorities at the large Institut Médical Evangélique (IME) in Kimpese was in 1961. Workers there told Arkinstall and me that the Congolese did not have a good understanding of the nature of the contagion, and therefore did not practice isolation of the infected individuals. Thus, it was impossible to impose quarantine on them. Only with the eradication campaign mounted by the World Health Organization (WHO) in the 1970s did smallpox diminish in the Lower Congo. The last reported case in Africa, and on the entire globe, was in Somalia in 1977. The disease was officially declared globally eradicated in 1980.[3]

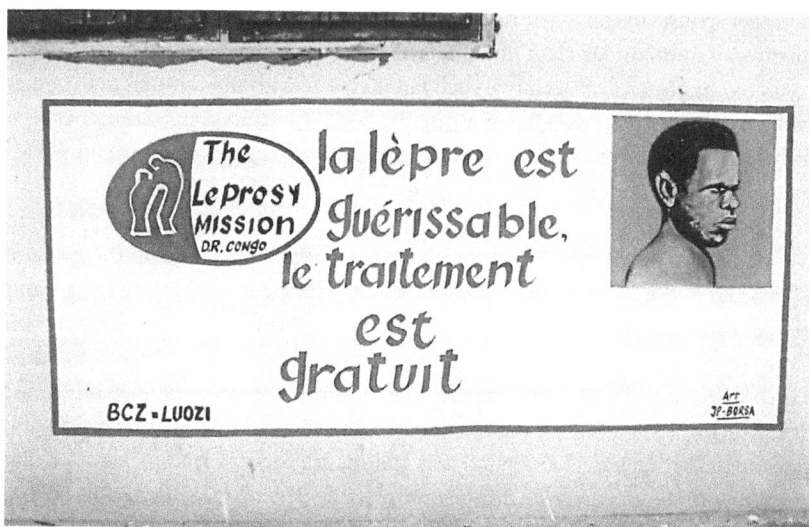

FIGURE 2.1. "Leprosy is treatable, treatment is free." Poster painted on the outside wall of the Luozi Health Zone, indicating generous financial sponsorship by the worldwide Leprosy Mission. Painting by artist Jean-Pierre Boursa. Photo: John M. Janzen, 2013.

Polio

Polio was another Lower Congo endemic disease spread by person-to-person contact, and therefore a candidate for a WHO global eradication campaign. Following the introduction of the health zone administrative structure in the DRC, antipolio vaccinations were included in routine campaigns. The outbreak of civil wars in the 1990s set back this effort. However, a national campaign was launched in 1999 that proved remarkably effective given the country's several regional wars. A blitz campaign was called for August 13–15. Health officials and diplomats negotiated a truce between warring factions to allow vaccines and portable refrigerators to be distributed to local health zones and committees. An amazing 80 percent vaccination rate was achieved in this manner, amounting to 10 million children. Kisangani, a city in the middle of the war zone, achieved 91 percent coverage of children (Hull 1999; Bush 2000). In the Manianga a 2008 campaign combined polio vaccinations with Vitamin A (Map 2.1). Luozi Health Zone staff reported a high rate of coverage, although they noted resistance to these vaccinations by adherents of the Bundu dia Kongo movement. Still, no cases of polio were reported by the Luozi Health Zone in 2013; nor were there any in our intensive sample. By midyear 2018 only isolated cases had been reported from the DRC and several other African countries. Thus, although the victory over polio was not complete like that over smallpox, the disease had effectively vanished.

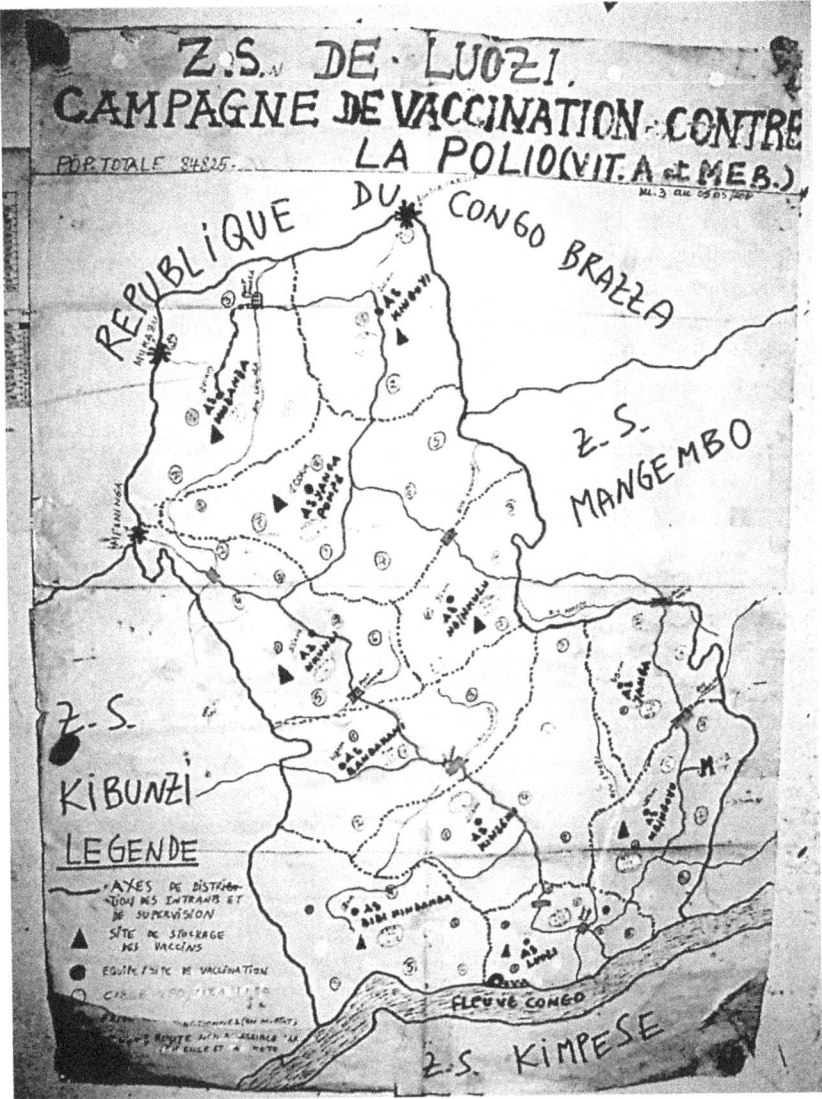

MAP 2.1. Polio vaccination campaign, Luozi Health Zone, 2008. Map shows supply route, storage points where refrigeration was available, and health posts where vaccinations were carried out. Vitamin A was also distributed at this time. Photo by John M. Janzen of map on wall of Luozi Health Zone office.

Trypanosomiasis

"Professor Janzen, have you heard that your village Kisiasia was hit by an epidemic of sleeping sickness a few years ago? Many people were infected and died. Others fled. The villages are empty." This grim report greeted me on my return to the Manianga in 2013. The hope to sift fact from rumor was on my agenda when I traveled to the North Manianga in April with Célestin Lusiama, who had grown up in the area, as my guide.

Ethnographic accounts of illness and health should not only include the biological and medical facts but also illuminate the broader social and cultural context that brings events to life, that makes the perceptions and emotional charge around them visible and believable. This inquiry into a 2007 outbreak of sleeping sickness—African trypanosomiasis—provides a good case study of how an outbreak of a historically devastating disease is perceived, how it is dealt with when medical solutions and expertise are available, and how memory of it is shaped by deeper cultural memory from earlier decades.

Trypanosomiasis is caused by a parasite that is transmitted to humans by the bite of the tsetse fly, a large fly whose distinguishing feature is crossed wings when it is seated on a leaf or branch. Mammals may offer a cohost, including some wild animals that are immune to the disease and may thus be invisible carriers of the microorganism. The disease usually manifests in increasingly severe and debilitating phases that may last months. Infected individuals typically develop abscesses at the point of the tsetse fly bite, and go on to have a fever and to feel sick and experience other side effects. At a later stage the central nervous system is impaired, leading to slurred speech, "sleeping" behavior, unconsciousness, and ultimately death if not treated.

This 2007 outbreak menaced a number of villages in the Sundi Lutete/Kivunda area. Scrutiny for signs of the disease's presence continued until 2011. In Nseke Mwini, a small hamlet of the Kisiasia village, there were two cases, both of which were successfully treated, and those who had been ill were reported as being well at the time of our visit. In the larger section of Kisiasia, reports were of up to five infected. Here too, after treatment in Luozi, they were reported as being well. We met several of these individuals, and they confirmed this positive outcome. Several other infections were reported in surrounding villages. All were successfully treated in Luozi or at other centralized hospitals. We could find no reports of cases resulting in death.

These locally reported cases of successful treatment of sleeping sickness were the result of significant intervention by public health officials in two adjoining health zones, with treatment occurring at the hospitals at Sundi Lutete and Luozi, and being offered by a medical team from the IME in Kimpese. The effort was part of the WHO's major eradication initiative on human trypanosomiasis.[4] They took care of reporting of the cases of infection and installing tsetse fly traps, cone-shaped canopies from which the flies cannot escape, hung in trees that provide dense shade that attracts the flies. On order of the health zone underbrush was cleared in affected areas. Finally, people were ordered to kill the local wildlife, possible vectors of the spread of the disease. At the time of our visit, the prohibition on domestic animals remained in place.

Despite the span of two years since the last reported case, an undercurrent of suspicion remained in the populace that the outbreak had not really ended or been fully cured. Some felt that the authorities were keeping something hidden. They specifically mentioned the fact that the health inspection team had never returned to assure people that the epidemic was indeed over. Several families and individuals who had fled at the time of the outbreak had not returned.

The wider Lower Congo public could not be blamed for fearing sleeping sickness. For many, their ancestors of a century ago had suffered a catastrophic epidemic in connection with the late nineteenth-century transition from coastal slavery to the Congo Free State's incursions. Forced labor at the Free State's harbors, on the portage trails inland, and during the construction of the railroads had caused many to flee to the forests, where diseases raged and decimated many communities. Then there was the memory of extensive forced mass vaccinations in the post-World War II years with lomodine, the first widely available drug that served as a cure and for short-term prophylaxis, although not without side effects (Lachenal 2017, 29–34, 47–48).

In the early twenty-first-century outbreak, public fear, fanned by media coverage, far surpassed the minor statistical blip of the cases that were quickly treated. The flight of some people from the areas of infection and their refusal to return contributed to the public fear. Even locally, where survivors of the disease lived, suspicion swelled that hidden motives were causing the outbreak and continuing to perpetuate it. Lusiama spoke to one recovered victim about her conviction that she was continuing to be affected by these hidden causes. She mentioned her headaches from the time of her original infection, and the nonreturn of the inspection team. Additionally, she harbored the suspicion that her clan's former masters were using the sorcery—*kindoki*—of sleeping sickness to get rid of her and her group, their former slaves.

Slave ransoms continued in postcolonial Congo. As a legacy of the heavy precolonial coastal slave trade and the Belgian colonial policy of leaving in place slave group relations while fostering ransom negotiations, two prominent cases of slave groups seeking redress occurred in Kisiasia. According to Kivunda communal court records, most former Kisiasia slave clans had found redress and ransom in the 1940s, 1950s, and 1960s, and had moved back to their ancestral homes.

The two remaining cases of former slave clan fragments had processed ransom and redemption in court, and had then tried to return home in the postcolonial era. But what made these two cases unique was that the people in the two clan remnants had been rebuffed by their home-resident clan brothers and sisters. In their desperation to secure permanent homes, both groups had gone to court and sued their former master clans for rights to the land they had cultivated while closely intermarrying with these same former masters. One group had used as their main evidence in court the alleged verbal promise of a former clan head to grant them occupancy of the land in perpetuity. The current clan head told me that this had been a serious mistake. He accused the court of lax standards when the judge had simply taken the former slave clan's statement at face value and declared it the new rightful owner of the land. In the case of the woman claiming ongoing symptoms of sleeping sickness, her clan remnant had also sought court redress to gain rights to the land they had occupied as slaves. Now, she suggested, these former masters were using the *kindoki* of sleeping sickness to make them sick, and thus to get rid of them in order to regain the land.

The 2007 outbreak of sleeping sickness was like a genie that has escaped its bottle. Prompt public health measures, reflecting a century of scientific research into the nature of the trypanosome; its insect, animal, and human vectors; and the efficacy of drugs, vigilant monitoring, and the use of fly traps, have achieved effective suppression of the actual biological disease. However, diseases have a social and material history that enters into the conscious, even the semiconscious, memory of the community.

Principal Diseases of Twenty-First-Century Manianga

Despite these public health victories, many of the diseases that have caused the people of the Manianga and Western Equatorial Africa so much grief in the past continue to be present, although now they are mostly held at bay by general knowledge about their signs and symptoms, methods of avoidance and prevention, continuing popular education by the health zones and schools, access to hospitals, tracking of patterns of infection, and the availability of medicines and skilled personnel to treat outbreaks in individuals and larger publics. This section offers a cursory ethnography of these principal maladies in the Luozi Health Zone, including how they are addressed, singly or with groups, the human and environmental ground within which they persist, their incidence, their relative rise or decline, and their consequences and meaning.[5] The statistical information in this section comes from the Luozi Health Zone (table 2.3) and from the intensive sample (table 2.4). The zone's diligent staff work with the local animation teams to carry out vaccination campaigns and to collect population figures (births and deaths), and incidences of diseases treated at the posts, centers, and referral hospitals.

One way to assess these principal diseases is to take note of their incidence during the most recent decade that the health zone has documented cases seen in the health posts, centers, and referral hospitals. Malaria is by far the most frequent and

TABLE 2.3. Principal diseases, Luozi Health Zone, 2003–2012

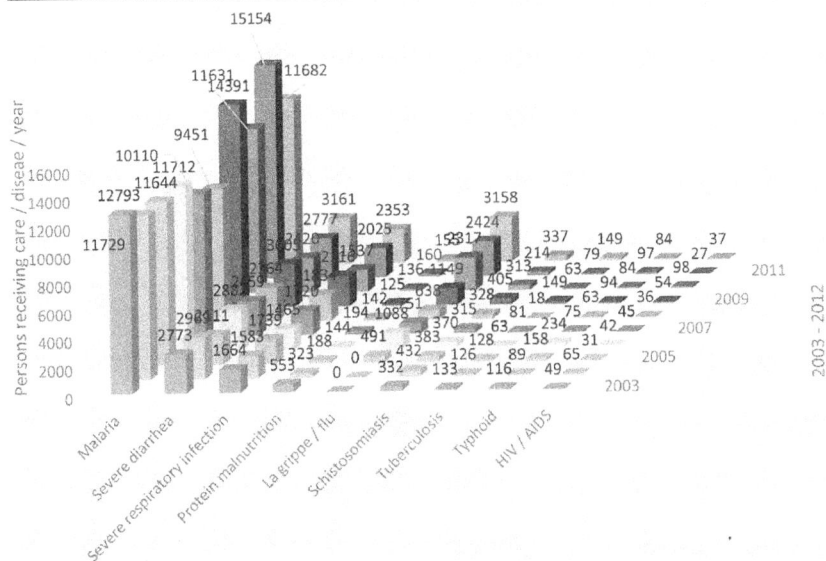

SOURCE: Luozi Health Zone records.
NOTE: Major diseases recorded by Luozi Health Zone as having been seen and cared for in all health posts, health centers, and the referral hospital, 2003–12.

serious of the diseases. It shares the dubious qualification as a steady state disease, along with schistosomiasis (bilharzia), HIV/AIDS, tuberculosis, and typhoid fever. That is, its overall frequency remains about the same from year to year, and it is a chronic disease. We must also take note of the diseases that are either on the decline or have been more or less eliminated due to vigilance in immunization or other interventions. This group would include polio, sleeping sickness, protein malnutrition, and childhood disease such as measles, diphtheria, chicken pox, and whooping cough. The lowered incidence of these diseases could be said to represent public health victories, or at least relative successes compared to earlier years. A third group of diseases are those that, unfortunately, are chronic and on the increase. This group would include severe diarrhea, severe respiratory infections, and seasonal flu (la grippe).

Malaria

Malaria is by far the most prevalent principal disease in the Manianga, Lower Congo, and Western Central Africa. Although its characteristics as well as its prevention and treatment are well known, malaria has proven difficult to deal with, not to mention eradicate. The Luozi Health Zone reports in the past decade that

TABLE 2.4. Disease episodes in intensive sample, by venue and treatment

Episodes per disease	Diseases, conditions	Luozi General	Luozi Catholic	Sundi Lutete	Other hospitals, clinics	Health posts	Self-medication w. pharmaceutics	Self-medication w. herbals	Healer-prophet-diviner
	Total episodes per venue	55	40	60	24	21	119	34	22
	Diseases, conditions								
137	malaria	32	9	25	3	12	47	6	3
51	grippe (seasonal flu)	6	10			1	31	3	
31	schistosomiasis (bilharzia)		1				21	9	
23	stomach pain (gastritis)	5	4		2	2	4	3	3
17	appendectomy	1	2	14					
17	rheumatism, pain in joints	3			2		3	4	5
15	hypertension "excess de sang"	2	2	3		3	1	1	3
15	fever		3		2	1	7	2	
13	hernia	3		7				2	1
7	ovarian cyst	1		6					
6	filaria						2	2	2
5	tuberculosis	2	1		2				
3	hemorrhoids							1	2
3	varicella (chicken pox)						2		1
3	earache		3						
3	"miome" (adenomyosis)		3						
2	headache, asthma, cardiac insufficiency, trypanosomiasis, kidney, eyes, diarrhea, urinary infection	2	3	7			2		1
1	fracture, weakness, miscarriage threat, amoeba, curse, anemia, meningitis, toothache, pneumonia, angina, protein malnutrition			2	6		1	1	1

NOTE: Disease episodes were reported in intensive sample in 105 households, with 579 individuals. The interviewer asked household heads to recall such episodes within the past year.
SOURCE: Intensive sample, 2012–13.

annually between 13 and 21 percent of the population have experienced episodes of infection serious enough to have visited a recording health post, center, or hospital. But malaria affects everyone. Indeed, most of our acquaintances during the four months in Luozi were "down" at least once with malaria or "fever." Malaria accounts for 137 episodes in the intensive sample, nearly half of all reported illnesses. Of those incidents reported, nearly half were self-treated with pharmaceutical or herbal medications, suggesting that the number of actual cases is at least double that recorded in the health zone figures. Though my wife, Reinhild, dutifully took prophylaxis, she came down with a serious case that was successfully diagnosed and treated by Doctor Rose Ndoda Kumbu and her staff at the Luozi Catholic Hospital.

Malaria, named for *mal aire*—"bad air"—was for centuries thought to be caused by a combination of swamps, muggy air near swamps, and spirits lurking in various kinds of bad air. The link between mosquitoes, the spirochete, and the disease's symptoms was only established in the early twentieth century. The exploration team lead by Henry Stanley thought his near-fatal bout with fever and chills at Manianga was caused by the sudden chilling winds that came through the river canyon after a hot day. Lower Congo residents' preferred habitations were atop the hills that figure prominently in the landscape because they were considered healthier than the lowlands near the rivers. Breezes kept the insects to a minimum, and with the help of shade trees, the air was coolly comfortable.

Transmitted by several subspecies of the *Anopheles* mosquito, after "the sporozoite (the parasite form inoculated by the female mosquito) of *Plasmodium falciparum* invades a liver cell, the parasite grows in 6 days and produces 30,000–40,000 daughter cells (merozoites), which are released into the blood when the liver cell ruptures. In the blood, after a single merozoite invades a red blood cell, the parasite grows in 48 hours and produces 8–24 daughter cells, which are released into the blood when the red blood cell ruptures" (Janzen 2017, 94, citing the CDC). Infected individuals will develop fever and chills, which occur in waves that may last several hours and continue to recur with increasing severity. In children this can lead to severe anemia and death. In youth and adults it contributes to chronic weakness and inability to perform intellectual or physical tasks, and is overall very debilitating.

The red blood cell ruptures produce the fever and generate a more rapid replacement of the cells. When the *Plasmodium falciparum* became endemic around the time of the beginning of food cultivation in West Africa four to five thousand years ago, a condition that came to be known as sickling of the red blood cell conferred an adaptive advantage on populations living in the emerging malaria zones. The genetic mutation that developed created several predispositions in offspring in relation to malaria: a resistance to malaria through a kind of normal sickling behavior (seen in offspring of heterozygous parents); extreme sickling, resulting in anemia attacks (seen in offspring of homozygous parents); and no resistance or anemia, thus susceptibility to malaria attacks. Sickle cell anemia is a fairly common condition in the Manianga; its presence may produce a series of children who die early in childhood. The condition is extremely hard on women in a pronatalist society such as this, and results often in divorce.

Methods of treatment have taken several directions, each with partial and temporary success, but yielding no long-term, permanent solution. As a cure, quinine continues to be a dependable treatment. But it does not confer immunity, and if taken in overly large doses for too long, it causes ringing in the ears and may result in temporary mental dissociation. Generations of other drugs have come and gone, with some degree of efficacy and usually with side effects if taken for long periods of time. One of the greatest difficulties in combating malaria has been mosquitos' ability to resist and adapt to methods to eradicate them. DDT became a favorite method of mosquito eradication in the 1950s and 1960s. Tropical cities such as Kinshasa were saturation sprayed from airplanes. But this chemical proved disastrous from two perspectives. It was highly toxic for all wildlife and humans, especially affecting reproductive capacity. Furthermore, surviving mosquitoes developed resistance to the chemical. Thus, extensive spraying produced a superior bug. Drug treatments and prophylaxes were plagued by the same phenomenon: genetic adaptation and resistance by the mosquitoes and the spirochetes.

Currently researchers are experimenting with medicines and protection methods that take into account the evolutionary process of the target. The medicated mosquito nets that everyone in our survey used, courtesy of the WHO, Ministry of Health, and the health zone, have reportedly reduced malaria incidents somewhat, but many people are still bitten in early twilight or in the morning before mosquitoes withdraw for the hot sunlight hours. Pharmaceutical experimenters have discovered that synthetic drugs designed around a single chemical property or process are more easily adapted to than chemicals with complex structures, as in the case of natural products like quinine. Manianga pharmacist and drug manufacturer Batangu Mpesa has built his products for prophylaxis (Manadiar) and treatment (Manalaria) around a particular plant he has found and now grows commercially for drug production purposes.

Many Maniangans use a range of local traditional products and methods that have not yet been studied systematically. Some people rub themselves with a poultice of several plants before they go off into the bush, or when they happen to walk by such plants. They say that the aroma of the plant repels mosquitoes. About a third of the households in our survey mentioned keeping the yard around the house free of grass and sweeping it daily to keep mosquitoes away; there is some evidence that these households reported fewer incidents of malaria than those not mentioning this technique. However, no one seemed to be concerned about large, water-filled potholes in streets, and pools of water in ditches close to human traffic.

No preventive vaccinations have been given. Malaria is so pervasive in the region that people consider it to be normal. Cures and prophylaxes are available, whence the high numbers frequenting medical institutions for this disease and self-medicating with medicines purchased in pharmacies. Yet reinfection occurs routinely. The challenge remains of how to break the cycle of transmission via the female *Anopheles* mosquito carrying the sporozoite *Plasmodium falciparum* from one infected person to another.

Severe Diarrhea

One of the waterborne diseases especially dangerous in infants, severe diarrhea has been the focus of much attention by the international health community in recent decades. The worldwide advent of simple-to-administer oral rehydration therapy, along with maternal education, has contributed to an impressive decline in infant mortality rates and an overall decline in mortality rates. However, a generalized concern with clean water for drinking and food preparation has also contributed, worldwide and in the Manianga, to this decline in infant and overall mortality rates. Health zone tracking indicates a 2–3 percent (reporting) incidence of severe diarrhea from 2003 to 2012. Figures from the Aire de Luozi—the town and surrounding villages—shows an incidence of half that of the larger zone. This is confirmation of the impact of the Luozi clean water system on the health of the community. The figure is quite probably even lower within the city where access to clean water is nearly total. The *aire* includes a periphery of households that depend for domestic use on a variety of springs, pumps, rainwater, and streams, which may be infected with waterborne disease agents. Our intensive survey shows no episodes of severe diarrhea in households with access to the city water system.

But by contrast, in the entire zone severe diarrhea showed a slight increase, occurring mainly in children, and a great risk for infants. The increase in reported cases may be due to the lack of maintenance of clean water installations that exist in most villages and towns in the region. In our visits we noted that a number of these installations—wells, cemented in springs—were broken and lacked available repair parts or budget for upkeep (Territoire de Luozi, *Rapport Annuel*, 2012). In these circumstances, I was told by several witnesses, people have no recourse but to go to rivers where they know the water is infested. This also happened when people did not pay their water bill. Their faucets were rendered dysfunctional, and they had to use river water.

Tuberculosis

Tuberculosis, a well-known bacterial infection usually of the lungs, has been treated effectively worldwide with antibiotics, and thus until recently has been considered a conquered contagious disease. Reasons for its reappearance in the Manianga and worldwide are several. The first has to do with the manner in which tubercular nodules that are present in treated and recovered cases reopen and reinfect under stressful and compromising conditions. This would be the case in the Manianga, where, I was told by health zone authorities, these cases are easily treated with antibiotics in clinics at every level. There was concern, however, that unreported cases existed and that the community volunteers were not vigilant enough in getting patients to the clinics. Still, the relatively low morbidity and very low mortality rates suggest that although tuberculosis is resurgent, it is largely under control. But the second cause for its resurgence worldwide is more worrisome: the emergence of drug resistant tuberculosis, which the Manianga Health Zone workers assured me was not present there—yet. Traces of tuberculosis that resists conventional antibiotics have been found in populations across the world—including the United States—in places such as prisons and homeless shelters, and in people who have HIV/AIDS. People in these circumstances often are living on the edge, are physiologically stressed, and have begun but not completed antibiotic courses of treatment, and thus serve as hosts to the mutation of antibiotic-resistant superbugs.

Typhoid Fever

Typhoid fever is usually characterized by high fever, stomach cramps, and diarrhea. It is specific to humans who are infected by and carry the bacterial microorganism *Salmonella Typhi* in their intestines and blood stream. Typically, it is spread through food or water that carries fecal material or sewage. A small number of persons who are infected and recover on their own become carriers and can spread the disease without being aware of it. Treatment with antibiotics until all traces are gone is the conventional treatment. Vaccinations exist, but they are not 100 percent effective.

Typhoid fever was first identified by the Swedish medical teams early in the twentieth century in regions where people had fled their homes to escape colonial labor recruiters. It has been present on a continuing basis ever since. Great strides in limiting it have been due to the introduction and near universal use of pit latrines in villages and towns.

Severe Respiratory Infections

Bacterial or viral pneumonia, asthma, and a variety of lung infections are tracked by the health zone separately from seasonal influenza, or grippe. The northern, mountainous, region of the Manianga has a cool dry season from June to September that people generally do not like. Since houses are not equipped to be heated, and much living is normally out of doors, they retreat to kitchens where fires smolder to provide just a bit of warmth through the cold night. Furthermore, the dry season is dusty, and smoke from many grass fires fills the air. As a result, many people develop respiratory tract infections at the time of dry-season brush burning. The increase in such infections may be due to increasing economic hardship, deteriorating housing for some, and generally more adverse living conditions.

Grippe/Flu

On the other hand, seasonal influenza—commonly referred to by the French *grippe*—is the local version of the annual global flu that demonstrates the global linkages of the epidemiology of this region. This is the annual flu for which northerners are supposed to get their yearly shots. It is not clear whether the annual recurrence in the Luozi Health Zone is due to fresh global spread and infection, or whether it is a locally evolving species of virus. This is always a viral infection and cannot be quickly treated with antibiotics. I am not aware of any campaign for annual flu shots, nor of anyone receiving the inoculation that drug companies produce, nor that an inoculation was even available. So people generally just suffer, stay at home, and if sick enough find a clinic or hospital. This disease represents the unpleasant reality that new infectious diseases require constant monitoring, and that a legitimate infrastructure of public health, available materia medica, and competent personnel are required to deal with this dimension of health.

Schistosomiasis/Bilharzia

Although schistosomiasis is rarely fatal, infection with the microscopic worms causes damage to the liver and other internal organs, skin eruptions, weakness, diarrhea, fever, interference with growth and maturation in children, and a range of other debilitating chronic conditions. Next to malaria, schistosomiasis is the most severely debilitating tropical condition common in the Manianga. The cycle of life of the schistosomes alternates between humans and other mammals, and snails that inhabit the shaded edges of watercourses. Eggs in the water hatch, and their larvae enter and reside in the snails. Successive generations of sporocysts live in the snails, eventually becoming free-swimming cercariae (microscopic worms) that enter the skin of humans who swim or bathe in, or have contact with infested water, usually on river edges. Once these microscopic worms enter the skin, they become schistosomulae and enter the blood stream. Some lodge in the liver or other organs, and paired adult worms reproduce in the liver. Their eggs migrate to the bowels or bladder, then are released into the water, where they repeat the cycle.

Treatment nowadays is a simple single dose of medication. But reinfection will occur if the patient reenters the same water where infection occurred. In our health survey we intentionally visited fishers along the river. This accounts for the thirty-one cases in a single group of households; there were no cases in the other groups. These riverain residents were acutely aware of their problem and expressed the desire for clean water sources for their domestic use.

Protein Malnutrition

Also known as kwashiorkor, protein malnutrition affects mainly children whose diet is chronically short of protein. They are recognized by their reddish hair and distended stomachs. Common causes include a diet of starchy, carbohydrate-heavy manioc, with very few greens, groundnuts, or meats. Most people recognize this condition and associate it with poverty and the difficult economy of the Congo. They realize that children with kwashiorkor do not thrive: they do poorly in school, and their growth is often stunted. The most readily available protein source in the Lower Congo is usually fish or small livestock such as goats or chicken, but even these are costly for some budgets. A cold storage locker in Luozi has been opened to import fresh meats and make them easily available to the population, but for a price. The health zone has sought to raise consciousness about this condition, and incidence has diminished in the decade covered from 553 in 2003 to only 155 in 2012.

HIV/AIDS

No stranger to the Lower Congo, HIV/AIDS is not considered the death sentence it was thought to be a few years ago, at least in the West. Posters abound in Luozi warning people about unprotected sex. But it was not something many people talked about, at least not in our presence. The incidence shown by health zone statistics is also underwhelming: less than 1 percent of the population. When we pointedly asked a hospital lab technician how many HIV/AIDS cases they had worked up in the past year, he asked his colleagues, who were seated at stools checking malaria slides. Together they responded with "Oh, perhaps two or three."

The health zone workers with whom I discussed the matter said, "It's an invisible, hidden disease." Yes, it is stigmatized, and there is denial. People resist testing, not wanting to know if they are infected, for fear that it might be true. Among all the young adult students in Luozi, the rural youth are most afraid of AIDS, and this, to a degree, keeps them from experimenting sexually. The urban youth, on the other hand, tend to believe that AIDS is a myth, and they act accordingly.

Congolese AIDS physician Joseph Kapita Bila, a big name in Kinshasa HIV/AIDS research circles, is known for having discovered the disease and for having first noticed the danger of infection while giving nursing care, which some Western researchers dismissed (Bila 1988). Bila is from Luozi and has maintained a clinic in his home village of Kinsemi, west of Luozi. So the professional consciousness about HIV/AIDS is keen in the region. As if to follow through on precautions in a region with such consciousness, condoms are widely available, but our contacts in the health zone said that no one really knows how many people are infected.

DISEASE AND TREATMENT IN THE INTENSIVE SAMPLE

The health zone figures of disease incidence (see table 2.3), when compared with the study's intensive sample responses to the question "For which disease in the household have you sought or taken treatment in the past year?" (table 2.4), reveal many similarities, as well as some significant differences. In both, malaria represents by far the highest incidence and number of cases: over half of the health zone episodes and a third of the intensive sample episodes. The two registers correspond on the incidence of grippe, or seasonal flu, as a rising-incidence disease in the health zone report, and as the second-most-significant disease in the intensive sample (at 41 of 375 episodes). Schistosomiasis has the third-most-numerous episodes in the intensive sample, while it is only a minor figure in the health zone report. This may be explained by our intentional seeking out of riverain individuals, professional fishers, in our sample. Virtually all fishers and their families were infected. Oddly, the childhood diseases—protein malnutrition, severe diarrhea—barely show up on the intensive sample. It may be that parents consider these conditions so routine that they do not recall them from over the past year. The absence of HIV/AIDS in the intensive sample may well be explained by the disease's lingering stigma; an individual may find it embarrassing to report it to a community member and a foreign professor.

An important feature of the intensive sample is that nearly half of the episodes reported were handled at home with self-medication. This was especially true of malaria, schistosomiasis, and seasonal flu, suggesting that the overall incidence may be significantly higher than that recorded in the health zone figures. This feature also implies that pharmacies are doing a booming business, and that the sick may be avoiding the larger institutions because of clinical costs or other factors.

CONCLUSION

The population figures and related disease profiles in this chapter provide a background for the central topic of this work: the persistence of these diseases in the face of growing scientific and medical expertise regarding their treatment. All the illnesses on the principal disease list are well known, their causes are understood, and methods of avoiding and treating them are equally well understood. The Manianga region enjoys the presence of at least twelve physicians and numerous health experts, as well as healers of other types. Granted, most of the diseases are rooted in tropical environmental conditions, and the majority of people in this study are exposed daily to the vectors and settings of the diseases—going out into their fields, forests, and rivers to cultivate, collect, and fish.[6] But the rising incidence of some of the diseases is also caused by a declining quality of life or inadequate public services, as for example the water-borne diseases, or those associated with inadequate housing. Then too the factor of globalization may be seen in at least one disease, seasonal flu.

Each of these plausible background factors in the explanation for the persistence of well-understood diseases supports the hypothesis of this work: that the crisis of institutional legitimacy and the history of repeated and continual institutional upheaval and change have weakened the effectiveness of those institutions that exist at any one time to carry the load of addressing basic needs.

PART II

The Social Reproduction
of Health

3

Health in Household,
Family, and Clan

Tata Luyobisa and his wife, Mama Bakima, came to our guesthouse one evening
to see the videos I had taken of the ceremonies in a recent worship service of the
Communauté du Saint Esprit en Afrique. When we saw them walking down the
road, they were carrying a container of some kind. Upon arrival, they proudly gave
us its contents, a small portion of their groundnut harvest, fresh from the field.
They knew that Reinhild loved freshly roasted groundnuts, or peanuts. Luyobisa
had stored that in his mind and was quick to offer a gift of friendship when the
opportunity arose. Groundnuts are a cherished food staple, as well as an integral
part of the economy in Manianga society. The various dishes made with them—
including *muamba nguba* (groundnut stew with chicken)—figure in kinship relations. They are a much desired cash crop because they keep well and are easy to
transport to distant markets, where they fetch a premium.

Groundnuts may be traced along the contours of society. As a token of society's
resources, they are controlled by social classes and power centers, and moved
through institutions of greater or lesser scale to meet perceived need. They are
given meaning and symbolic definition, and they are reproduced as society sus-
tains patterns of care, healing, and well-being. This chapter lays out the role of
domestic institutions and practices in health and health care in Manianga society.

The World Health Organization's guidelines for health in a community include
adequate food, good water, sewage treatment, housing, safe living conditions, and
the assurance of a cushion of customs and social relationships to ensure these
standards are met. By whatever definition, where part of society is decidedly less
healthy than another, this hierarchical condition is a reflection of power and class
relations—the control or lack of resources needed to enjoy good health. The social
reproduction of health combines the health definitions and terms of the society

itself and of outside evaluations with a society's ability and ongoing set of practices and potentials to define, maintain, or restore health where ill health is present.

THE SOCIAL REPRODUCTION OF HEALTH

Social reproduction, a standard concept in the social sciences, is the notion that over time groups of people and social classes reproduce their social structure and patterns of living to preserve their advantage (Bilton 1996, 670).[1] It has been applied to globalization studies and to the manner in which huge gaps between haves and have-nots reemerge in the worldwide shifting of capital, labor, and commoditized goods. In the African setting it has included the study of the expansion of colonial and global capitalism, and the often very uneven access to global resources (Ferguson 2006). The rights and privileges of which nations once assured their citizens seem to have come undone for many, especially for children, whose parents face an increasingly desperate struggle on their behalf (Katz 2001). All these observations hold true in the historical context of health in the Lower Congo. It was already true of the impact of the precolonial mercantilist trade, which included the slave trade. It was true of labor-extractive colonialism, of both the Congo Free State era and the Belgian colonial era. It remains true in the present weak-state neoliberal global economy, in which many realms of life are defined by commoditized goods and services that are to be had only with capital gained through the sale of marketable produce or people-demanding services.

Anthropologists no longer refer to the impact of colonial capitalism on far-flung societies of the world, or to the current structures and effects of globalization, as relating to separate traditional and modern sectors of society. Rather, the impact of colonial or global capitalism and the commoditization that accompanies globalization is evident within households, lineages, and local societies as they reproduce themselves through daily labor, and in rituals and gift exchanges that provide or reinforce local well-being and identity.

Anthropological writings on social reproduction usually begin with the domestic household as their primary unit of analysis, and, within that, family and wider kin groups like lineages and clans. The household harbors the resources, symbols, persons, and practices that are strategies of well-being (Meillassoux 1964; Bourdieu 1977; Murray 1981).[2] Household is defined to include persons who reside together and may or may not be related as kin. Usually those residing together in this close way share the tasks of daily living and caring for each other. It is possible to observe quite closely the manner in which resources are generated by those productive members of the household and shared or redistributed to those who are dependent. Thus, the household is the social unit most likely to "produce health" (Berman, Kendall, and Bhattacharyya 1989, 1994).

Over a longer term, for a society to survive and persist, its productive members must produce adequate surplus resources—however these are defined—to take care of their own needs as well as the needs of the dependent young, elderly, and sick. These needs may also include educating and socializing the young and ensuring a meaningful worldview. Furthermore, there need to be adequate institutionalized channels of redistribution beyond the household to coordinate this redistributive activity over time from the productive members of society to the dependent ones for a society to survive—that is, to "socially reproduce" itself (Meillassoux 1964, 1981).

Anthropologists studying the reproduction of local society within a broader global economy became more interested in the concurrent articulation of domestic and global processes and flows of resources and symbols.[3] As an example of this type of analysis, Robert Foster (1995) identified two kinds of social reproduction in the Tangan society in Melanesia, one based on replication, the other on multiplication of forms, practices, and resource uses. Replication occurred in mortuary rituals that honored the lineage dead, in stimulated exchanges, and in the performance of ceremonies. This type of social reproduction sealed off a domain of culture that the Tangans recognized as *kastam* (custom) from more open-ended commercial transactions that they came to call *bisnis* (business). However, some aspects of replication displayed practices of commodity production and exchange. The contrast between replication and multiplication suggested that the process of commoditization had taken different trajectories in different Melanesian settings (1995, 17). A more significant distinction between replication and multiplication was that the exchanges of *kastam* that are found in mortuary rituals promoted egalitarian relations, whereas the transactions of *bisnis* introduced hierarchical relations. In sum, Foster sees tensions between the two types of reproduction: replication promotes identity and valorization of local society; multiplication fosters the accumulation of wealth in global currencies at the expense of the local community (1995, 18).

A later section of this chapter will examine this process of ensuring a resource base within the household while at the same time engaging in production and commerce within the wider economy. The final section of this chapter then examines the manner in which households in the intensive sample meet or don't meet their health care needs from their perch within the neoliberal economy that is the Congo.

Although anthropologists have often focused their analytical lenses on social reproduction within such a sealed-off realm of culture, they find that today households in modern society encounter a new, more "rapacious capitalism" (Katz 2003), in which ever increasing dimensions of the family and household are commoditized, requiring those who wish to cope with this situation to work ever longer hours just to keep up. The sealed-off domestic realm of the household has been eroded to almost nothing and has itself become a site of speculation and profit. This is true of many households in the Lower Congo.

Another way a dimension of the economic base may be sealed off to support the marginal, sick, or otherwise afflicted is through self-help networks and communities of the afflicted as they bring together knowledge about their condition, a common identity focused on that condition or its resolution, and the ritualized membership procedures that funnel resources into such a distinctive group. Some well-known examples in the Western world include Alcoholics Anonymous, Weight Watchers, sufferers of heart attacks, parents of dyslexic children, and parents of children lost in school shootings.

In Central and Southern Africa, *ngoma* networks and cells are focused around particular self-identified disability groups—women with reproductive troubles, parents of twins, troubled elite merchants fearful of their kinspeople's envy of their wealth, urban immigrants with diffuse troubles. These communities of the commonly afflicted follow a typical format for the identification of their affliction: diagnosis by a diviner, initiatory therapy with a healer-master, counseling and ritual activity while in a novice state, and eventual graduation to healer status or continuing semichronic suffering of the condition. Social reproduction here "refers to the maintenance of a way of life and the commitment of resources to relationships, institutions, and support organizations" (Janzen 1992, 159). Wounded healers emerge from the ranks of the sick to reach out to others similarly wounded. This network model thrives in stateless, segmentary societies in societies with weak states, in social sectors at the periphery of state societies, and in contemporary urban settings. Where states are at the center of addressing affliction, the social reproduction of health obviously takes on a more centralized profile. Professional organizations and craft guilds may also serve the purpose of sealing off a segment of society from global market forces.[4]

In the contemporary setting of globalized postindustrial society, a social reproduction of health perspective needs to look at the infrastructure of health and health care with a keen regard for conditions that create privilege—better care and conditions for some, and worsening circumstances for others. In modern industrial society, access to health care is often shaped by a subject's health insurance. Residents of the United States range widely in this regard, from enjoying extensive coverage to having mediocre coverage, to being entirely without health care support, at the mercy of a merciless marketplace. In most modern industrial nations medical coverage is universal, with some gradations of additional service provided to those who pay privately.

Lower Congo social reproduction of health most resembles the situation for uninsured United States residents, who are at the mercy of their own productive powers within a highly class-divided setting. Lower Congo residents may have limited access to clan treasuries for health crises, or they may be members of rotating credit-sharing networks. But for the most part they find themselves facing a health care situation in which most practices and drugs are commoditized, with prices corresponding to the global market.

Studies of health-seeking behavior on the part of uninsured Americans might thus be helpful in understanding the pressures felt by most Congolese. The wealthy have access to more and better services. In the Lower Congo setting this may mean the ability to hire an ambulance or even an airplane to transport the patient to the best facilities at the best hospital in the capital or to the regional medical center, rather than having to depend on the health zone. At the lower end of the economic scale it may mean that one cannot afford life-preserving surgery. Risk assessment therefore becomes a critical dimension of seeking care.

Studies of the uninsured in the United States have shown that short-term, crisis-related solutions are taken over longer-term and more widespread solutions.[5] In one study it was established that subjects with insurance (that is, with means) tend to opt for biomedical solutions, whereas those without insurance tended toward body image-affecting solutions.[6] In another study of children's health in the United States, those parents with good insurance tended to have access to a "proximal care provider"—that is, someone who was situated within the medical network and who had access to many available resources (Antonelli and Antonelli 2004). Parents of children without health insurance tended to lack knowledge of the system and tended to delay seeking treatment. In the Lower Congo, where no one benefits from such insurance, there may be a corollary to the latter, uninsured group, in the widespread "therapy managing group" provided by most families and clans. This perspective is essentially that adopted by critical medical anthropology, which concerns itself with the corollary of health inequality and health disparity.[7]

These studies suggest a more precise methodology for the study of the social reproduction of health. First, this inquiry must be based on an understanding of the social arrangements and institutions through which health exists and health care is made available, including the scale of such organization. Second, it is important to understand the economic mode—ritual or labor exchange, fee-for-service, centralized provider—by which resources have been generated and have been put through these institutional arrangements. Third, it is important to understand the symbolic capital and the knowledge that has been generated within this social and economic framework, and how the symbolic capital and knowledge are legitimized. Finally, it is necessary to take note of the political energy or will that has been asserted to ensure that a particular program is actually carried out and sustained. Who are individuals or group of individuals who really make a program happen?

NORTH KONGO SOCIAL AND ECONOMIC ORGANIZATION

The basic unit of social organization in Manianga society, as everywhere else, is the household, an arrangement for meeting the most practical human needs: shelter; sleeping; storing food, clothing, and tools; and sometimes food processing. It is therefore also the minimal economic unit in the society. Who resides together in a household may reflect many factors, including kinship or common descent.

But the household need not necessarily consist of individuals who are so related; for example, a group of young adults may share a dwelling. Thus scholars differentiate the residence and these practical activities of the household from the family, which is usually defined as individuals who are related by common descent or by marriage. In this work we are interested in the economics of the household and how it supports the basic social unit, those who live together.

This household or family must be seen also as existing within time—that is, the social time of the cycle of birth, maturation, aging, and death of the individuals constituting it (Fortes 1971, 1–15; Goody 1976). Some societies have households that persist through time, but in Kongo society, much as in Western society, the household comes into being with young adults, expands as children are born and need to be raised, and then reaches a kind of plateau as they grow up and the parents again live by themselves; the household is dissolved upon their death, and usually the physical house is left to disintegrate. Figure 3.1 shows this flow of the household cycle and the resultant range of residential types in the North Manianga village of Kisiasia.

The dynamic life cycle of the Kongo household or family involves the active exchange of goods, gifts, symbols, and bodies to constitute the new household—the socially appropriate, newly created core of society. A household is generally formed by the marriage of a man from one family unit with a woman of another, based on the deep value in Kongo thinking that marriage is a union between individuals of different descent communities, or clans. This deep value accentuates exogamy, thus avoiding the society's understanding of incest, or mating within one's own group. Kongo society is therefore grounded in the fundamental importance of the reproductive potential of a fertile woman, situated within a negotiated relationship between her family and her suitor's family. This negotiation results in establishment of the bride price, which represents payment and gifts from the groom and his family to the bride's father and mother and her mother's lineal relatives. Failure to meet expectations of either side of the agreement results in hard feelings and further complications.

Let us, somewhat arbitrarily, begin our tracking of the lifecycle of the household when a young man decides to seek a young woman in marriage. Although Kongo youth fall in love like youth elsewhere, the elders have a great interest in the protocol of kinship reckoning, establishing the bride price, and the transfer of the goods and payments. Many couples enter into a common-law relationship until the families make the requisite negotiations and transactions of the gifts and payments. In any case, the young woman usually goes to live with the young man at his house. He will have already made the move to an independent household either in his matrilineal village, where he works, or in a city or foreign country. To the extent that the families cooperate, the groom and his elders assemble a substantial bride price of clothing, money, food, drink, and nowadays gadgets

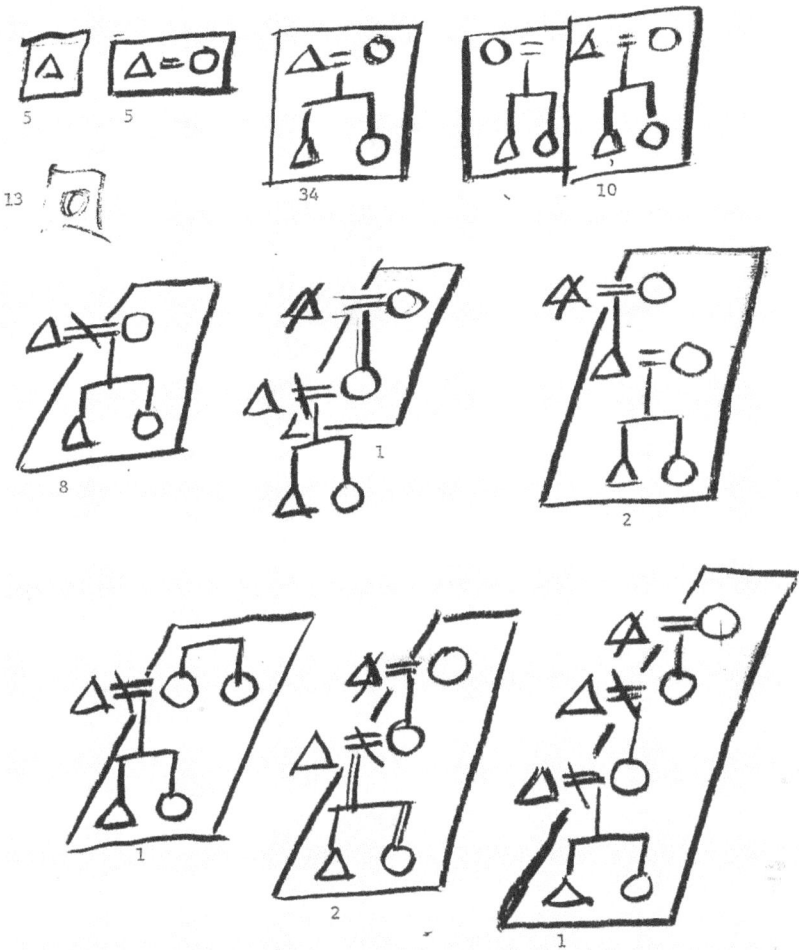

FIGURE 3.1. Kisiasia household residence patterns and frequencies in the Kimbanga clan section, Kivunda sector, Luozi Territory, 1969. These represent: single young adult males having moved from their parents' home to their matrilineal village (numbering 5); single females, mainly widows or divorcees, often of advanced age, living in their matrilineal home or remaining in the community of their late husbands (13); young couples with no children (5); married couples with children (34); polygynous—two or more wives—households with children (10); matrifocal households of divorced women with children (8); and a variety of matrilineal extended households (1, 2, 1, 2, 1). *Source*: Janzen Fieldwork Survey, 1969.

for the bride's parents and grandparents, and particularly the bride's mother and matrilineal aunts.

Social production and reproduction happen within this set of linked units. It is within this linked household or family that biological reproduction occurs, and in which the social and economic support needed is available for women becoming mothers, their new dependent offspring, the dependent elderly, and the sick. Economically a society must be productive enough to be able to cover these nonproductive individuals with the resources assembled by the actively producing adults.

Social science literature and folklore usually describe Kongo society as matrilineal, meaning that individuals are members in their mother's descent community. This is only partially true. Individuals are filiated with—that is, their identity is derived from—their mothers. They may also live in a community some of whose members are descended together from a common maternal ancestor along matrilineal lines. Such communities, if landed, may have good soil for cultivation, streams for irrigation and drinking and bathing water, and a cemetery where the community members are buried when they die. The dominance of female lineal identification in some older and deeper Kongo communities has been explained as a function of the mercantile era's preoccupation from the seventeenth to the nineteenth century with the accumulation of "people wealth" (*bantu mbongo*). Thus, entrepreneurially minded headmen and merchants were intent on breeding as many slaves as possible to further their economic ambitions in the regional economy.[8]

But Kongo society has other kinds of ties that filiate members with their fathers and their fathers' fathers. It is thus helpful to characterize Kongo society as bilateral, meaning that an individual is considered to be descended from both father and mother, plain and simple. Or it may be that an individual carries identity markers—like a name, rights such as access to property or land, or spiritual inheritance—from one or the other. Another possibility is to characterize Kongo society as double unilineal or bilineal, meaning that such inheritance of identity, rights, or other markers occurs along both the male-to-male and female-to-female line. Individuals in Kongo society identify with both parents and gendered lines, and opportunistically use whichever ties seem most advantageous.

The historical—and even present-day—importance of marriage politics cannot be emphasized enough in terms of its impact on the social structure of North Kongo. Matrilateral cross-cousin alliances were used to tie the slave-remnant matrilineages in a community to their masters, thereby solidifying the hierarchical status of descent groups. Alliances between free lineages took on the contrasting form of a series of patrilateral cross-cousin marriages, which created father-child bonds and a community of patrifilial children—the *bana bambuta*—who formed the core of a community's potential for political consolidation.

The Kongo society I witnessed in 2013, as represented in the town of Luozi, its villages, and other urban centers of the Lower Congo, included an array of patterned variations which had their roots in both historical formations and particular identifiable functions. One of the most significant structural features I perceived was a sharp divergence between the landed village and other settlements. This difference was expressed not so much in household or residential features, but in the nature of the ownership of land on which most people depended for their food production. In the landed village communities, like Kisiasia near Kivunda and Sundi Lutete, matrilineal estates held most of the land that was cultivated by members of these communities and their married-in affines. Ownership rested on the matriclan leadership's ability to link contemporary members to their lineal ancestry and the *makulu* cemetery at the center of such a landed estate (map 3.1).

In Luozi, as in cities across the Democratic Republic of the Congo (DRC), a completely different pattern of access to land depends on private ownership and titles registered with a cadastre service administered by civic authorities (map 3.2). Although this system of land tenure and property ownership was introduced by the colonial government, postcolonial aspirant landowners find it very attractive. Many of Luozi's inhabitants have purchased and own title to land parcels within walking or short driving distance from their residences in town. Some of them, such as Tata Luyobisa and Mama Bakima, have one foot in each legal system, private parcels and the use of clan lands.

The common feature of—and the link between—these two forms of property ownership within Kongo (and wider African) jurisprudence is the principle

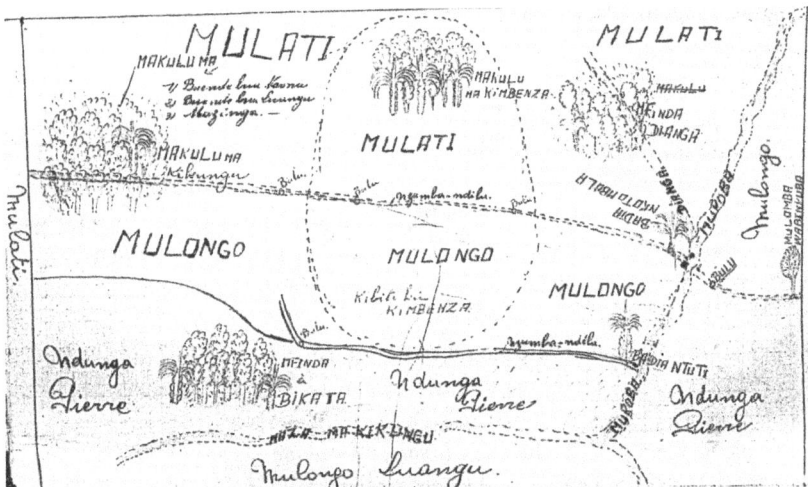

MAP 3.1. Land case map drawing by judges, Kivunda sector court, 1965, identifying hillside names (e.g., Maloti, Mulongo, Ndunga) and clan names (e.g., Buende, Mazinga, Kimbenza) with ancestral cemetery (*makulu*), and ordinary forest groves (*mfinda*). Photo of map by John M. Janzen, 1965. Source: Kivunda Communal Court.

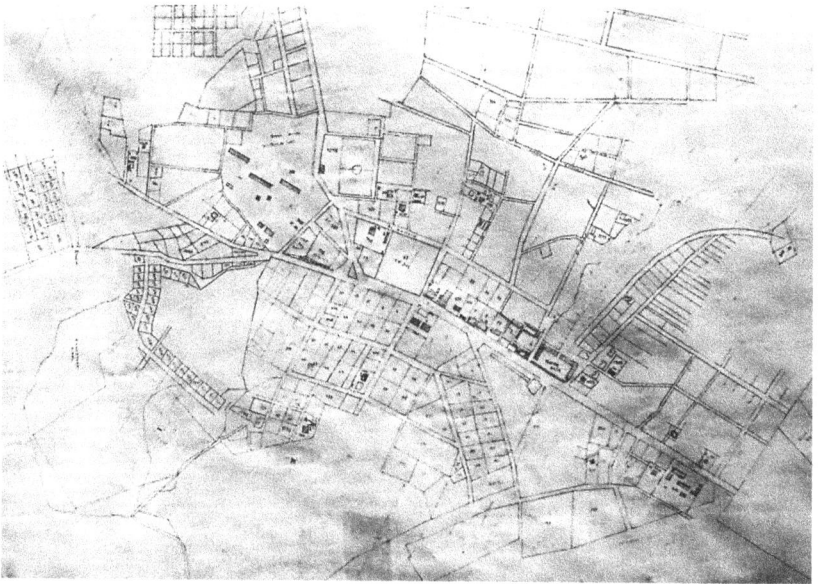

MAP 3.2. Luozi city land registry (cadastre) map; diagonal street across middle is Avenue du Commerce (Kasa-Vubu Ave); clusters of lots indicate development permits. The map dates to the colonial era but continues to be used. The legal codes that make this scheme official are being extended to the seven villages surrounding Luozi as negotiations with land chiefs continue. Photo: John M. Janzen. Source: Original map in Cadaster Office, City of Luozi.

of use-right (usufruct in Latin Western law), whereby land held in perpetuity by a corporate owner may be used by another party for a fee or periodic gift. This principle was implicit when the local landowners of Kilemba agitated against Commander Buffalo of the Congo Free State until he negotiated a deal with them. Similarly, some Luozi citizens who have access to local land have negotiated use-right from the clan land chiefs (*mfumu za nsi*) in the villages surrounding Luozi.[9]

But a further dimension of individual ownership of land in Luozi and other centers has to do with the legal codes that make this the default system once land enters the cadastre records. Individuals like Batangu Mpesa, the founder and CEO of the Centre de Recherche Pharmaceutique de Luozi now has title to the land he acquired from a clan land chief for a nominal gift. Such lands can be sold and title conveyed to further individuals or corporate parties. The longer-term claim of a land chief to such transferred or sold land depends on the political and legal circumstances of each party. Suffice it to say that many enterprising individuals who wish to create a capital fund for themselves, to educate their children, or to pay for medical services try to obtain urban or near-urban land that will appreciate in value over the years.

This is the case with two middle-aged professionals with whom I became acquainted. They had obtained ten hectares and planned to create a banana farm for marketing in the cities of the Kinshasa-Matadi belt. They were intent on getting a bank loan to purchase a used truck in Europe, ship it to the Congo, and within a year begin to have a return on their investment. In my conversations with these men they were keen to learn about life in America, but especially the inner workings of the American family farm: how one dealt with family members and how one reinvested earnings in the business to make it thrive and be lucrative.

Meanwhile, the clan estates like those in Kisiasia, in the north of the Manianga, and those elsewhere in the historic clan land system, were perpetuating the use-right to land by matrilineal clan members and their affines. The Nsundi estate of Kisiasia that I knew best in the 1960s had nearly to a person been replaced by the next generation, except that Nkebi Victor—who, with his wife, Sidoni, had hosted us earlier—had become the clan head. Yes, they said when asked, they had enough land for all the nephews and their families, the widows and divorcees with and without children who had come from elsewhere to their legal home. However, the childless widows were often not so welcome, he said, because they needed to be cared for, and they brought neither the ability to cultivate fields nor the daughters who could bring a good bride price to enhance the treasury.

A further complication for the clan land system, much discussed in 2013 and a headache for clan land chiefs, was the return of former slave remnants to their former masters' estates. Each of the major hamlets of Kisiasia—the Nsundi of Nseke Mwini, the Kimbanga of greater Kisiasia—had experienced this phenomenon. In the case of the Nsundi, the Buende remnant, whose history went back generations and perhaps centuries, had been explained to me in the 1960s as "they are part of us"; "we are together," as two branches of the same estate. Yet in the meantime the Buende had sought to return to their original home, and had found themselves unwelcome. So they returned to Kisiasia and claimed the land that Nkebi's predecessor had "promised them." There was a long history of intermarriage between the Nsundi and Buende, so the latter could claim all kinds of rights. When the Nsundi resisted a straightforward transfer of land to the Buende, the Buende took their former masters to court again. In a judge's ruling in the district court in Luozi, the predecessor clan head's word and the intermarriages prevailed. Today the Buende have their subhamlet down the road a few hundred yards from the main Nsundi hamlet. In greater Kisiasia, the story was the same with the Kikwimba, who occupied an entire wing or ridge of this large village.

This bifurcated legal system—landed matrilineal estates and independently titled parcels, sold or purchased—perpetuates itself at both ends. The clan estate operates like a social security system to ensure rights to land and well-being not only of the lineal descendent men and their wives and children, but especially of the dispossessed and dependent: widows, divorcees, and former slaves who are rejected by their erstwhile fellow clansmen. The urbanized individual property system attracts those who wish to invest in businesses and advance their enterprises and their middle-class families. As long as land is the capital and social security for most people, the production and social reproduction of health will rest on a foundation of households in both property arrangements.

Subsistence and Capitalized Household Production

A grasp of the relationship between subsistence and capitalized production in Manianga households is essential in order to understand the true cost or value of health and health care. The capitalized realms that concern most Maniangans are schooling for their children and health care in time of emergencies. Yet to take only the cash income of a household as the total income is inappropriate, since most households, even urban ones, and those whose earners work as professionals, have one foot in the agricultural sector. They have fields or gardens that they intensively cultivate for their immediate food needs, and from which they sell produce to pay for their capitalized expenditures. The model of an agricultural household economy that follows is based on figures and examples provided by Luyobisa in 2013.

Luyobisa and Bakima work together. In addition to their residential parcel in Luozi, they have a small garden nearby. The main parcel they cultivate is five hectares in Bakima's clan lands at Yalala village, several hours walk west of Luozi. This is in a classic clan estate with an old ancestral forest, *makulu*, of the Mazinga clan. Yalala also includes a second Mazinga clan, as well as the Kindamba, Kinanga, and Buende clans. Luyobisa is Kindamba from farther away, so he does not cultivate in his own clan estate. Luyobisa and Bakima practice shifting cultivation, if possible, but they do not use the traditional *mazala* mound of grass piled and burned before planting. They use commercial fertilizer if they can acquire it. Luyobisa estimates that the two of them spend five days a week in the fields, seven to seventeen hours each day—thus up to 85 hours per week, for a total of 4,420 hours per year or 884 hours per hectare.

Their main crops are groundnuts, manioc, and beans, although they also have gourds, peppers, tomatoes, cabbage, *nsafu* fruit, and other fruits and vegetables. They raise small livestock such as goats and have beehives for the production of honey. They also have orange trees that are not yet bearing. The first three crops produce a significant surplus, which provides them with cash to cover especially medical costs and the school fees of their teenage children. Groundnuts and beans can be cultivated for two crops per year, but that requires a lot of hard work of tilling, cultivating, weeding, and harvesting. The agricultural year runs from March through February, with field preparation, planting, cultivating, and harvest (table 3.1).

TABLE 3.1. Annual climate and agricultural cycle in Manianga, Luozi region, by seasons

	March	April	May	June	July	Aug.	Sept.	Oct.	Nov.	Dec.	Jan.	Feb.
	rainy	rainy	rainy	drier	dry	dry	dry	rainy	rainy	rainy	rainy	dry
	hot	hot	hot	cool	cool	cool	cool	warm	warm	warm	hot	hot
	Ndolo			*Sivu*			*Luangu*			*Mwangu*		
	time of plenty—nsafu, groundnuts			winter, cold, hazy			time to burn mounds			time of hunger		
Groundnuts, cycle 1												
	prepare field	plant w. manioc & gourds, weed	cultivate & weed	harvest								
Groundnuts, cycle 2												
							prepare field	plant w. manioc & gourds		weed	harvest	
Beans, cycle 1												
	prepare field	plant	cultivate & weed			harvest						
Beans, cycle 2—must be new soil												
							prepare field	plant	cultivate & weed			harvest
Manioc—single annual cycle												
	prepare field	plant stalks	cultivate & weed						begin harvest if desperate for food			normal harvest

new varieties produce tubers in 6 months if leaves are not taken; growers are returning to old varieties that require up to 18 months, produce tubers even if leaves are harvested earlier

SOURCE: Tata Luyobisa and Mama Bakima; Janzen fieldwork.

Luyobisa and Bakima are a good example of the professional-aspiring couple who have had to return to their agrarian base to make a living for themselves and their six children, all of whom also aspire to professional status. Luyobisa grew up in a home where the head of the household, his father, was an uneducated polygynist villager and non-Christian until just before his death. Luyobisa, however, attended both Catholic and Protestant schools in North Manianga. He had an aptitude for learning and a gift for pastoral counseling. Early on he came under the influence of the prophets of the Church of the Holy Spirit in Africa (DMNA) and its spiritual head, Mangitukwa Luc. However, the Protestant elders encouraged him to attend seminary. So he pursued both with the awareness of both. He was in seminary during the school year and with the prophets in vacation. He was already married at this time, so Bakima was with him at seminary and benefited from the acquaintance of a wider circle of people. She has held major positions in women's organizations.

After seminary graduation, Luyobisa and Bakima served the prophet church in the major urban centers of Kinshasa, Kimpese, Matadi, and Boma. It was in these cities that they raised their family of six children, who today are in their teens and twenties. Two boys are off in university—studying medicine and computer science—and the others are still at home. A grown daughter, married with two children, is temporarily at home while her husband, a chauffeur-mechanic-pharmacist, finds a niche in Kinshasa or elsewhere.

During their postseminary urban life, Luyobisa and Bakima were at least partially supported by the DMNA church, which had several prominent businesspeople and wealthy merchants as members. Two had fleets of transport trucks that regularly brought agricultural produce from the Manianga to Kinshasa and the cities of the Lower Congo. Another was a nurse who had branched out into the lucrative automotive parts business in Kinshasa. When all three of these wealthy underwriters of the DMNA church died during the financial crisis and civil war in the DRC in the 1990s, this support withered. Luyobisa and Bakima decided to return to Luozi to establish themselves within working reach of their clan lands. He shifted his church and pastoral duties to the Luozi congregation, and they found a house to rent. Later they bought a lot on which they built their own house. They purchased a garden plot nearby and arranged to cultivate five hectares on Bakima's clan land west of Luozi. This is the situation I found them in and which they agreed to share with me. Table 3.2 presents the relationship between capitalized cash cropping and noncapitalized subsistence agriculture and consumption. Both sectors of household production are important to the family: they need food they can grow themselves, and they need cash for the increasingly commoditized economy around them, including especially school fees for their children and payments for medical emergencies.

TABLE 3.2. Household and commercial allocation of produce, 2011–2012

Item	production	yield	domestic use	surplus	Market costs	Net cash income
Groundnuts, 2 harvests	Seed, own & hired labor	15 sacks or 1,650 verres	3 sacks or 330 verres	12 sacks, 1,320 verres	Carry to local market Luozi	99K FC $120.
Manioc	Stalks, labor	58 sacks *fufu*	8 sacks	50 sacks	Ship to Mbanza Ngungu 235K FC	705K FC $849.
Beans	Seed, labor	1,500 verres	300	1,000 verres minus seed	Carry to local market Luozi	300K FC $361
Honey, goats, vegetables, fruits	labor				Luozi market and direct sales	290K FC $350
Total surplus earnings in Congolese francs (FC) and US dollars for household for year						1.538K FC $1,680

SOURCE: Tata Luyobisa and Mama Bakima; Janzen fieldwork.

The cost accounting that is represented here has existed in the Manianga since at least the seventeenth century, when producers of foodstuffs, textiles, metals, and slaves needed to figure out how to relate to the markets like Manianga and Mpumbu, and ultimately to the European factories on the coast. Conversion rates were regularly calculated and used by everyone in a trading or ritual exchange network.[10] Luyobisa and Bakima, however, were not in the practice of sharply calculating the currency worth of their household consumption. The first time we discussed this project and my interest in a total cost accounting of their household, I was given only the cash cropping and monetized portion on a neatly columned sheet of paper.

When I asked for the subsistence portion and amounts, Luyobisa was able to give approximate figures in the measures he used, the *verre* ("glass") and the sack, rather than kilograms, and Congolese francs and US dollars. He estimated that domestic consumption of groundnuts, manioc, and beans was about a fourth of the total production. Then he kept remembering additional foods the family had produced for consumption—tomatoes, peppers, *nsafu* fruit, and so on—and that they also had beehives and sold honey, and oh yes, they had raised some goats that they had sold, and there were fruit trees—like oranges—that would soon provide a good cash crop. Their energy in cultivation, their joy at harvests, and their excitement over their children's careers was palpable, no doubt contributing to their success at the back-to-the-land life they were leading. The outside observer and reader of this account should not romanticize this situation unduly. It is clearly an adaptive response, a coping strategy, for dealing with the collapsed state and the neoliberal economy that prevails.

The pivot between subsistence household production and selling for the commodity market is an important issue in social reproduction theory and ethnography. Producers' ability to manage this divide to their own advantage is critical for keeping their control over their affairs and their fate. Their ability to control this boundary determines whether and to what extent they have sealed off a sector of their household economy (Foster 1995) from the dictates of the neoliberal market that would commoditize and extract every last bit of value. Luyobisa tacitly recognized the dangers of overdrawing credit from the household when he noted, without my soliciting the comment, that "if you are desperate for food," you can begin to harvest manioc tubers as early as November instead of January, but you will sacrifice the size and quantity of your ultimate harvest. This echoes the "time of famine" and the balance between food and productivity that Audrey Richards observed half a century ago in Zambia (Richards 2004).

Demonstrating the facile mental calculations that many Congolese make these days, Luyobisa explained his marketing decisions for the season. They had sold six sacks of groundnuts in Luozi, where there was a ready demand, thereby avoiding marketing and transport overhead. Manioc, on the other hand, had been ground into flour (*fufu*), and fifty sacks of the fifty-eight produced had been shipped to an urban market at Mbanza Ngungu, where the demand is great. The markup was significant, but the transportation fee of 235,000 Congolese francs (CF), or $280, had been very costly. They sold beans locally, avoiding further overhead expenses. These three commodity sales had yielded $1,330, just enough to cover the costs for the children's school fees of $1,250 and medical fees of $50, leaving just $30 "in the *caisse*." There was some wiggle room in Luyobisa's calculations. Normally he could have counted on two groundnut harvests, thus doubling that income source. He could have also, with labor invested in opening a new field, doubled the bean harvest, although that would have required more hired labor. His calculations allowed for some slack in that not all commodities produced were either consumed or sold; there was a reserve, but he couldn't cut into the seed base for the following year's planting. Farming is always a risky business and one must therefore plan for the unforeseen exigency.

A big risk factor in their household calculations was health care costs. During the year they were fortunate to avoid some of the big-ticket items that other families have faced—appendicitis (75,000 CF), extended hospitalization with grippe or malaria with convulsions (30,000 CF), or even just several malaria treatments (at 2,500–5,000 CF). Rather, they had only one episode in the family that required payment, their eldest son's dental work in Kinshasa (12,000 CF), and two other episodes that were handled by prophetic healing, including a sore arm. But one can quickly see the hit a household budget might take if there were widespread malaria that needed cures and vitamins for recovery, several surgeries, or a complicated birth.

The commoditization of everything in the DRC and the absence of insurance and other publicly funded social services means that one is totally at the mercy of the resources and support that the household, wider family, and clan may offer. Luyobisa suggested that the clan network might be able to cover 25 percent of the cost of a major medical episode. In cities the regional associations also sometimes step in, but they tend to operate mainly as burial mutuals that come to the aid of families who seek to honor and bury a loved one on a moment's notice.

PATTERNS OF CONSULTATION AND THE COST OF HEALTH CARE

We have seen which principal diseases individuals are likely to encounter and the intensive sample listing of types of illness episodes and their frequency (tables 2.3 and 2.4). The intensive sample reveals a pattern of consultation confirming that there is a fan of medical resources that range from home care with traditional medicines, to home treatment with pharmacy-purchased medications, to consultations with healers, to visits to primary health care centers, to visits to hospitals in the health zone system, and finally to elite private care that usually requires travel to the capital, Kinshasa. Which of these options, or combination of options, is selected depends on the individual or family's perception of the case's severity, held against the household's means.

Although the health zones and the medical departments that coordinate the health care institutions have established rates for various types of treatments and medications, each case is unique and may require a different combination of care, institutionalization, and medication. An overview of episodes of malaria provides one glimpse into the structure of care and cost. Home care for malaria fever and chills with a drink of the lata plant may be entirely gratis. But if the cycles of fever and chills, diarrhea and weakness persist, a visit to a health center or hospital is warranted. A round that includes a lab test of blood, a brief consultation, and a cure will cost between 15,000–35,000 CF, or $13–28. This was the routine Reinhild received at the Catholic Hospital in Luozi. It cost 15,000 CF and even included a consultation with the doctor Rose Ndoda Kumbu.[11]

The cost and complexity of a malaria treatment increases if the patient has experienced anemia, which is common in children, and a course of vitamin A needs to be added to the treatment, or a blood transfusion for severe anemia. These added treatments involve hospitalization, which may last several days. The top cost for a full malaria regimen will approximate 70,000 CF ($65). A household or family whose members all experience one or two rounds of malarial infection in the course of a given year can expect to pay several hundreds of thousands of Congolese francs (or hundreds of US dollars). Seasonal influenza infections with complications and respiratory infections, especially those resulting in pneumonia, were generally as costly as the more serious malaria treatments.

Many households also experienced one or several big-ticket medical expenses in the year. These included surgeries like appendicitis, hernia, ovarian cyst removal, tubal ligation, and childbirth, which each cost approximately 130–150,000 CF ($120–134). The first two items seemed to affect cultivators more than others. It was explained to me that the hard physical work required of these people resulted in ruptures. Ovarian cysts were common in elderly women and were removed because of the women's susceptibility to cancer. A household or family that needed to deal with at least one round of malaria medication per individual and also pay for a major surgery would clearly exhaust its available resources or become unable to pay for the procedures.

Although we do not have a precise and systematic accounting of the financial burden of health care in the households of our intensive sample, in relation to their income as seen in the single case study in this chapter, it is apparent that many households were pressed to their limits in covering medical costs. The medical department of the Protestant church published an average household income figure for the Manianga of $1/person/day, or $720/household/year (Communauté Evangélique du Congo 2012). The above typical scenario of each member of a family experiencing one round of malaria or flu or respiratory infection per year, would easily cost half of the average income, as estimated by the medical department.

Health care costs of the society's elite present a somewhat different picture. This is most visible in our intensive sample households of top administrators, executives, and merchants. These households report not fewer, but more diseases: the conventional ones, as well as diseases that do not appear in the other cases. Here we encounter mention of hypertension ("too much blood," or simply "tension"), diabetes (although no cases were actually reported), along with the conventional diseases of malaria, flu, and so on. Among the elite of the Manianga there is a clear awareness of the rise in their circles of what have been called diseases of civilization. Here is a pattern of lengthier hospitalizations and of traveling to the city to consult private clinics or top physicians and medical specialists, at far more expensive prices. A further pattern seen in these elite households is the continued support of adult children in their twenties and thirties. The total reported outlay for the most recent annual medical expenses in one such household in Luozi was $2,766.

The production and reproduction of health is also evident in preventive measures. All households confirmed that they used medicated mosquito nets and washed their hands with soap after visiting the toilet. Fully a third of the households were explicit in their mention of sweeping the yard daily to ward off flies, mosquitoes, and other insects. But there was only one household of the 105 in our intensive sample that had no illness episodes whatsoever to report for the previous year. I noted that they had an expansive, cleanly swept yard, curtains over the windows, and well-constructed kitchen and outdoor toilet buildings that matched the house in baked-earth brick construction with metal roofs. Public health and medical authorities should encourage all preventive measures possible, because they measurably minimize financial costs for households with limited means.

Among the few diseases for which the health zone, the state, or NGOs like the World Health Organization may cover costs of care are HIV/AIDS, trypanosomiasis (sleeping sickness), and polio. These are considered dangerous diseases on the national or global front, or diseases that have a public perception of being horrific. It is ironic that malaria, the far most debilitating disease to most inhabitants of Western Central Africa, and costly in numbers of lives lost and work energy sacrificed, is not in any way covered by public funds. Nor is the second most debilitating disease, schistosomiasis—bilharzia—addressed by public funds. These diseases are so common that they are regarded as normal, or invisible. They are neither stigmatizing, like HIV/AIDS, nor highly contagious.

CONCLUSION

The social reproduction of health allows us to see the contribution of society's institutions to the well-being or illness of individuals in a community. The concept has been applied here to the main domestic unit of Kongo society, the household, and to the more inclusive kin institutions that organize households over time and across generations. Households in Kongo society, as everywhere, are the main channels of resource flows as food, material goods, cash, favors, and labor are exchanged within and between them. This flow is the life blood of the society. It is also the means by which the health of individuals is ensured however health is defined.

The sealing off of the domestic realm from the wider economy is an important dimension of the means to health and health care in the Lower Congo. This was as true during the mercantile period as it is today in the neoliberal economy that is the Congo. When everything is commercialized and commoditized, there needs to be careful cost accounting of the means to preserve the household—food, housing, clothing, and other essentials—as well as some sort of income to afford those essentials that cost cash: education, health care. Both in the theoretical literature and in the case study of Luyobisa and Bakima's household, the dividing line between subsistence for survival and capitalization for commoditized needs becomes noteworthy.

The case study reveals a family and household that works very hard and is reasonably successful in covering all their bases, at least in the year 2013, when Luyobisa and Bakima agreed to contribute to this anthropologist's data. Yet all around them were illustrations of households that did not make ends meet, because of crop failure or job loss or unanticipated health crises.

4

Public Health and Health Care Institutions, Reconfigured

Our land does not do well at helping people live. It is difficult to pay hospital costs and fees to get children through school.

—Peasant couple (intensive sample interview, 2013)

The health zone system . . . is possibly the only system in the country still recognizable as a nation-wide quasi-state structure. And even with critically little or no support, it commands allegiance and support from health workers, despite years of war and turbulence that have had a catastrophic effect on health care in Congo.

—World Health Organization, "WHO/UNICEF Joint Mission, DR Congo (18–29 Jun 2001)"

The visible daily signs of the unique constellation of public health and health care institutions, agencies, and networks in Luozi were the vehicles that regularly drove around town. There was the van of the Département des Oeuvres Médicales (DOM) returning late in the afternoons from inspection and supply trips to outlying health centers and health posts. The public health *animateur* and a colleague could be seen riding on their Chinese motorcycle out to distant villages and health posts, or returning after a campaign or data-gathering trip. There was a flatbed truck hauling a huge load of firewood, roaring through town with several "boy-chauffeurs" atop it. This firewood was used not to cook the evening meal but to heat the large vat at the Centre de Recherche Pharmaceutique de Luozi that processed the artemisia leaves harvested from a nearby plantation. There was the station wagon that several times per week brought a big canister of artemisia concentrate to the river beach ferry for shipment to Kinshasa, where it would be transformed into antimalaria pills for both cure and prophylaxis. Finally, there was an ambulance that occasionally brought patients to the Catholic hospital or to Luozi General

Hospital, although most patients came on foot, by bicycle, or on some kind of stretcher. The fact that this infrastructure had vehicles at all, and fuel to run them, while so many people moved around by walking or hitching rides indicated the relative support it received.

This chapter features the reconfigured public health and health care institutions as I found them in the second decade of the twenty-first century, following the 1990s collapse of the Congolese state. At the outset of this work I characterized this reconfiguration as a phoenix rising from the ashes. Here I explain just what a reconfigured or risen-from-the-ashes institution might look like in relation to its previous manifestation.

For illustrative purposes, let us consider the colonial or early postcolonial medical mission entities that were often operated within the framework of churches and headed by expatriate specialists. These were nationalized under Mobutu and integrated into a national structure within a multitiered hierarchy under the Ministry of Health. When that state-centric hierarchy crumbled in the late 1980s and early 1990s and the health zone became the centerpiece of the new configuration, the ecclesiastical medical institutions that emerged were now completely staffed by nationals, without the international financial support that the missions had enjoyed. Also, the decline in state influence in the coordination of public health and health care created a power vacuum that was not immediately replaced by anything else. The increasing emphasis on the health zone as the regional entity around which all public health and health care would be organized meant that new administrative boundaries and networks were drawn that did not correspond to the preexisting governmental or ecclesiastical entities. Thus the phoenix was a different color and different shape from its predecessor; it still resembled a bird, and it could sort of fly. That is, it was focused on health and health care.

The Social Reproduction of Health in a Neoliberal World

The post-1960 postcolonial transformations to public health and health care in the Democratic Republic of Congo and the Manianga may be seen in roughly four historical phases. First, from the late colonial era until a few years into the Mobutu era that began in 1965, the foreign missions—that is, the churches—and the state shared responsibility for both public health and health care. Protestant missions continued to cover their regions, the Catholics theirs, and the state the major cities and the gaps between. Second, beginning at independence in 1960, and with greater intensity with Mobutu's military coup in 1965, government policies and actions of the single political party, Le Mouvement Populaire de la Revolution, moved the country, renamed Zaire, toward nationalization of all major institutions, including public health and health care. Expatriates remained in some prominent positions, but increasingly Congolese nationals replaced them as they completed their professional training. The national university flourished, with campuses in Kinshasa, Lubumbashi, and Kisangani, and complementary faculties and research institutes in these centers. The postal service continued to function, domestically and internationally, producing brilliant stamps for collectors. Roadways were improved and expanded. A national airline moved people between major cities. This phase lasted into the 1970s, corresponding to a time of relatively good copper prices and sufficient funds to develop infrastructure and maintain centralized state agencies and services.

The third phase—the time of economic crisis and shrinking national means—began in the 1980s. Copper prices plunged, inflation soared, and national institutions began to wither. The postal service stopped functioning in all but some urban centers; there was no replacement. The national university collapsed, to be replaced by dozens of private universities with disparate funding sources and varied standards. The Free University of Luozi, an outgrowth of the Centre de Vulgarisation Agricole, was an example of this trend. Remaining businesses owned by expatriates were confiscated by the government or simply closed. A major palm oil refinery north of Luozi experienced just such a demise, with disastrous economic consequences for the region. The crisis deepened. The Kinshasa riots in 1991 expressed the growing frustration of many citizens, the depth of which was evident when the army joined the looting. The pillaging of the Ministry of Health and the abdication of its officials was the death knell of centralized medical and public health administration.

The fourth phase in the reconfiguration of institutions began well before the 1991 riots and the collapse of government functions. This phase was characterized by neoliberal globalization and the search for viable institutional remnants that would serve the purpose of managing public health and health care. The global market replaced the Congolese economy. The US dollar became the de facto currency, alongside a rapidly inflating Zaire. Those millions who did not have their fingers in the flow of dollars or other international currencies were driven into destitution. Many educated Congolese professionals emigrated. In the Manianga—the Territory of Luozi—this fourth phase represented a deep crisis, as it did everywhere. Budgets were slashed, infrastructure deteriorated, and personnel disappeared or continued their professional work while earning a living in subsistence cultivation or petty commerce. Privatization was the order of the day. Fee-for-service financing and local taxation replaced the now all but invisible national budget. Most major NGO donors abandoned the Congo, at least for a time.

Looking at the progression of these four phases, one can see the institutions that persisted and those that came to the fore and in some way carried public health and health care forward. My list of such institutions, as I encountered them in 2013, is more inclusive than what most public health and health care analysts would offer. It is an anthropologist's overview that incorporates the entire range of efforts at maintaining life, addressing disease, and producing and reproducing health. It includes, most locally of all, the villages and clan communities of the landed estates, each with at least one land chief, *mfumu nsi* (plural, *mfumu za nsi*), in charge of the most precious resource of all, cultivable land; as well as local governments like the villages and sectors, extratraditional jurisdictions like the town of Luozi, and, in larger cities, the communes and to some extent the territorial administrations. It also includes the health zone system, implemented in the 1980s according to models developed by public health planners, and jump-started to new significance by the Congolese Protestant Council's Santé Rurale du Congo (SANRU) program, which began to create and administer public health zones across the country. This program was given a big boost in 1985 by the World Health Organization's primary health initiative, with which it dovetailed. The health zone structure was progressively adopted from 1992 on as the framework for the new public health system.

Also on my list are Catholic and Protestant health services that replaced or paralleled the Ministry of Health as a central coordinating body for hospitals, clinics, and health posts; parastatal organizations such as Régie des Eaux (REGIDESO), the waterworks seen in towns and cities, which are now being privatized; and the shifting coalition of the region's power brokers that coalesced around particular projects, such as the ferry across the Congo River at Luozi and the creation of the town's waterworks. Also included are NGOs: Congolese NGOs, like the numerous educational institutions and development organizations that brought into being institutions of higher learning to educate students in the sciences and liberal arts; and international NGOs that care for special health conditions, in particular the World Health Organization (WHO) and its various agencies and focused campaigns, as well as NGOs that focus on HIV/AIDS and the regional medical teams that deal with disease outbreaks. The private sector also makes the list: businesses such as pharmacies that both produce medications and import drugs that they sell to the public; and prophet-healers and herbalists who provide a broad-based popular service that is trusted but is also pricey, including plant-based medicines, divination of the causes of misfortune, and protection from spiritual and temporal aggression. Finally, what remains of the shadow government provides a nominal coordination of services, some legal cover for professionals, and occasionally funding for special projects, amounting to less than 1 percent of all health care expenditures.

The question now is, in our research on public health and health care in the Lower Congo, how do we understand these hybrid structures that assumed the vestigial functions of the state? What is their relationship to each other?

LOCAL GOVERNMENT AND HEALTH

As an anthropologist interested in the societal forces that shape a range of important services—conflict resolution, local schools, rudimentary public health and health care, roads, and so on—I have noted the pivotal role of local administrators, such as chiefs and mayors, in jurisdictions that have been variously called *chefferies, groupements, collectivités*, communes, or sectors. The officeholders of these jurisdictions have the paradoxical status of being representative of local populations, often elected by popular ballot, while at the same time being the lowest officials in a bureaucratic hierarchy and thus expected to speak for and act on behalf of higher authorities. They are often chosen in elections or directly appointed in crises because of their success in some other, previous role or career that gives them a reputation for wisdom, wider understanding, and some degree of connectedness with the world beyond. Several of the more effective mayors I met had been teachers. In office, they were expected to be all things to all people; they were in charge of ensuring public order, good health, fiscal prosperity, and the availability of varied services. But where and when did these local governmental institutions originate?

Urban and rural communes represented the final stage of local government reforms at the end of Belgian colonial rule in the late 1950s (Brausch 1961, 43). The Pax Belgica had adjusted existing local and regional political institutions into a uniform model of the *chefferie*, on the assumption that all African societies had—or should have—chiefs, and that the customary institutions of authority could be rationalized or civilized and brought under the mantle of colonial government (Sohier 1954). In most regions the final colonial local units were consolidated into sectors, zones, and territories; elsewhere kingdoms or regions were recognized and incorporated into colonial government (as in Rwanda, or Katanga, or in the Kuba kingdom of the Kasai). But by 1957, under the inspiration of former Minister of Colonies Louis Franck, the urban communes and rural sectors were given fuller autonomy and made into modern administrative units complete with a secretariat, a treasury, a court and police force, road maintenance services, an agricultural staff, primary schools, one or more dispensaries (sometimes even a maternity ward, a social center, and a farm settlement scheme. These units had their own budget, their own taxes, and a degree of self-government.

This framework of local government experienced remarkable staying power in the postcolonial context. Wherever I traveled in the former Belgian colonial empire during the postcolonial period from the 1960s to 2013—the Lower Congo, Eastern Congo, Rwanda, and Burundi—the local commune or sector continued to display most functions on my list. Health-related features included pit latrines and pit refuse dumps in all village and commercial centers. Drinking water sources—springs in the gentle valleys lined with palm and other fruit trees—were cemented in to protect them from contamination. Primary and secondary schools were available in all the areas, as were medical centers and sometimes hospitals. Markets were regularly inspected and taxed. The public health infrastructure of Belgian colonialism dovetailed nicely with the primary health campaign of the 1980s, which featured the hierarchical network of local health clinics, health centers, and a referral hospital in each health zone.

Even though people resented the paternalistic nature of Belgian colonial government, and for a time after independence local government was boycotted, many of the structures and services of local colonial government became the backbone of postcolonial local government. Despite the autocratic tone of the Mobutu-era national government, local democratic traditions prevailed, giving citizens strong ownership in local government.

Later, from the mid-1990s on, major health disasters and horror stories of epidemic outbreaks (such as the Ebola crisis in Kikwit and the cholera outbreaks in the eastern Congo) were accompanied, even caused by, political upheavals, massive population displacement during wars, and the squalor of life in emergency shelters and refugee camps. These situations usually demonstrated that the local administration had been overwhelmed by forces it was hardly designed to deal with. Yet the mayors with whom I spoke often recognized that the embryonic sources of the bigger crises were in day-to-day conditions in their communities.

Local Government and Public Services

Although elections sponsored by the Kongo party ABAKO in May 1960, a month before independence, effectively terminated what one person called "a thousand years of Belgian colonization," the machinery of government available to the new regime was largely that which had been formulated by the Belgian colonial presence, itself a makeover of precolonial western Bantu governing traditions. But now, because the mayors or chiefs were democratically elected after independence, they had increased authority. On the other hand, local government struggled with higher government and bureaucracy over which policies were permissible for the enhancement of local life and infrastructure, and above all over control of taxation and tax revenues.

Because they were popular, sector chiefs became more powerful figures than their colonial-era predecessors had been. Their office and their person became the point of contact with national and provincial government for the local people. They presided over the court (at least until 1964), heard palavers, acted as chair of the council meetings, and occasionally toured their constituent areas on foot. Mbuta Yoswa Kusikila kwa Kilombo was the new chief in Kivunda. He was re-elected in 1965 and again in 1968, and he served until 1972, leaving a strong legacy of good governance. His popularity and status took on overtones of mystical qualification that began to circulate in his regard. A teacher by training and not prone to self-adulation, he nevertheless recalled incidents to me in which he had been considered a healer (*ngunza*) for effective arbitration of disputes. Others confided to me that he probably possessed the positive witchcraft powers (*kundu*) of certain historic chiefs. His mother told me that she had dreamed prior to his birth that he would become a great leader. He told me in 2013 that when he reluctantly agreed, against his better judgment, to be renominated for office, the people celebrated his acceptance with gun salvos and dancing. His even-tempered good judgment was greatly appreciated. I revisit his rule in chapter 6 and elaborate on his philosophy of governance.

The second development in postcolonial local government had to do with the vertical relationship with higher governmental bureaucracy. Whereas at first local chiefs and their councils had been free to propose projects and programs, later on, with the advent of Mobutu's Revolutionary Popular Movement a much stronger, autocratic government emerged. This squelched local initiatives for infrastructure improvements. Road projects and educational and health facilities were often proposed but then vetoed.

The issues of taxation and allocation of revenue were at the heart of the tension between the commune or sector and the higher levels of government. Nearly 60 percent of sector tax income was forwarded to the provincial and central government. In theory financially autonomous, the sector was supposedly free to levy any tax it saw fit, subject to approval by higher-level jurisdictions. In 1962 the Kivunda sector conceived a plan to install a gas pump for the benefit of merchants and as a source of tax revenue. The territorial government denied this proposal on the grounds that "government should not engage in commerce." Failing this, the sector in 1963 quietly levied a supplementary 80 francs per person (then $1.60) to the head tax to pay for road repairs, which brought in an additional revenue of 69,000 francs that year ($34,500 at the time). The local council agreed that the tax could become permanent and the sector could keep the roads fit without imposing public work on everyone. However, the territorial office ruled this tax illegal after the fact and ordered the sector to refund it person by person, which it did not do, arguing instead that residents could simply reduce the next year's taxes by that amount. Simultaneously the sector received orders to increase the conventional head tax for the following year.

In the face of these persistent impediments to problem solving through local government, the less courageous sectors gradually became the passive lowest instance of an increasingly repressive central government, while those with more resilient personnel came to believe, as one sector chief put it bluntly, "The authorities are crazy! You think up a conceivable tax and it is illegal. Yet nothing ever comes from above by way of improvements. How are we to improve the local condition at all?"[1]

Electoral Politics, Sorcery, and
Military Intervention by a Fragile State

After independence local government had rising responsibility for conflict resolution. I offer two examples of such conflicts to show the place of the local officials in either resolving them or being overcome by them.[2] A third factor in postcolonial sector change was the growing politicization of relations between various regional, professional, and status groups, and, above all, political parties at the time of national elections. The mayors or sector chiefs usually had a strong hand in arbitrating disputes, whether through their official courts or informally in the traditional manner of the big *lukutukunu* circle.

Mbuta Kusikila, the postcolonial mayor of Kivunda, ran for reelection in 1965. His main opponent was a candidate from a predominately Catholic district. When the ballots were counted and Kusikila was announced the winner, his competitor lodged a complaint of electoral fraud with the election commission. As incumbent mayor, Kusikila called a traditional large, circular *lukutukunu* conference into session near the communal offices. He and his opponent each hired advocates (*nzonzi*). The *nzonzi* introduced the affair. The communal council, also elected, steered the process forward. In a further round of conversations, through his *nzonzi*, Kusikila threatened to withdraw his name if the accuser refused to accept the ballot results. After several more rounds of claim and counterclaim, the public reiterated support for the original ballot count, thereby legitimizing Kusikila as the winner. The accuser withdrew his complaint and accepted a small fine. This procedure showed the genius of traditional Kongo court procedures and their efficacy in modern political dispute resolution.

A second conflict emerged in the 1990s to 2000s and still simmered in early 2013. It was also election related, climaxing in the run-up to the local and national elections of 2010. This conflict illustrates local government being overwhelmed by fractious forces beyond its control. This conflict pitted the existing local, regional, and national governments against the ethnic-nationalist party Bundu dia Kongo ("Church of Kongo" or "Kongo Union"; BDK), led by Muanda Nsemi. Unlike the other regional parties that were backed by Uganda and Rwanda, controlled the northern and eastern regions of the Democratic Republic of the Congo (DRC), and by 2007 had a stake in the provisional interim government, Nsemi's movement had no army and no backing from another country. But his platform was radical, seductive, and destabilizing. He argued that the BaKongo, the descendants of a famous historic kingdom, inhabitants of prime northwestern regions of Angola, the western DRC, and southwestern Republic of the Congo (Congo-Brazzaville), were being marginalized in their own land.

The centerpiece of Nsemi's campaign was the promise to take the Kongo region out of Angola, the DRC, and the Republic of the Congo to form a new independent nation-state. At the heart of this new state would be the energy-industry crown jewel, the Inga Hydroelectric Power Station on the Congo river between Matadi and Luozi. Nsemi's base as the self-appointed leader of the movement was among the less well educated, disaffected youth and adults. His version of cultural nationalism stressed a rejection of Christianity and a return to the customs of the forefathers. This struck some as an extremist pipe dream, but many others found it compelling. His promise of economic prosperity through control of the region's and subcontinent's electricity, so close geographically to the people, had obvious appeal, especially in light of their total lack of electricity from a source so close, just across the river from the Manianga. Nsemi eventually won the parliamentary seat that included the Manianga, and his followers were energized by events in 2007, when they took things into their own hands, in part by playing fast and loose with sorcery accusations. The Luozi territorial administrator began his 2008 annual report on security: "It was toward the end of the year 2007 that the bitter taste of demands by the BDK began, timidly at first, then reaching a climax the 24th and 25th of February 2008, dates on which two persons were burned alive."[3]

Here I offer a summary of the report:

On February 24 Jean-Marie Lusende, a seventy-year-old married man and father of several children, was accused by an *nganga ngombo* (diviner) of being a sorcerer. He was burned alive at the public square at the headquarters of the Kinkenge sector, right beside the sector administrative building, facing the official residence of the sector chief. On February 25, Nestor Mansanga, alias Tshamala, an eighty-year-old, was similarly accused of being a sorcerer, and was burned alive in the village of Betelani, sector of Mbanza Ngoyo, twelve kilometers from the territorial capital. These were only two of the actions committed by the movement, others of which also led to the loss of human life and the physical damage of property in the population.

For these reasons, on February 28, 2008, Operation Restoration of State Authority was launched in Luozi Territory, formerly the bastion of the BDK. Since then, calm, order, and tranquility reign. The territorial agent traveled the length and breadth of the territory during the course of the year to make the population aware (*conscientisé*) of the need to conserve the peace and to restore calm following the restoration of state authority across the totality of the territory. The population was called on to accept the former members of the BDK and to restore them to their villages after their time in flight in the bush or elsewhere. Everywhere in the ten sectors we have awakened the conscience of the population so they will no longer be tricked as in the past by those who go fishing in troubled waters. According to the administrative letter and the ministerial decree,[4] the BDK movement is outlawed across the entire Democratic Republic of the Congo. As a consequence, its political party has ceased to exist this year. The movement's founder and leader, Nsemi, denies any role in the violence against Manianga civilians in 2008.

The local police, the national police, the Rapid Intervention Police and the Unité de Police Integritée undertook this action at the request of the territorial offices on orders of the provincial and national government. They came to reinforce the commissariat of Luozi, whose means were inadequate to deal with the situation. Once on the scene, the military units remained in the barracks near Kilemba and caused no further issues between them and the population.[5]

The territorial administrator's 2008 report on the BDK is the local government's account of state security in action. The last of the troops were still residing in their barracks in 2013. We were told to avoid them; local citizens were evidently fearful of crossing them or even of meeting with them. As far as "Operation Restoration of State Authority" was concerned, eye witnesses and local citizens provided a more graphic description. They confirmed that the two men burned to death had been identified as *bandoki* ("sorcerers") by an *nganga ngombo* who was engaged to investigate—*fiela*—other local deaths. The local authorities tried to put a stop to these actions, but they were overwhelmed and could not control mobs of more than 500 people. When the national police arrived in Luozi, BDK militants, who were concentrated in one of the poorer quarters of the town, set fire to one of the police vehicles. The force retaliated, killing a number of people. The media reported that twenty-two people were killed, but my sources estimated the number to be higher.

Has this action, the banning of the BDK, and the territorial agent's invitation to the population to reintegrate these people into their ranks, brought the agitation to a close? One of our interlocutors had this to say: "On the surface things are calm, but the sentiment of resistance and resentment continues beneath the surface." At the time of this writing in early 2018 Nsemi is still a deputy in the national Parliament. Although he continues to dissociate himself from the events of 2008, he has not set foot in the Manianga since then. Under another organizational name he continues to issue antigovernment pronouncements and to publish similar pamphlets, which can be seen in the hands of youth in Luozi.

Challenges and Successes of Postcolonial Local Government

Singly in particular instances, and collectively as a group of officials across the vast landscape of Western Equatorial and Great Lakes Africa, including the Lower Congo, communal and sector mayors and chiefs have tried to meet the expectations of sociability and governance, resource identification and allocation, and maintenance and perpetuation of legitimacy of their offices and their authority— often through the sheer force of their personalities. These are the hallmarks of social reproduction identified earlier as the measures of effective governance.

All the mayors struggled with the high degree of politicization of their offices and jurisdictions. As occupants of the lowest elected office in the party hierarchy, they needed to satisfy party superiors to be nominated and elected. But thus elected, they continued to be beholden to their constituents as well. Kusikila struggled with the repressive character of higher administrators and how they disregarded his initiatives and humiliated him. His periodic threats to resign in frustration evoked reactions of support from his constituents. Thus his political adroitness saved the day, although it drove him nearly crazy, as he conferred simultaneously with a Kinshasa psychiatrist and a local prophet-diviner over how to deal with the arrows of envy and antagonism, and the contradictions of his office.

The mayors, their councils, and local leaders have become much more sophisticated and innovative in identifying resources and organizing financial support for desired public projects. Merchants, as in precolonial trading networks, have become innovators in local and long-distance commerce. In the Great Lakes, this remained within the better-functioning spheres of the state. By contrast, in the Congo, state legitimacy and function have in large measure collapsed except at the local level around the mayors, who with the merchants, the churches, and other creative individuals restore public institutions as best they can.

The mayors often oversee maintenance and improvement of the public health infrastructure, which includes both formal institutions (hospitals, clinics, and periodic inoculation campaigns) and informal processes that contribute to health and well-being (such as clean water sources, private and public sewage, and conditions of schools and other public facilities).

The Origins and National Spread of Health Zones and Public Health

Following the withdrawal of the federal government from active management of health in the 1980s and 1990s, the decentralized regional health zone became the effective framework for both public health services and the coordination of health care institutions. Some of the five hundred health zones that had been established across the Congo dissipated as wars broke out, personnel fled, and buildings were destroyed. Yet the survival of the Congolese health zones is a remarkable story that needs to be told. It features local and regional leadership, as well as international coordination. Ecclesiastical medical directorates were established in 1992 by the Congolese Protestant Council's medical department to operate health posts, clinics, and hospitals in selected health zones. Within a few years a comparable national Catholic medical directorate was formed to administer other institutions within health zones. WHO's primary health care program dovetailed with this emerging structure.

The roots of the health zone system that emerged in the 1980s and became the dominant structure of health and health care services in the Territory of Luozi and the DRC generally in the 1990s and beyond are found in several disparate earlier initiatives. The idea of a public health district dates back to efforts by colonial authorities and mission medical personnel to deal with the serious diseases of a century ago. For example, the Swedish mission tracked and treated sleeping sickness, and the colonial government, through Fonds Reine Elisabeth pour l'Assistance Médicale aux Indigènes du Congo Belge (FOREAMI), identified pockets of declining population and low natality. The idea of health zones—regions where serious public health efforts could be organized in communities by local people—was put into action in a selected number of localities in the 1960s and 1970s, including Vanga, Kimpese, Karawa, Wembo Nyama, and Nyankunde.

A second source of the health zone as it emerged in the 1980s lay in the government's empowerment of national bodies for the churches: Catholic, Protestant, and Kimbanguist. Although this initiative was taken in order to control the churches, church leaders and the ecclesiastical structures that emerged had a longer life than the government's regime and ended up serving entirely different purposes. The Église du Christ au Zaire (later renamed the Église du Christ au Congo, or ECC) and its medical directorate became the real source for the independent national public health system in Congo. Catholic medical services, as well as remaining state medical structures that survived the government crisis of the 1990s, would merge within the national framework. WHO's primary health care program buttressed this already-emerging structure in 1985.

In 1975 the medical offices of the ECC and the office of the national Catholic Church cosponsored a major conference in collaboration with the Ministry of Health (Kintaudi, Minuku and Baer 2013). The conference established a consensus for decentralized health zones and primary health care as priorities for the direction of public health in the country. Leon Kintaudi, Felix Minuku, and Franklin Baer, who were participants at this conference and in subsequent joint initiatives, note the extraordinary foresight of this national planning three years prior to WHO's 1978 launch of its Health for All by the Year 2000 campaign at the Alma-Ata conference.

Due to the faltering trend of government agencies by the 1980s (Young and Turner 1985), outside funders of health and development began to favor increasingly direct work through national or regional NGOs. Thus, in 1980 the influential United States Agency for International Development (USAID) invested major funds in an initiative to create fifty health zones across the country. With the endorsement of the Ministry of Health, the ECC was selected to manage this multimillion-dollar, bilateral project, called the Basic Rural Health project, and later to become known as Santé Rurale du Congo (SANRU) (Kintaudi, Minuku and Baer 2013). Shortly after the launch of this program, further health zones were organized around Catholic, government, and various NGO-managed hospitals. SANRU quickly became a national umbrella organization that succeeded in establishing 306 health zones across the country by the time WHO's primary health care campaign was implemented globally. The working nature of this national effort is reflected in the following description by Kintaudi, Minuku, and Baer:

> The existing network of ECC hospitals provides a good infrastructure for the management of decentralized health zones. The presence of a functional referral hospital, office space and equipment, a garage and maintenance facilities, housing and gardens, electricity and fuel, supply line for medicines, teaching facilities and schools attract and retain competent staff even in isolated rural areas. This infrastructure helps these health zones to quickly develop. It also established a critical mass of

developing health zones and a national momentum that spread rapidly throughout the country. (Kintaudi, Minuku, and Bear 2013)

In the 1980s SANRU became the national clearing house and conduit for international funding agencies into the new and highly lauded public health system in Zaire, which was up and functioning earlier than many other national systems worldwide, thanks in large part to the preliminary work by model health zones. By 1987 the funding base was extended to include other faith-based agencies, such as the Jewish Organization for Rehabilitation by Training, as well as further USAID support. A second round of funding and initiative launched SANRU II and further development of additional health zones.

This upbeat picture of public health and health care ended within a few years. The outbreak of the HIV/AIDS epidemic, the challenging economic picture, and then in 1991 political chaos in the country, led to an abrupt end to investors' enthusiasm, or even ability to continue their work. Following the riots of 1991, USAID withdrew its personnel and funds. Many expatriate workers and experts, and a good number of national medical personnel, fled the country. This was followed by the rebellion in Eastern Congo in connection with the Rwandan genocide of 1994, the all-Africa war that engulfed the Congo by the late 1990s.

Despite the flight of outside funding and the departure of many professionals, the ECC/SANRU initiative persisted within the country as its name changed from the Republic of Zaire to the old term Democratic Republic of the Congo. During the difficult decade from 1991 to 2001, the ECC/Department of Medicine extended its work to additional health zones with the assistance of MAP International (in 1992), the World Council of Churches (1993), the World Bank for urban health zones in Kinshasa (1994), the US Office of Foreign Disaster Assistance (OFDA) for displaced persons (1994–1995), and Solidarise Protestante, a Belgian NGO (Kintaudi, Minuku, and Baer 2013, 2).

During the Ebola outbreak in Kikwit, the capital of Bandundu Province east of Kinshasa in 1996, SANRU offices and the ECC became the coordination center for all NGO and governmental agencies, organizing training and surveillance in collaboration with the Centers for Disease Control, handling radio and email services, and coordinating the receipt and distribution of two US Department of Defense planeloads of medical materials (Kintaudi, Minuku, and Baer 2013, 3).

The ECC's medical work and the more inclusive SANRU's efficacy during the chaotic decade of the 1990s set the stage for SANRU III (2001-6), a five-year initiative jointly coordinated by Protestant, Catholic, and public agencies to assist and rebuild many health zones that had suffered during the all-Africa war, mainly in the east of the country. This initiative was funded by USAID at $25 million. It included national campaigns of basic health services, including distribution of Vitamin A to children, provision of insecticide-treated mosquito nets, preventive treatment for malaria, HIV/AIDS blood testing, and vaccination coverage for children. By 2010 SANRU was finally registered as a national NGO in the DRC and providing annual support to public health valued in the range of $10 million (Kintaudi, Minuku and Baer 2013, 3).

At the time of this writing (early 2018) the SANRU agency, now an independent national NGO with multiple partners both Congolese and international, continues to draw significant international funding in ever more areas of public health. For example, Global Fund provides malaria and HIV/AIDS assistance for more than two hundred health zones, and SANRU serves as the principal conduit for childhood vaccinations from Gavi, the global vaccine alliance.

Luozi Health Zone: A Close-Up View

The Luozi Health Zone, following the prescription of the WHO global primary health care program coordinated with SANRU, was divided into health circles (*aires de santé*), each with at least one *centre de santé* and one or more *postes de santés* at the lowest, most basic level, plus one central *hopital de réference*, or referral hospital. Table 4.1 lists the major medical institutions in Luozi, Kibunzi, and Mangembo. Map 2.1 shows the health circles and health posts.

The public health agency of the Luozi Health Zone operated out of a modest building facing the Luozi Referral Hospital. Its official name, painted on the wall facing the street, was Zone de Santé Rurale Luozi Bureau Central (figures 4.1 to 4.4). The building housed a reception room and several meeting rooms on either side of a long corridor. There was no running water in the building, but there was a pit latrine around the back. In each of these meeting rooms was a table with chairs and, along one wall, shelves or cabinets holding folders and reports. On free walls were taped large paper sheets covered with the names of the various *aires de santé* on the left, and numbers in titled columns with flowing across the sheets: population and cases treated, vaccinated, seen or not seen. These were the handwritten progress reports of various campaigns of recent years: Polio Vaccinations 2008; Maternal and Child Health Indicators 2011, and so on.

This record keeping and monitoring by the health zone office reflected the extensive tracking of diseases and conditions reported at each of the three levels: the sanitary post, the health center, and the referral hospital. Periodically each health post needed to fill out a basic report of its activities, including number and type of patient visits, diseases or conditions shown, medications or treatments given, and results. The Luozi Health Zone did not possess a computer, so all these reports and calculations needed to be made manually and entered on the big paper sheets or into notebooks. This information was passed to the provincial level and ultimately provided WHO with the basic information for its global reports. As the goal of Health for All by the Year 2000 (WHO 2000b) came and went, the same reporting techniques and compilation formulas continued to be used.

TABLE 4.1. Major Manianga medical institutions, with bed capacity and resident physicians

Health zone	Locale, institution[a]	Affiliation	Bed capacity	Physicians
Kibunzi	Kibunzi Referral Hospital	CEC Protestant	70	2
	Kinkenge CS, PSs	CEC Protestant	60	1
	Kingoma CS, PSs	Catholic	45	1
	Kimuaka CS, PSs	Private	47	0
	Other CSs and PSs			
Mangembo	Mangembo Referral Hospital	Catholic	50	2
	Sundi Lutete CS, PSs	CEC Protestant	60	1
	Sundi Mamba CS, PSs	CEC Protestant	20	1
	Other CSs and PSs			
Luozi	Luozi Referral Hospital, 9 PSs	State	110	2
	Luozi Catholic Sisters CS, PSs	Catholic	68	1
	Nkundi CS, 8 PSs	State	54	1
	Kingoyi CS, 1 PS	CEC Protestant	55	1
	Mbandakani CS, 3 PSs		N/A	0
	Bidi-Kindamba CS, 9 PSs		N/A	0
	Kinsemi CS, 2 PSs	Private	N/A	0
	Mbanza Ngoyo CS, 6 PSs		N/A	0
	Muzana CS, 7 PSs		N/A	0
	Nganda-Nkulu CS, 3 PSs		N/A	0
	Yanga CS, 2 PSs		N/A	0
	Yanga Pompe CS, 8 PSs		N/A	0

SOURCE: Health Zones of Kibunzi, Luozi, and Mangembo.
[a] CS = centre de santé; PS = poste de santé

In some senses the health zone staff functioned as the eyes, ears, arms, and legs of the entire medical establishment. Ngemba Jeanbenoit, *animateur communautaire*, and Mansinsa Dianzenza Delvin, *infirmier superviseur*, would go off on their motorcycles to visit far-flung health posts and centers and check up on the resident nurses, encourage them, monitor supplies, follow through on campaigns or consultations, and collect records of their accomplishments. Mbasani Veronique, their secretary, stayed at the office to record the documents they brought back from their trips into the health zone hinterland. They sometimes commented that a particular series of figures was the result of their own field trips and surveys where they thought the existing record keepers were not finding and counting everyone. I noted that the mortality rates of the health zone were far lower than those reported in the territorial annual reports, whereas the birth rates were comparable. Every health post had a group of volunteers who were charged with encouraging the local community to use the post for their health concerns and to

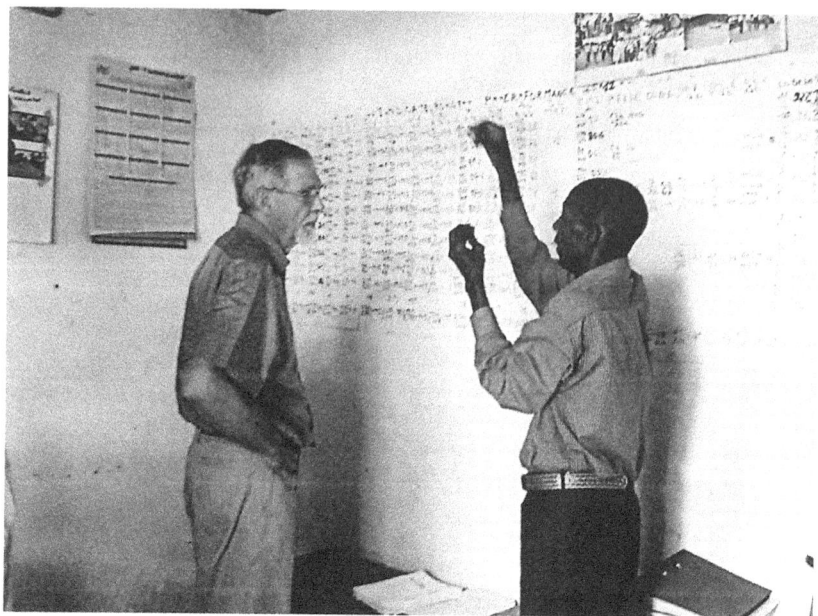

FIGURE 4.1. Record keeping at the Luozi Health Zone. Jeanbenoit Ngemba, chief *animateur* of the Luozi Health Zone, explains to Janzen the record keeping method on a large sheet of paper attached to the wall of the meeting room. Photo: Reinhild Janzen, 2013.

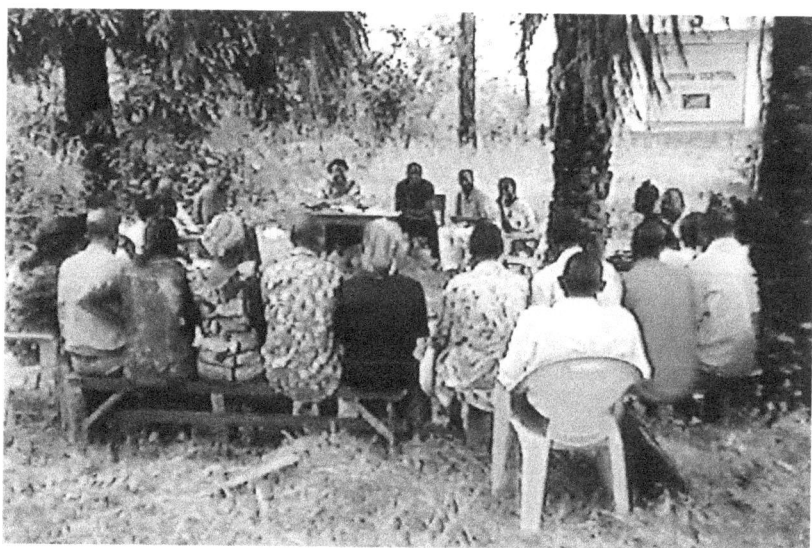

FIGURE 4.2. Public health volunteers receive instructions. A periodic meeting of health post community members receiving training from a public health official on the shady grounds of the Luozi Health Zone. The local citizens committee that oversees their health post is a central feature of WHO's original concept of primary health care. Photo: John M. Janzen, 2013.

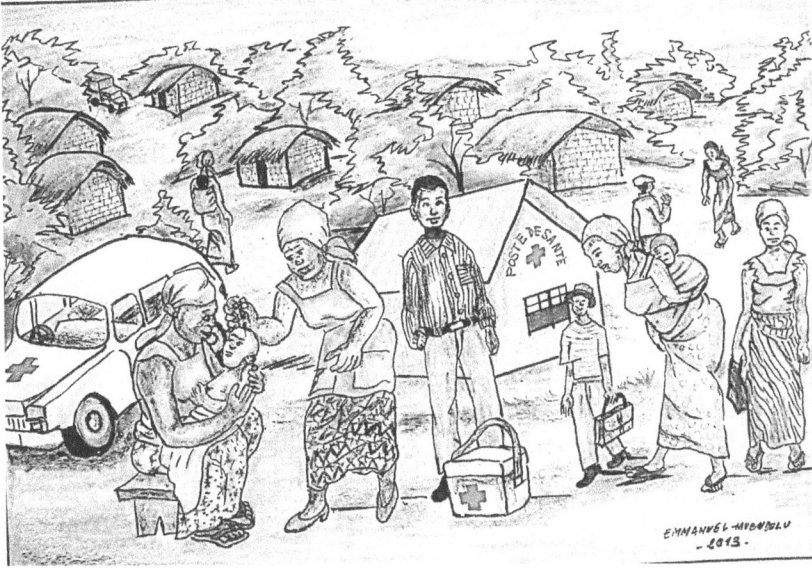

FIGURE 4.3. The health post. This 2013 drawing by artist Emmanuel Mvibidulu for the Janzens highlights maternal and child care.

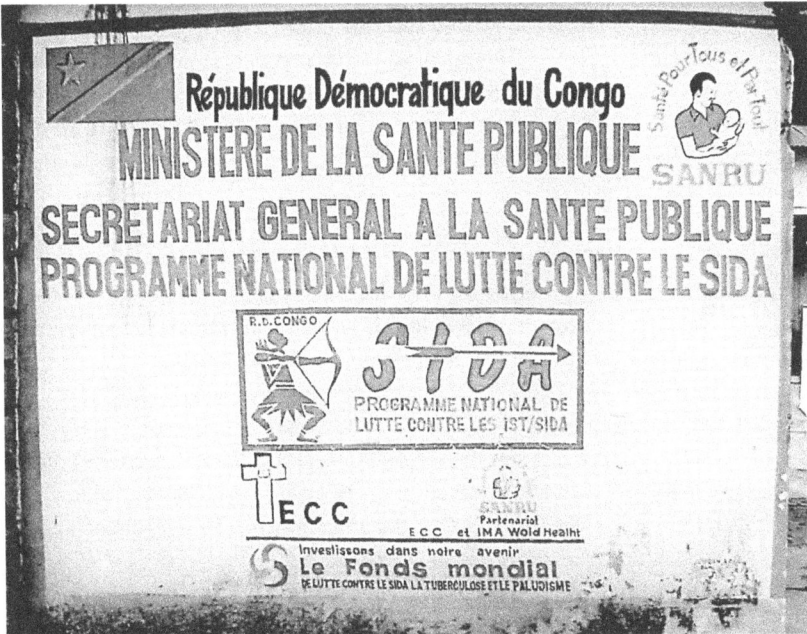

FIGURE 4.4. Ministry of Health sign at the Luozi Health Zone featuring logos of organizations sponsoring HIV/AIDS campaigns: the Congolese Fund, the Église du Christ au Congo (ECC), Santé Rurale du Congo (SANRU), and Le Fonds Mondial (World Fund for the struggle against HIV/AIDS, tuberculosis, and malaria), 2013.

report births and deaths. WHO's experience with grassroots participation in public health campaigns had led to the incorporation of local volunteers into the primary health care structures already in 1984.

The Luozi Health Zone public health program, like the WHO program in general, emphasized the health of women and children. Childhood vaccination campaigns constituted an important part of their outreach. Children's nutrition was a further important feature of the entire complex of practices: maternal health visits, birthing, neonatal care, inoculations, and nutrition. Ngemba and Dianzenza were particularly concerned that the Vitamin A supplement be properly administered and that children be protected from the anemia that often accompanies malaria attacks. Through the health zone, medicated mosquito nets were distributed to everyone. Everyone with whom we spoke said they used the nets in their bedrooms, but we heard stories of them being sold and of fishers using them as fishing nets.

WHO and ECC/SANRU statistical expectations included recording the percentage of the population that participated in various campaigns. These figures became part of the indicators-of-health scores that measured progress toward health development. Health zone personnel in general were sensitive regarding nonparticipation in vaccination, child care, nutrition, and supplement programs, and they engaged volunteers as much as possible so people could benefit from them. However, there were naysayers, principal among them the Bundu dia Kongo nationalists, who saw any and all programs that injected, instilled, or encouraged the adoption of outside materials or ideas as a conspiracy to control and dominate them.

Health Zones as a Framework for Institutional Reconfiguration

In the Manianga and many other regions, the collapse of the Zairian state brought back into the business of managing health care the only remaining corporate structures with any substance and scale—namely, the churches. But the institutional platform for this resurrection was the recently created and much heralded health zone infrastructure. During the era of postcolonial national institutions in the 1970s and early 1980s, a number of public health initiatives served as prototypes for the more systematic national program of primary health care initiated under WHO in 1984. The first health zones were launched in various parts of the country, at both Protestant and Catholic institutions.

In Manianga (the Territory of Luozi) Protestant and Catholic medical departments were organized in 1991 with semiautonomous status and responsibility for administering health care institutions within one or across several health zones. Although this move seemed to restore church-related medical work to a status similar to that of the missions of colonial days, there was a big difference. Whereas previously, before independence and in the early postcolonial period, many professional personnel had been expatriates, now all or almost all personnel were Congolese. Also, the medical directorates did not take charge of the zones in the overlapping, sectarian, and competitive manner of the colonial era. Across the DRC, in this new arrangement, about half of the health zones were administered by church organizations. The rest were state-administered. In effect, these ecclesiastical organizations were substituting for the state. The state-private-church partnership model prevailed in many respects in all Congolese health-related endeavors, as was evident in the institutional affiliations of the three health zones of the Manianga.

Thus, out of the shambles of nationalized institutions, old buildings and organizations were resurrected to create a viable, if uneven, system of public health and health care. Institutions from all orientations—state, religious, and private—were folded together into a single regional entity based on the three-tiered system: local health posts, health circles or health centers, and a single referral hospital per zone (see figures 4.5 to 4.9 for scenes of Luozi Catholic Health Center and Sundi Lutete Health Center).[6]

In the Southwest, the CEC Protestant health department administered the Kibunzi Health Zone, into which were incorporated the Kibunzi referral hospital and the health centers of Kinkenge, Kigoma, and Kimauka. These institutions had

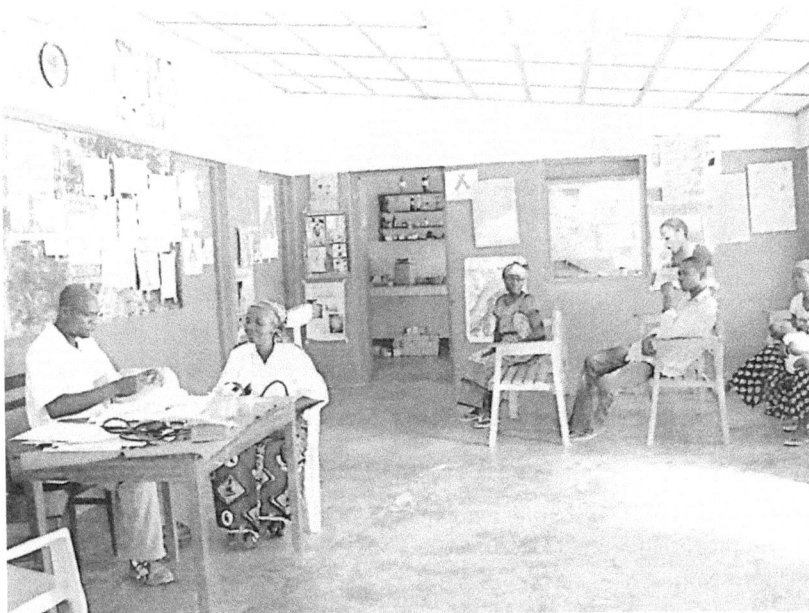

FIGURE 4.5. Catholic Health Center Luozi waiting room. Patient registration on the left; waiting patients on the right; door to the lab in the center; examination offices through the doors along the left-side wall. Photo: John M. Janzen, 2013.

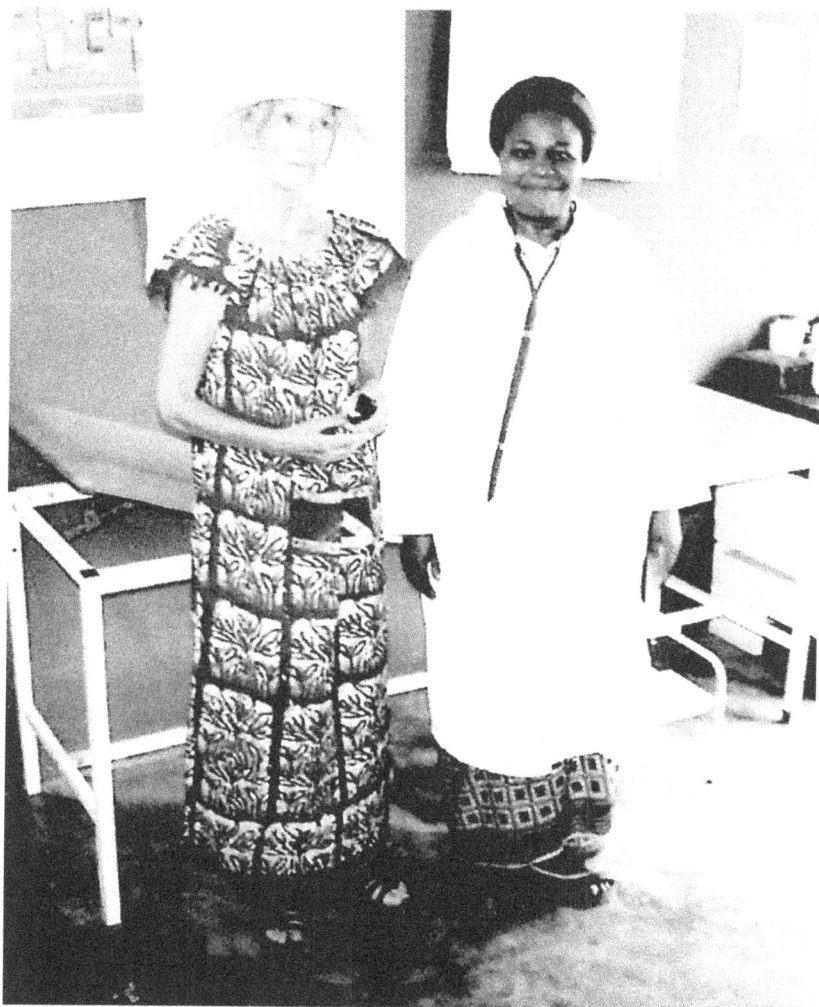

FIGURE 4.6. Reinhild Janzen and Dr. Rose Ndoda Kumbu, after Reinhild's checkup following her bout with malaria. Photo: John M. Janzen, March 2013.

a total capacity of 184 beds, with four physicians and many more nurse practitioners, nurses, pharmacists, and lab technicians.

In the Northeast and East of the territory, the Catholic Church's medical service administered the Mangembo Health Zone, which incorporated the Mangembo referral hospital, the Sundi Lutete and Sundi Mamba health centers, with a capacity of 140 beds, and the presence of four physicians, as well as nurse practitioners, nurses and other aides and technicians.

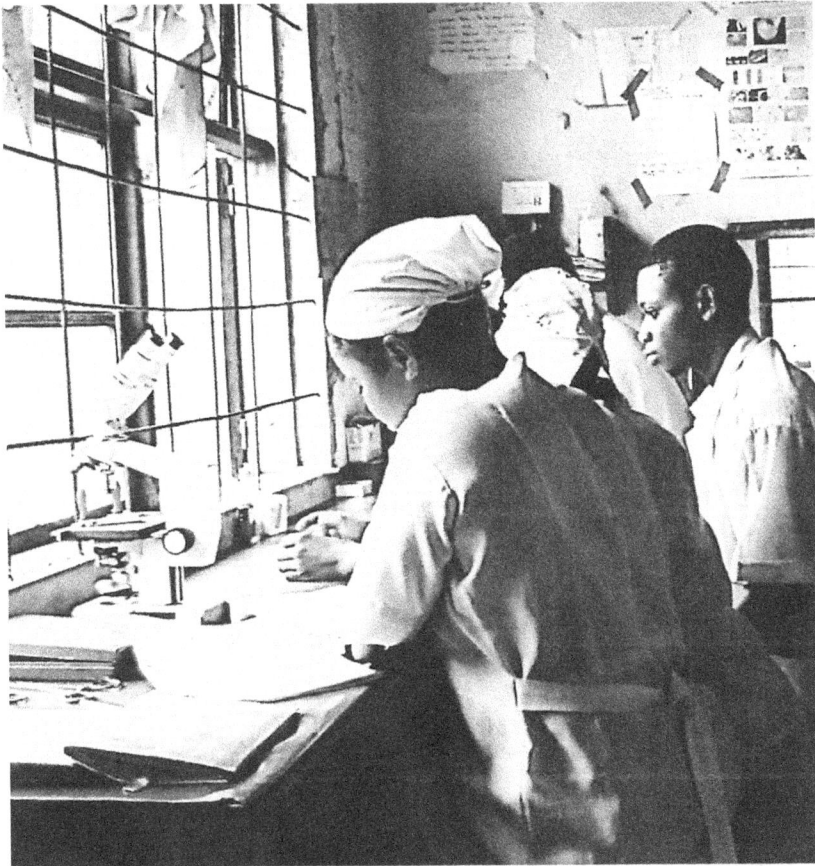

FIGURE 4.7. Lab technicians, Sundi Lutete Medical Center. In the absence of regular electricity, the bright, sunlit windows are essential to effective laboratory examinations. Photo: John M. Janzen, 2013.

The Protestant CEC health department also administered the Luozi Health Zone, which incorporated the Luozi General Hospital, the referral institution of the zone, and the health centers of Luozi Catholic, Nkundi, and Kingoyi. These had a total capacity of 249 beds, and four physicians and the other technicians and aides.

The challenge of these ecclesiastical, state, and private medical agencies was to coordinate historically well-funded institutions, with all their buildings and personnel, with a fee-for-service income and whatever could be raised from independent donors or obtained through the national SANRU sources. In the DRC there was very little public funding—government contributed only 0.9 percent of overall health and health care expenditures. What small public funds there were

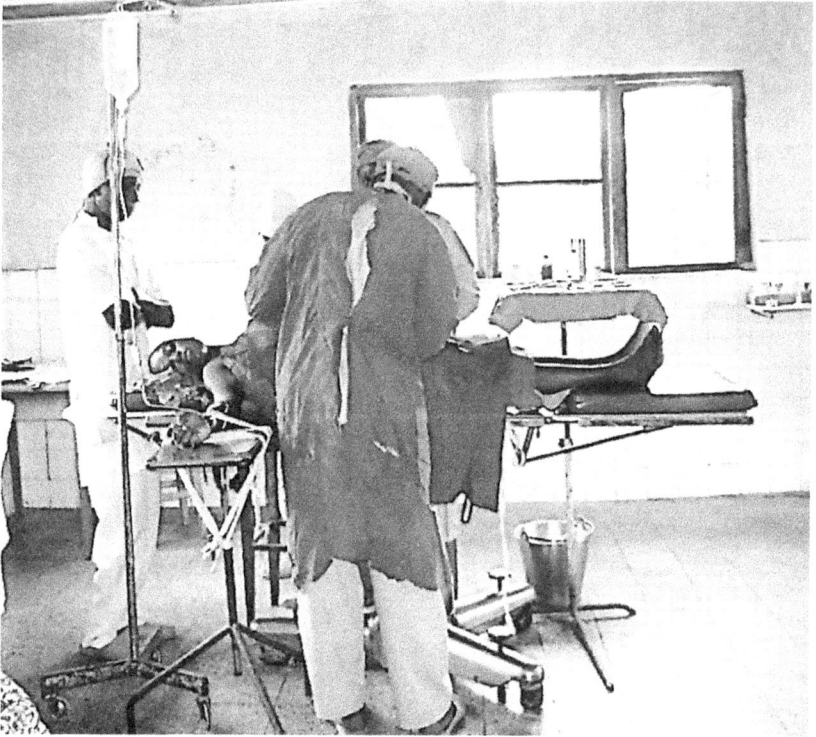

FIGURE 4.8. Surgery without electricity, Sundi Lutete Medical Center. Photo: John M. Janzen, 2013.

went for childhood vaccinations, HIV/AIDS campaigns, sleeping sickness, and a few other "dangerous" diseases. This meant that everyone was financially strapped. All other medical care in hospitals and centers was charged to users. This resulted in a paradox of widely available services and medicines, offered at prohibitive prices, leaving many communities only partially or inadequately covered. At the personal or household level it meant that a large piece of the annual pie was spent on medical emergencies. At the institutional level it meant that all vigilance had to be exercised to extract operating funds and salaries from patients or from other sources as each institution or service could find them.

Hospitals, NGOs, and Churches:
Tapping the Most Rigorous Resource Base

It is ironic that the phoenix-like post-state resurrection of faith-based medical institutions occurred in the face of the nativist BDK revival of pre-Christian Kongo customs of misfortune. Yet both conditions were brought on by the collapse of

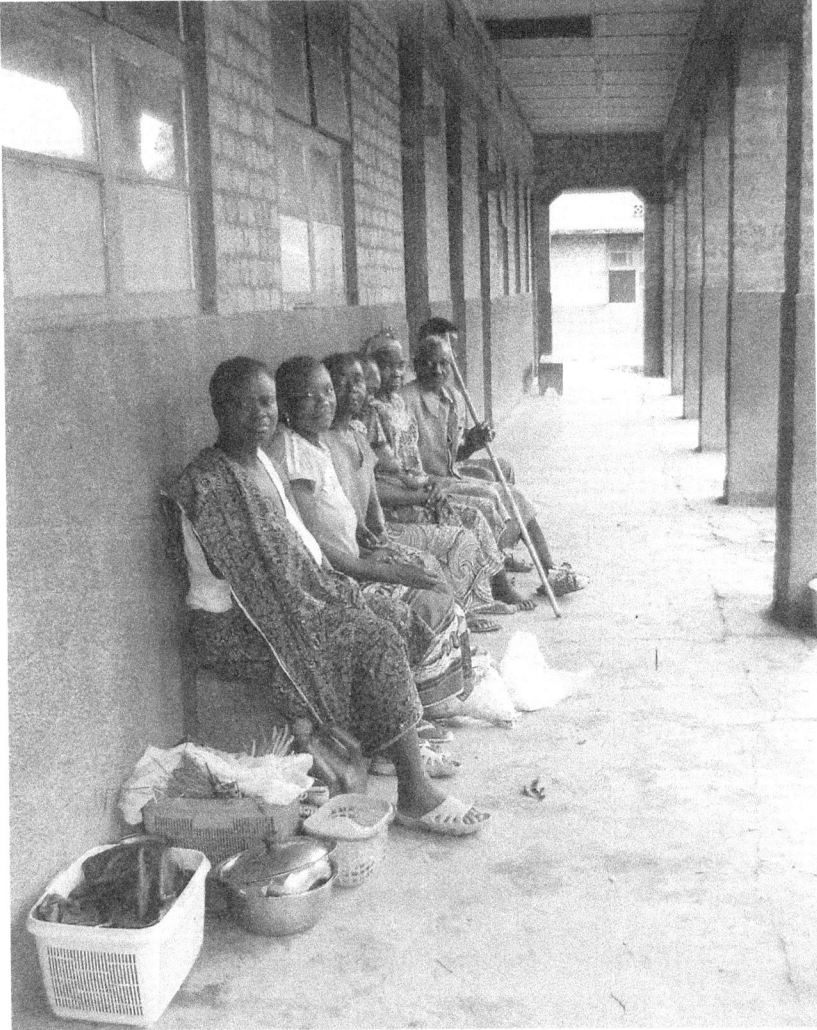

FIGURE 4.9. Patients convalescing on veranda, Sundi Lutete Medical Center, 2013.

authority structures in state and society. Public officials and the religious community alike did what was most possible: they marshalled the remaining existing institutions with human, infrastructural, and financial resources. Thus the regional Catholic and Protestant ecclesiastical authorities reconfigured the church medical agencies that had existed in colonial and early postcolonial times to back up the fledgling, much-heralded public health zones that had been introduced in the 1980s.

In the Territory of Luozi the major player in health care was the CEC's Department of Medical Works (Département des Oeuvres Médicine, DOM). The CEC was previously called the Eglise Evangélique de Manianga et Matadi (EEMM), the Protestant church that succeeded the Swedish Covenant Church mission Svenska Missions Förbundet (SMF) in 1961. From its administrative offices in Luozi, the DOM administered the medical institutions in the health zones of Luozi and Kibunzi to the west. Its Catholic counterpart administered the Mangembo Health Zone from the hospital at Mangembo.

Headed by Doctor Alfred Monameso from its headquarters in Luozi, the DOM staff included a financial assistant, a technical assistant, an accountant, an assistant for logistics, a pharmacist, a secretary, and a chauffeur. The DOM administered two general referral hospitals (Luozi and Kibunzi), five health centers (Nkundi, Kingoyi, Kinkenge, Sundi Lutete, Sundi Mamba), 36 health posts, and two medical technology institutes. Further, in Matadi it administered three medical centers, and in Kinshasa two medical centers. It was responsible for 329 employees, including 14 physicians, 41 nurses, 74 nurse assistants, 80 auxiliary nurses, 16 laboratory technicians, one radiology technician, 54 administrative staff, and 49 maintenance personnel. The DOM directly administered institutions in two health zones and had institutions and services in four others.

The historical background of this impressive medical organization is rooted in more than a century of medical work by Swedish doctors, nurses, and other medical scientists who established the first biomedical work in the Manianga. The DOM was officially organized in its present form in 1991 in order to assume responsibility for the health zones. Although the medical work had continued from 1965 to 1991 under government supervision and control, little infrastructure maintenance and development was done during that time. In 2013, the DOM was just launching its five-year plan, which is spelled out in its document *Vision 2017: Plan Stratégique 2013–2017* (Communauté Evangélique du Congo 2012). This strategic plan began where the emergency intervention following the collapse of the state medical system had left off.

In 1991, a series of initiatives were taken to restore the buildings, equipment, and stocks of the institutions under DOM responsibility. From 1991 to 1996, under the project PROSAN III, at a cost of $419,714, six hospitals (Luozi, Kibunzi, Kingoyi, Nkundi and Sundi Lutete) were freshly equipped, forty health posts were constructed and equipped, and all medical personnel were given a medical refresher course (Communauté Evangélique du Congo 2012, 7–8). Also beginning in 1991, the project PROHOPITAL, which cost $283,428, was undertaken to rehabilitate or construct a medical internist pavilion, a dispensary, a pediatric pavilion, a sanatorium, and toilets. This project included the purchase of an ambulance, fifty hospital beds and mattresses, and one electrical generator. At the same time project PROVEHICULE, for $76,000, purchased two vehicles for Kingoyi and Kibunzi hospitals, one motorcycle for Luozi, and ten bicycles for health posts. The funds for these initiatives came from a combination of local, national, and former mission churches, as well as several foreign aid programs, including USAID and Swedish foreign aid. They were administered through a SANRU program to bolster faith-based institutions.

In 1994 and 1995 further initiatives were taken, including the construction of residences for physicians in Luozi ($24,571) and for the medical director of Sundi Lutete ($58,515), and the construction of a nursing school and institute of medical technology in Luozi ($33,285). In 1996, there were further purchases of a generator, two stabilizers, and electrical wiring at Kibunzi ($50,000). In 1999 a pharmacy in Matadi was equipped and medical stocks were purchased ($24,857).

From 2000 to 2002 eleven hospitals and medical centers in the Territory of Luozi were equipped and units created to deal with malnutrition and nutritional rehabilitation ($156,817). In 2000 pharmaceutical stocks were purchased to resupply hospitals and health centers ($42,861). From 2002 to 2004 health centers at Nkundi and Sundi Mamba were rehabilitated and equipped, an ambulance was acquired for Nkundi, and a motorcycle for Sundi Mamba ($248,714). Taking advantage of the urgency of the era, from 2003-10 project PROLUSIDA focused on an educational campaign regarding sexually transmitted diseases, particularly HIV/AIDS, and blood transfusion security ($770,724).

DOM is increasingly self-conscious of its image among the public it is serving (70 percent of the Territory of Luozi), and how well it is doing vis-à-vis its competitors (Communauté Evangélique du Congo 2012, 10). In the Manianga these are the Catholic Medical Service; the Salvation Army, which has some parallel institutions not tied in to the health zone structure; the healing churches (*bangunza*); and the traditional healers (*banganga*). The DOM has begun to look a little like a North American health care corporation. In its most recent synodal meeting a decision was reached to develop a logo for better identification and name-brand recognition. DOM is also explicit to its supporters and boards about which services create loyalty among clients. Apparently prenatal, postnatal, and child nutritional and care services, as well as childhood vaccinations, are regarded as loyalty producing. Surgeries, too, have this effect when the outcome is successful. However, these services that people want, and that draw them to loyalty to these institutions, do not pay for themselves. Among the most lucrative are the sale of medicines, maternity services, and laboratory services (Communauté Evangélique du Congo 2012, 10).

DOM administrators and directors are well aware of risks to the organization and its successful future in the niche it has occupied since 1991 (Communauté Evangélique du Congo 2012, 11). Only seven of fourteen physicians possess liability insurance provided by the state. The state supports only sixty-nine out of the total of 329 personnel. Buildings are in need of general repair. Seven health centers are in a condition of "advanced dilapidation" (Communauté Evangélique du Congo 2012, 11). Five of nine vehicles are broken down. The Congo River is a big barrier to easy travel to and from the rest of the region. The population is impoverished, earning less than a dollar a day.

Threats to the work of the DOM include weak participation of the state in the financing of health; lack of financial support for the work of DOM, other than direct fees for service; lack of structural partners; a population that often first consults traditional medicine; weak purchasing power of the population; elevated illiteracy in the population; resistance to mass health campaigns (such as vaccination campaigns and distribution of Vitamin A supplements) among adepts of the Bundu dia Kongo; disruption of supply of basic and generic medicines in the central pharmacy; inadequate means of transportation and communication; a convention for billing in the Mangembo Health Zone that reduces income in the health centers DOM operates, especially in Sundi Lutete; and the inaccessibility of some medical establishments, making it difficult to communicate, to follow their activities, and to provide them with medicines (Communauté Evangélique du Congo 2012, 14).

The directors of the DOM consider its administrative and financial structure to be unstable, and anything but permanent. It is serving a public that must pay for all services rendered, yet those services do not cover all costs. The sources of foreign funds that have supported some initiatives are not guaranteed. This is the case with the Swedish Gemensam Framtid, which supported some recent major initiatives. The Congolese state is a partner that could guarantee direct and indirect support: allocations for certain personnel, support for electricity, water, and other resources; indirect support in the form of tax relief, subventions, and much more. Since about 2005 there is again a Ministry of Health, which may be lobbied to increase its support for the work of the DOM.[7] In the strategic plan the DOM commits itself to augment its negotiations for contractual arrangements with the national state administration and with these funding sources abroad.

A final feature of the strategic plan is to promote health and wellness (Communauté Evangélique du Congo 2012, 18). This will be done by social marketing to the community, specifically in schools, to women and families, and to youth. Institutional and community leaders must be sensitized to the issues that are critical. Public health education will be offered in areas of hygiene and cleanliness, trash pickup, water usage, and sewage disposal. Finally, health mutuals will be encouraged to share the costs of health and health care.

RISE OF THE INDEPENDENT PHARMACIES

The large number of self-care episodes in this study's intensive sample of 579 persons in 105 households suggests the importance of pharmacies and herbal remedies in Maniangans' management of their health and health care issues. Approximately two-fifths (153) of all episodes (375) reported needing attention were taken care of through "self-medication," 119 with commercially available medicines, and 34 with "indigenous" remedies (see table 2.4). A high rate of self-medication holds true even of episodes of the principal diseases, such as malaria (53 of 137 episodes), schistosomiasis (30 of 42 episodes), and seasonal flu (34 of 41 episodes). If this ratio of institutional care to self-care were projected onto the health zone annual reports of incidence of these diseases, the total episodes of malaria, schistosomiasis, and seasonal flu would be nearly doubled. In the case of malaria it would mean that nearly half of the population experienced infections serious enough to require medication or a visit to a specialist or clinic.

The pharmacies of the Manianga and of the DRC at large are an extremely varied lot. They range from commercial pharmacies that hire or are operated by a university-trained pharmacist, to enterprises that resell medicines they buy from such pharmacies or other suppliers, to market stalls that sell commercial medicines without any pharmaceutical competence whatsoever. These latter establishments are part of the reselling phenomenon of a neoliberal economy. The open and free economy of pharmaceuticals is both a blessing and a bane to the society— a blessing because the market promotes the distribution and availability of drugs; a bane in that there is no control over who can or cannot buy drugs and no indication of how they are to be used, short of instructions that may be on a package. In a society where there is a rich history of available herbal remedies and most individuals have access to fields, streamsides, and forests, a robust use of commercial medicines is not surprising.

Intensive sample participants from along the rivers all suffered from schistosomiasis and treated themselves with the commercial drug Biltricide, which apparently relieves the pain of the infestation. They also registered strong appeals to the authorities to do something to clean up their streams. Malaria sufferers who self-medicated, or their elders who cared for them, were able to obtain the drug Fansidar, as well as old-fashioned quinine to treat both the symptoms and the disease. Locally produced Manadiar and Manalaria were also commonly used to treat malaria. The history of high levels of disease and the rich lore in indigenous medicine, as well as historic acquaintance with coastal trade, translated into widespread use of commercial pharmaceuticals.

Another feature shared by these independent pharmacies in Congo—and in Africa in general, and in many countries of the world—is their catchy names, alluding to trendy images or with sacred or magical allure. Luozi names included Sacred Hand Pharmacy, Blessing of God Pharmacy, Eureka Pharmacy, Thanks Be to God Pharmacy, Wisdom Pharmacy, and Modern Pharmacy. The titles suggest that these pharmacies may not only provide drugs but offer the comfort of a church, and that the druggist may not just be a scientist but also sometimes double as a pastor or priest.

Standing in sharp contrast to these pharmacies is the Centre de Recherche Pharmaceutique de Luozi (CRPL) (figures 4.10 to 4.12). Its operation is as thoroughly scientific as its name suggests. The work of the CRPL, begun and owned by Batangu Mpesa, a university-trained pharmacist, research chemist, parliamentarian, educator, and above all entrepreneur, contributes mightily to the image of pharmacies in the Manianga (Janzen 2012, 122–24; 2015b, 51–52; 2017, 102–8). Early on after his pharmaceutical training in Canada, Batangu Mpesa opened a pharmacy in Kinshasa. While there, he launched his research enterprise by collecting and analyzing several dozen plants used by *banganga* of the region and distilling the best of their materials for the development of his malaria medications. Avoiding intermediaries or the trap of selling his patent to a first-world developer, he became his own financier and gradually established the Manadiar and Manalaria lines in the Congo, manufactured from locally grown artemisia.

The rapidly evolving world of materia medica in Western Central Africa rests on the careers of both small trader merchants reselling drugs and pace-setting research scientists like Batangu Mpesa. Many of the drugs sold by independent merchants and pharmacists are the same as those stocked on hospital shelves. But the former are largely independent of the latter, selling what they can for a profit, often with the implicit caution that the buyer should beware.

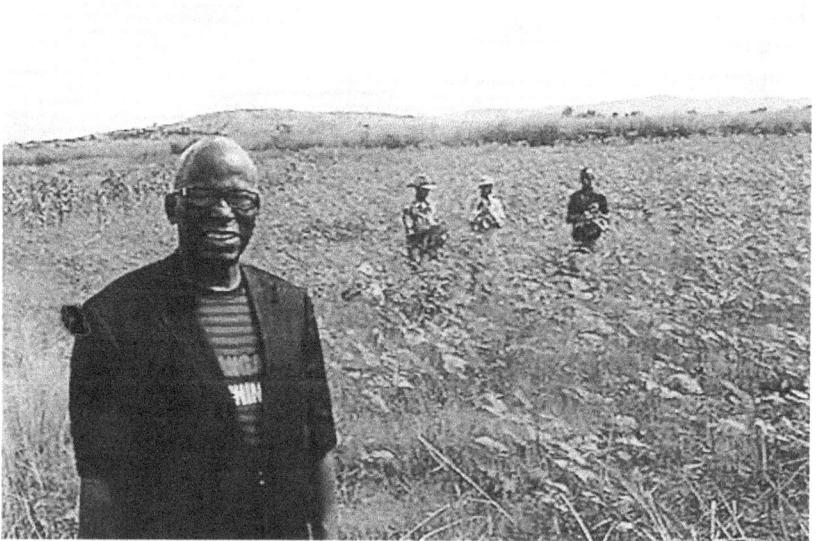

FIGURE 4.10. Pharmacist Batangu Mpesa in artemisia field, near Luozi. This plant was selected as the key ingredient in the malaria medications Manadiar and Manalaria. Photo: John M. Janzen, 2013.

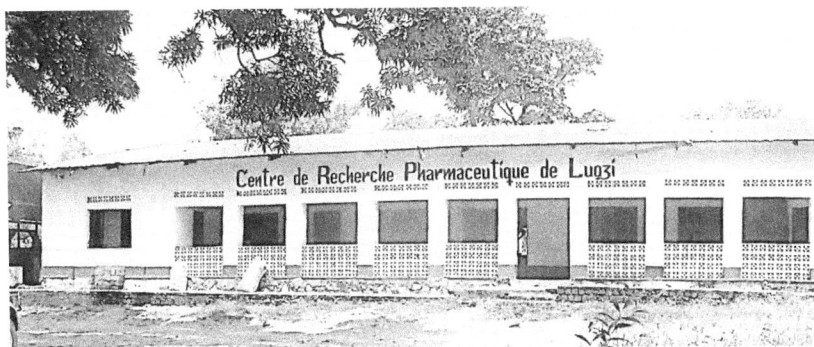

FIGURE 4.11. Centre de Recherche Pharmaceutique de Luozi (CRPL), where plant leaves are processed into extracts, and where original and continuing laboratory analysis is carried out. Photo: John M. Janzen, 2013.

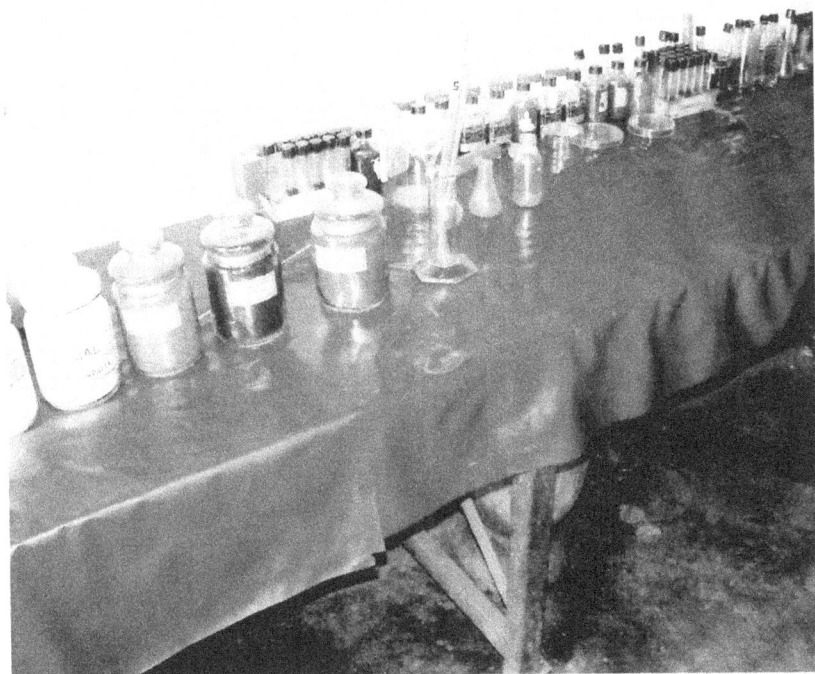

FIGURE 4.12. Plant extracts and compounds in CRPL Lab. Photo: John M. Janzen, 2013.

Banganga, Prophets, and Healing Churches

The market in Luozi featured a small section devoted to "indigenous medicine"—the usual mineral products, animal parts, shells, skins, and dried plant materials. In the intensive sample questionnaire, in about one-twelfth of the reported health episodes (22 of 375) the individual resorted to the use of indigenous materia medica or consulted a healer or prophet. Both physical treatments and more psychic or spiritual issues were involved, as is reflected historically in Lower Congo traditional medicine. The pattern of consulting all medical traditions that was identified in the *The Quest for Therapy* (Janzen 1978) appears to have persisted, although I did not follow multiple cases in depth as I had in that earlier study. For many Maniangans, traditional treatments are an option alongside biomedicine and its pharmacopeia.

The underlying dichotomy between afflictions or misfortunes that originate in natural (or "of God") circumstances, and those that are human-caused continues to drive the search for ill-willed agents if a condition persists or if there is clear evidence that someone harbors ill will toward another who is experiencing suffering or misfortune. The great degree of insecurity in current economic conditions prompts many families and individuals to seriously entertain the possibility that they are bewitched, or that someone is causing them harm. Specialists in various kinds of divination offer their services. The unrest associated with the Bundu dia Kongo brought to light someone who claimed to be a *nganga ngombo*, a user of the historic divination basket widespread in Western Equatorial and Southern Savanna Africa. Prophetic divination is also practiced by some of the healing churches. This level of insecurity also leads to a common search for mystic and spiritual protection from the sources of aggression one fears.

Luozi's Waterworks and Other Public Health Services

Public health structures and responsibilities such as domestic water provision, sewage disposal, and trash pickup are often handled differently from medicine and other aspects of public health. In the Lower Congo the fragmentation of institutions, structures, and services is visibly evident.

In the course of interviewing Luozi *chef de cité* Matondo Lufinama, I learned that it is his city hall that annually does an inspection of the pit toilets, one of three buildings usually found on a residential parcel (in addition to the house and the kitchen, and sometimes a work shed, or hangar). A city ordinance requires all homeowners to have a pit toilet. Indeed, this seems to be the case in most villages of the Manianga, going back at least to the 1960s, although in the health survey of 105 households some reported "going to *matiti*"—the bush.

Trash pickup is less well handled, although the procedure is known. In the Luozi market, at the edges of streets, and in some residential parcels, one sees piles of debris. In the market these piles are conspicuously swept into the middle of sidewalk-like aisles between the market stalls, so people have to walk over or around them. Men with *puss-puss* carts are hired weekly, Matondo stated, to haul this trash to near the river, where it is dumped into the bush.

The big story of public health improvement is, however, the installation of the Luozi waterworks in 1993. Although the Luozi waterworks serves individual parcel owners, it is a public works project of major proportions that has a significant impact on public health. Taps are installed on private parcels that have been purchased by the owners, sometimes from the original land chiefs, sometimes from previous individual owners (figure 4.13). Sometimes concessions are purchased by developers. Renting from the land chiefs or from owners is also possible. City water is purchased by the parcel owner. Each hydrant has a meter that counts water used. If people can't pay, their hydrants are shut off and fitted with a pinched end pipe that was shown to the anthropologist as evidence that the residents neglected their health (or were simply too poor to afford the water rates). The water system covers most of the city, although Luozi's recent expansion has spread beyond the water lines. A few areas have communal springs or wells with hand pumps.

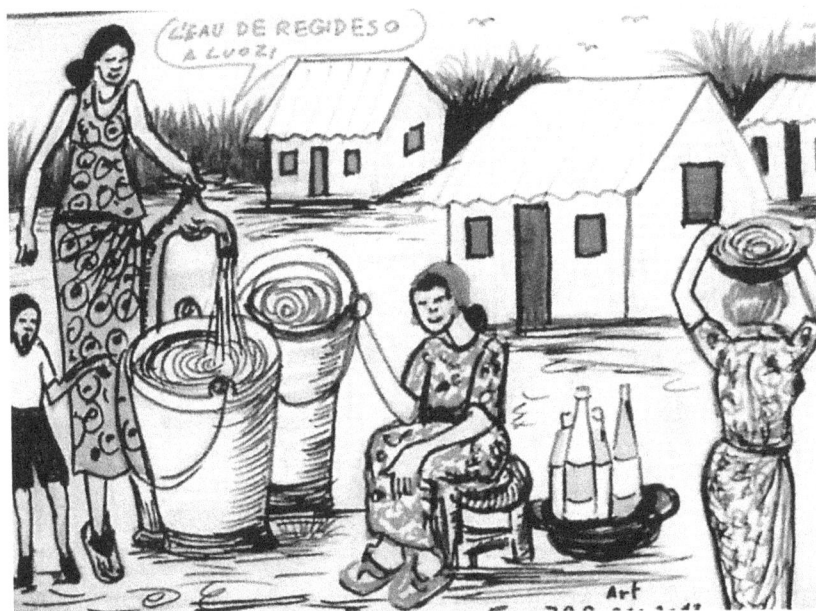

FIGURE 4.13. Women at the city hydrant. Drawing by J. P. Boursa, commissioned by John M. Janzen, 2013.

Urban waterworks in the Congo are usually created and maintained by the parastatal organization REGIDESO. This institution, like a few others in the DRC, has remained somewhat immune to the waves of corruption and dysfunction that have plagued the postal service (which has completely disappeared), the Matadi-to-Kinshasa railroad (whose last locomotive fell into a river), and Air Congo (which vanished in the 1990s). REGIDESO is now being privatized, as are all remaining state entities. In the Luozi project hydraulic engineers and construction experts discovered a big spring flowing into the river under the surface of the water. Workers tapped the spring, cemented in a pipe, and extended additional piping up to a tower and horizontally to the shore and to the pumping station (see figure 4.14). There, four pumps powered by diesel engines (figure 4.15) move the water up to the residential hydrants throughout the town.

The story of how this water system came into being includes major political strategizing and pressure on the government. Around 1988 the elite from the Manianga who lived in Kinshasa held a three-day meeting to identify priorities for improvements in their home area. The crocodile problem rose to the top of the list. Water for domestic use in Luozi was related to this problem. Too frequently someone going to the Congo River to bathe, to fetch drinking or cooking water, or to fish would be attacked by a crocodile. Luozi's inhabitants were terrified of this situation. Something needed to be done.

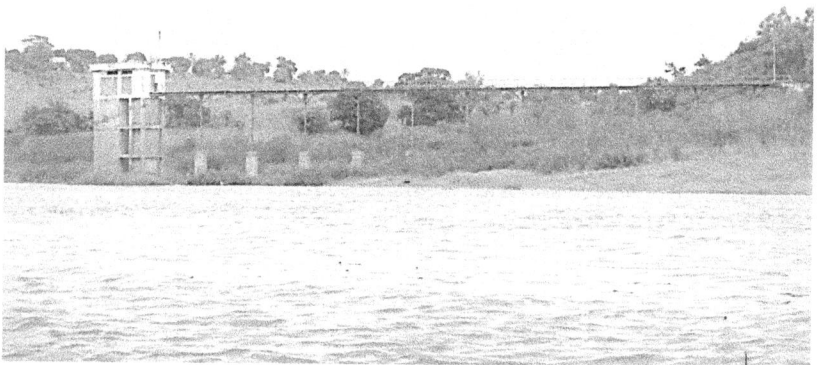

FIGURE 4.14. Luozi waterworks on the Congo River. The installation taps an underwater spring, from which distant pumps move it to taps in the city. This engineering feat was accomplished by the national utility REGIDESO (Régie des Eaux). Photo: Rhylin Bailie, 2013.

One outcome of the discussion among Kinshasa's elite was publication of Zamenga Batukezanga's adult comic book *Un Croco a Luozi* (1998). This was deemed interesting entertainment but not sufficiently compelling to move political will in parliament and government toward a solution. Kimpianga Mahaniah then wrote his book *La problematique crocodilienne a Luozi* (1989b). It offered a more compelling picture, including vivid case histories of one hundred persons killed by crocodiles (twenty-three in 1987 alone). He explained the environmental causes for the increase in the number of crocodiles (deforestation, loss of birds of prey to eat crocodile eggs, overfishing of big carnivorous fish that prey on little crocodiles), and discussed the folklore of croco-men and men with domestic crocodiles they send out to herd fish and occasionally to attack their human enemies. The construction of a water system at Luozi would solve multiple problems at once.

Furthermore, said Diallo Lukwamusu, executive director of the Free University of Luozi, the need for a water system in Luozi was very apparent because the water from the Congo River was polluted and nonpotable, and the Luozi River was dirty, sluggish, infested with bilharzia, and also dangerous because of crocodiles. The upcoming elections provided the people of Luozi with the opportunity to make

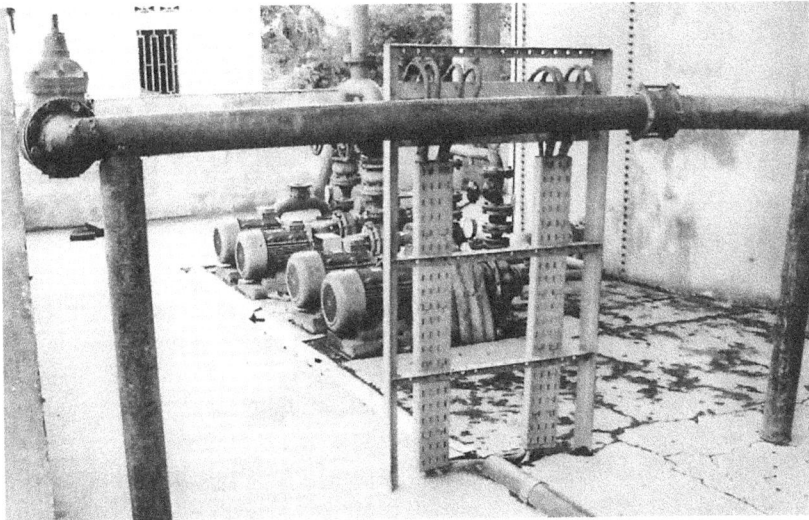

FIGURE 4.15. Pump turbines at Luozi waterworks. In the absence of electricity, the pumps are powered by diesel engines that require a steady supply of diesel fuel, trucked in from Matadi and transported by ferry across the two-kilometer-wide Congo River. The high-power lines from the big dam at Inga to Kinshasa pass within ten kilometers of Luozi, east of the Congo River. Plans are underway to bring electricity to Luozi from a smaller hydroelectric installation near Inkisi. Photo: John M. Janzen, 2013.

this their central cause, and the politicians chosen endorsed it. The REGIDESO project was financed by the central government, and thus was probably authorized by Mobutu or his lieutenants just a few years before the end of his reign.

Lukwamusu noted that the system is vulnerable to mechanical breakdowns and ferry outages, since all diesel fuel comes via truck over the ferry. This vulnerability may be resolved when Luozi and the rest of the region are electrified, although surely there will be issues of distribution, payment, and maintenance. The Manianga electricity initiative has begun, with construction of a hydroelectric dam under way on the Inkisi River at Zongo Falls. It is said that completion was anticipated in 2015, but the project was not finished at the time of this writing in early 2018.

The presence of a pure water system in Luozi, even though it is flawed and sometimes disrupted for weeks or months, has made a noticeable impact on the incidence in waterborne diseases, especially infantile diarrhea and dysentery, and also bilharzia. Within the town, where water is available, diarrhea infection rates are half or less of what they are across the Territory of Luozi. There were no incidents of diarrhea or dysentery in our intensive sample households residing in the town of Luozi.

Any narrative that seeks to present a clear-cut picture of structures and programs, and how they were shaped by the collapse of the state in the 1980s and 1990s, will miss some of the popular initiatives that were taken over the years. In March 2013, when I visited Mbuta Kusikila, former communal mayor of Kivunda, he volunteered a detail I had never heard, about the improvement of the spring downhill from Kisiasia village. This was the water source from which we—or rather our water carrier, Sylvain—had drawn our drinking water. I had visited the spring a few times and had noted the fine job someone had done of cementing in the spring with a pipe so the water was always clean and good tasting and kept us free of diarrheal infections (figure 4.16). I had failed then to ask who had done this. Now Kusikila told me that he had done it himself as a teacher with a few student helpers back in 1958, several years before he ever ran for office. He had taken this initiative because in his teaching he had become aware of the important role of clean water to health. Yet this act of public health had not been part of any official campaign; it was an outgrowth of the educational process at the leading secondary school where he had studied. No doubt his action had a ripple effect to other villages in the Kivunda region. Already in the 1960s many had similar cemented-in springs as their sources for drinking and cooking water.

On my tour of the hamlets of Kisiasia, I noted that both hamlets had hand pumps for water centrally located on the main streets—situated, I was told by someone at a European NGO, to relieve the burden on women, who would otherwise have to walk to the valleys to get water. But both pumps were broken. The villagers did not know what was wrong with them or who could repair them. The

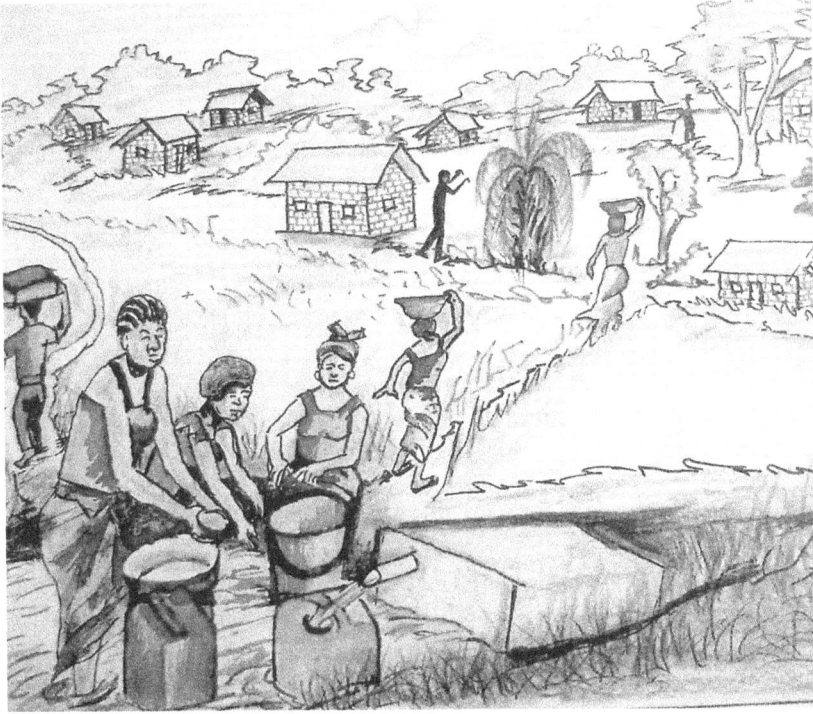

FIGURE 4.16. Women drawing water from an enclosed spring. Drawing by Emmanuel Mvibidulu, commissioned by John M. Janzen, 2013.

foreign installers apparently had not taught the people how to maintain the pumps or order repair parts. In his 2012 report the territorial administrator indicated that about half the pumps across the territory were broken and recommended that someone repair them. In Kisiasia, people once again used the cemented-in springs in the valleys, although that required about an hour's walk round-trip.

An acquaintance who works with a church NGO in the Congo explained why he kept coming back despite all the problems. He said he continued to be fascinated by this country full of promise, mysteries, and surprises. Kimpianga Mahaniah, Congolese visionary and an NGO organizer in the Manianga, observed after a pause over a Congolese meal that "defeat is never an option" in Congo. Both of these veteran observers of and actors in the Congo would nod, as if to prove their point, when they heard about the surprising development in this story of health in the Manianga. In 1993, the year when the directorate of the primary health care office in Kinshasa was pillaged, two years after the reinstatement of church-related medical organizations, and a few years before the outbreak of the civil war that would topple Mobutu, the town of Luozi inaugurated a pure water system.

CONCLUSION

Some observers and policy makers highlight the decentralized character of the reconfiguration of public health and health care after the collapse of the Zairean state, especially when they write about health zones as the centerpiece of the new arrangement and the fact that many of the zones are faith-based—that is, administered by ecclesiastical bodies. Although these features are important in an overview account of the reconfiguration, several equally significant features should also be noted.

The continuing absence of the state in shaping health and health care is fundamental to the reconfiguration. There appears to be no ultimate power broker in the mix, and this affects many people's perception of how they must go about shaping health and seeking health care. The strong persistence of local government in health infrastructure related to water quality and waste management is paradoxical in light of the state's relative fragility. Yet the case can be made that the two factors—the weak state and strong local government—are related, that they are two sides of the same coin. A less domineering central government allows for greater local responsibility.

Another important feature in the reconfiguration of institutions is the project-specific coordination of regional elites and power brokers to achieve particular ends, as exemplified in the development of the Luozi waterworks. The question now is how to ensure the institutional persistence of a facility like the waterworks, which depends on delicate infrastructural maintenance. As REGIDESO changes from a public to a private corporation, to whom will it be accountable when parts break down or diesel fuel is unavailable? Finally, the NGO sector of this reconfiguration of health and health care institutions needs to be considered—WHO and all the bilateral arrangements that channel funds, personnel, and services for specialized tasks like global inoculation campaigns. The reconfiguration of these institutions is a highly creative endeavor with unlimited potential. Yet as Monameso of the Luozi-based DOM noted, it is unstable. Any part can falter or fail at any time, imperiling the whole.

5

Rejoicing in Our Bodies

Popular Meanings of Health

C'est l'état complet de bien être physique, mental, social, mais ne consiste pas seulement de l'absence de l'infirmité [It is the complete state of physical, mental, social well-being, but does not consist only in the absence of disease].

　　—respondent, intensive sample survey

Mavimpi kima kia mbote kiena mu nitu kadi lenda baka ngolo mu sala bisalu [Health is a good thing for one's body; one can have force to do one's work].

　　—respondent, intensive sample survey

Someone has compared having "Good Health" to listening to "Good Music." Enjoying music requires good records (or CDs or MP3s) and a system to play them on. Similarly, "Good Health" requires good health interventions and a health system to play them on. However, too often the health system record player is broken. Meanwhile more attention (and funding) is concentrated on the intervention "CDs" rather than on repairing/maintaining the health system.

　　—Franklin Baer, "FBO Health Networks and Renewing Primary
　　Health Care"

The above lines are three disparate formulations of health, or good health. The first, by a lab technician in the referral hospital of the Luozi Health Zone, simply reiterates the World Health Organization's definition of health as enunciated in the 1970s launch of its primary health care campaign Health for All by the Year 2000. The second, by a Kongo peasant couple, focuses on health as the strength needed to carry out horticultural work in their fields. The third is a playful formulation by a seasoned public health physician who has devoted his career to the creation of health zones in the Democratic Republic of Congo. These three examples, and many more in this chapter, illustrate the public awareness needed to fashion health and health care.

Accordingly, this chapter examines some of the concepts related to health and health care that underlie the programs and institutions presented in the previous two chapters, as well as formulations of health that have governed health programs in Western nations in the past, and the scholarly perspective on health research. The centerpiece of this chapter is a closer look at the responses we received to several questions in the intensive sample "What does health/*mavimpi* mean to you?," "Are you satisfied with the health of your household?," and "Are there any further issues you would like to mention?"

Mavimpi is a word with multiple meanings, depending on the context in which it is used. It may serve as a greeting, as in *mavimpi maku*: health or well-wishes to you. But as the answers from the respondents in the study's intensive sample suggest, there are many nuances to the way individuals construe this quality of their well-being. Answers to the first question, "What does health/*mavimpi* mean to you?," fell into several thematic clusters reflecting occupation, education, and a range of convictions and preferences. Answers to the second question, "Are you satisfied with the health of your household?," revealed shortcomings in public health and health care provisions, as well as specific problems in the respondents' locales. The third question yielded laments about rising costs for children's school fees and medical care. Respondents' comments convey the sense that health-related aspirations are overwhelmed by economic and political crises. These responses, regardless of their variations and reflection of local circumstances, can provide a conceptual baseline for health educational campaigns and other health-care related endeavors. They constitute the first piece of evidence in the evaluation of the legitimacy of public health and health care institutions that is the topic of this work's later chapters.

Health in Anthropological Research

Thus far in this work I have used generic definitions of health that are tied to demography and epidemiology. The first of these involves the health implicit in rising birth rates, falling death rates, and population growth rates. The second is conveyed by both the incidence of diseases and the kinds of diseases that are prevalent—for example, whether they are contagious or related to old age. In this perspective, the general decline of both mortality and natality rates in the Lower Congo, alongside the recent population growth rate, suggests an overall improvement in health that mirrors worldwide trends. Yet the more nuanced responses to the question "What does health/*mavimpi* mean to you?" indicate a quite different popular perception, one fraught with economic pain in the face of frustrated middle-class aspirations. The gap between the objective, quantitative definitions of health and those that are more subjective and social reveals not only critical differences in the ways health is understood but also a range in the applications of these different definitions. The quantitative definitions are used by international health agencies to compare measures across continents and in national planning; the second are used in health education campaigns, in political and cultural portraits, and in community organization.

Anthropological and related social scientific studies of health have examined these different definitions of health and how they emerged in the history of societies, nations, and consciousness. The nineteenth-century rise of the modern nation-state brought to the fore biomedical notions about normalcy in a citizenry of workers, managers, and elites. The normal became the opposite of the abnormal or the marginal—health in contrast to un-health (Canguilhem 1966; Boorse 1977). It was the basis for priorities in building a national society of normal workers. Other nuances of health would be added to this construct. Health as both physical and social functioning emerged, with medical practitioners using what was considered normal functioning by age and cohort to determine whether one was meeting a collective norm in a host of areas, including weight, height, physical stamina, caloric intake, and sleep. Health as the absence of disease became the prevailing implicit definition in mid to late twentieth-century medicine as inoculations for contagious diseases became common, and surgeries, radiation, and chemical therapies became available for inappropriate growths of tissues in the body. By the mid-twentieth century a more ecological model of health began to emerge that incorporated the recognition that diseases were organisms and needed to be recognized in a larger framework as part of a community of organisms living together in competition for nutrition and biological space. In this model of health, adaptation of the human organism, or set of organisms, was often equated with health that was more than mere survival (Janzen 2002, 67–80).

The ecological perspective of health is foundational in the primary health care initiative. Launched in the 1970s by the World Health Organization (WHO) under the banner of Health for All by the Year 2000, primary health care was heralded as the path to better health in the world's poorer regions. It emphasized: "education concerning prevailing health problems and methods of preventing and controlling them; promotion of food supply and proper nutrition; an adequate supply of safe water and basic sanitation; maternal and child health care, including family planning; immunization against the major infectious diseases; prevention and control of locally endemic diseases; appropriate treatment of common diseases and injuries; and provision of essential drugs" (World Health Organization 1978).

Some dubbed this movement positive health. It would come to involve detailed analyses of the health of women and children and would identify the strong link between girls' education and fertility planning and control, and therefore better health for all. Thus, reproductive health became a part of primary health care.

Public health as seen in the primary health care movement, and as it was introduced in the Congo, including the Manianga, had a further feature. It viewed health care as a right, not merely a commoditized service available for a price. According to Nkoyi Bukonda, who invested an early part of his career in this program, public health "belongs to the people"; it is part of the commons that belongs to everyone, where risks should be shared and priorities set for the public good (Smith-Nonini 2006).[1]

HEALTH IN THE WORDS OF THE POPULACE

The intensive sample interviews, most of which were expertly conducted by Tata Luyobisa (figure 5.1), yielded a number of explicitly named values associated with health in response to the question *Wutu kamba mavimpi nki dieti songa?*—"What does health mean to you?" Responses reflected the diversity of participants' status, age, occupation, education, and religious orientation. Once respondents agreed to participate in the interview, they were offered a KiKongo or French set of questions, followed by an English translation. Here is a sampling of their responses, followed by the occupations of the respondents (first the husband's, then the wife's).

Living Well and Long

Seventeen percent of respondents noted that health meant quality of life, including the "education of our children."

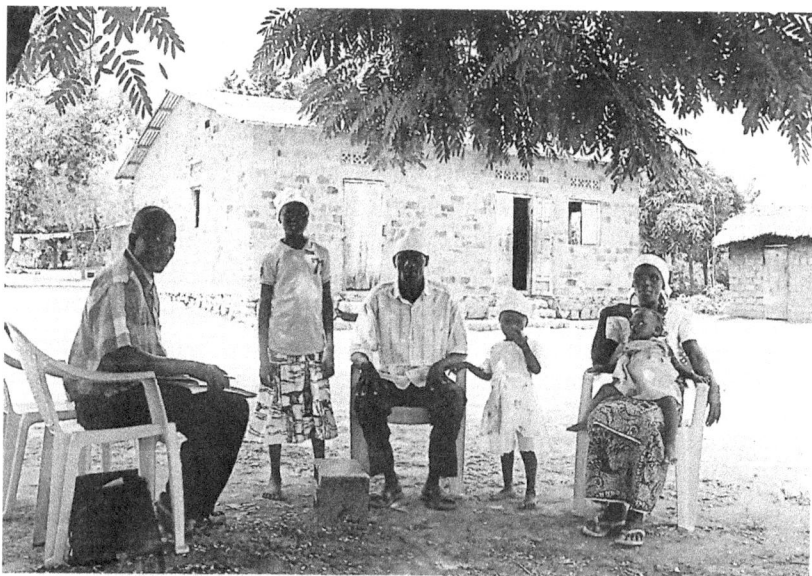

FIGURE 5.1. Tata Luyobisa administers one of 105 household interviews, 2013.

- *C'est une manière de bien vivre dans la vie*—[Health] is a manner of living well in one's life (university professor, teacher).
- *Mavimpi I luzingu lua mbote*—Health is to have a good life (fisher, seamstress).
- *Le bien vivre*—Living well (radio journalist, cultivator).
- *Mavimpi I ntomoso a nitu ye luzingu*—Health is the improvement of one's body and life (carpenter, cultivator).
- *C'est une bonne manière de bien vivre et de protection de la vie*—It is a good way to live well and to protect one's life (fisher-cultivator, cultivator).
- *C'est vivre en bonne état*—It is to live in a good state (or condition) (fisher, cultivator).
- *C'est bon moyen de vivre longtemps*—It is a way of living a long life (fisher, cultivator).
- *Mavimpi i mutula nitu mu bukindi ye mu lambula luzingu*—Health means to protect one's body in order to improve life (mason, cultivator).

Having Force in Your Body

Another 22 percent of respondents defined health in relation to the strength of their bodies, permitting them to perform their work. Many of these respondents worked with their bodies and hands as craftspeople or farmers. This feature has often been mentioned as a core belief of Central African religion. This may be true, but the following responses, with the prevalence of the idea that health equals the strength of one's body, also reflect a very practical understanding that if you wield a hoe, shovel, or machete all day you need to have a strong body.

- *Mavimpi mavananga ngolo mu nitu*—Health gives the body power, force (judge, cultivator).
- *Mavimpi meti songa vo muntu lenda sala bisalu bonso buka zolele*— Health means that a person can do his work as he wishes (carpenter, cultivator).
- *Mavimpi I mu kala nitu ngolo*—Health exists when the body is strong (both cultivators).
- *Idiambu dilutidi mu nena mu muntu, kadi vo wena mavimpi lenda sala dionso dilenda sala*—It is this that is the most important for a person, for with health one can do whatever work one wishes to do (fisher, cultivator).
- *Mavimpi kima kia mbote kiena mu nitu kadi lenda baka ngolo mu sala bisalu*— Health is a good thing for one's body, one can have force to do one's work (both cultivators).
- *Mavimpi I kima kia ntete mu zinitu zeto. Vo kuena mavimpi ko kulendi sala kima ko*—Health is the first thing required of our bodies; if one is not healthy, one can do nothing (both cultivators).

Being Clean and Pure

Another theme or value that emerged was that of cleanliness or purity: to keep one's body, the house, and the yard around the house clean and proper: *vedila nitu, vedila nzo*. Here are examples from this 7 percent of responses.

- *Mavimpi I mukukiba ba vedila*—Health consists in keeping pure and clean (both cultivators).
- *Mavimpi I vedila kua nitu*—Health is the purity of one's body (both cultivators).
- *Amelioration des conditions de vie; assenisement, propriété; aeration de la maison*—[Health is] the amelioration of the conditions of life; sweeping up, cleanliness; aeration of the house (retired administrator, assistant territorial administrator).
- *La santé pour une personne n'a pas de prix. Il est tres important de toujour garder son corps propre et eviter de consumer ni d'aborder des produits toxiques dans le corps. [On] risque de ruiner la santé et d'affaiblir les globules*—The health of a person does not have a price. It is very important to always keep one's body clean and to avoid consuming or being close to toxic products in the body. Otherwise one risks ruining one's health and compromising one's blood (city administrator, homemaker).

The ideas of purity (*vedila*) and pollution (*nsumununu*) have a ritual aspect in Kongo tradition. The terms have been adopted by linguists in the translation of the Bible to signify redemption and sin, respectively. It is therefore not surprising that other terms of this ritual complex—sanctity, peace, and benediction—emerge in discussions of health.

- *La santé c'est avoir un corps saint*—Health is to have a sacred, holy body (both cultivators).
- *C'est la paix du corps*—[Health] is bodily peace (cultivator).
- *Mavimpi I lusakumunu lutulambudi kua Tata Nzambi mu sala momo mu tuena nsatu*—Health is the benediction given by God to do the work that one wishes to do (pastor-prophet-cultivator, homemaker-cultivator).

Rejoicing in Your Body

A further 17 percent of responses interpret health to consist of rejoicing either in their bodies or in life in general, including having a spirit of hope. When I first heard this response, the visualization that came to mind was the energetic exuberance so apparent in singing and dancing.

- *Mavimpi dieti songa vo nitu yena mavimpi ngieti yangalala*—Health shows that the body is well, that I rejoice (domestic).
- *Kala kiese mu nitu*—[Health] is to have joy in the body (cultivator).
- *Mavimpi ma songele kiese mu nitu evo nkedulu ya mbote ye kiese mu zinga*— Health means rejoicing in one's body, or to have joy in one's whole life (tailor-healer, cultivator).
- *Vimpi dieti songa kiese mu nitu*—[Health] means rejoicing in one's body (industrial worker, cultivator).
- *Mavimpi I mu kala nitu kiese*—Health is to have joy in one's body (fisher, cultivator).
- *Mavimpi I mu baka luvuvamu mu nitu*—Health is to have hope in one's body (carpenter, cultivator).

Expressions of health listed thus far are rooted in Kongo tradition—strength, purity and sanctity, rejoicing—and applied to the exigencies of contemporary life. Each of these expressive categories or themes could be elaborated with further analysis and association with occupations, social roles, phases of life, or religious orientations.

Functionality, Normality, and Good Judgment

Other expressions of health clearly echo theories of public health and medical philosophy. In the primary health care definition of health, the words *function* and *normal* reflect the conceptual standards of modern medical diagnosis and therapy. However, the final three responses below are less clearly influenced by modern medicine. They appear to reflect self-conscious valuation of good judgment and independent thinking.

- *C'est l'état de bien-etre physique et mentale*—[Health] is the state of physical and mental well-being (administrator-bureaucrat, lab technician).
- *C'est l'état complet de bien etre physique, mental, social, mais ne consiste pas seulement de l'absence de l'infirmite*—[Health] is the complete state of physical, mental, social well-being, but does not consist only in the absence of disease (university student, lab technician).
- *Kala wa siama kondwa kimbevo*—[Health means] to be well without sickness (cultivator, librarian).
- *La santé est un état d'une personne d'ou les organs fonctionnent bien*—Health is the state of a person whose organs function well (teacher, cultivator).
- *Avoir un corps normal*—To have a normal body (both cultivators).
- *Mavimpi I diambu dilenda tuvana nduenga mutina bimbevo*—Health is something that gives us the intelligence to avoid sicknesses (both cultivators).

- *Mavimpi dieti songa vo muntu lenda kala ye nitu ya mbote, lenda vanga mamo meti vanga muntu; nduenga zandi zena za mbote*—Health means that the person has a sound body, that he can do all that he wishes, and that his intelligence is in order (mason, cultivator).
- *Mavimpi dikutuvananga ngolo mu yindula*—Health gives us strength to reflect (both cultivators).

Ambiguities and puzzles remain in this cross-section of expressions of the meaning of health/*mavimpi* in Manianga thought, as represented in the intensive sample of 105 households. The three final responses may have their roots in Kongo thought, although they clearly incorporate the common recent Western idea of the desirability of individual agency in health. The emphasis on agency suggests the importance of taking control of one's destiny with regard to health, healing, and the creation of a healthy environment.

I was surprised to see no evidence of several of the central ideas about health that I gleaned from healers in the 1960s. Where was the idea of balance between humans, and between the human world and nature? What about the notion of flow (or blockage) of fluids, food, and social exchange? How would Nganga Nzoamambu's theory of the person, of the heart as the head of the person in health and sickness, fit this picture (Janzen 1978)?

TAKING ISSUE

The final question in section 5 of the intensive sample questionnaire asked respondents to offer any further issues they wished to raise: *Nkia mpila mampasi ma sidi mu kubika?*—What kinds of issues remain to be dealt with? The previous question had asked if they were satisfied with health in their household, and almost all had said they were very pleased. The outpouring of comments and complaints in response to the final question was therefore surprising. The 105 narrative responses we received provide a rich source of opinion, conviction, and critique regarding issues of health and public affairs.

Our informants raised concerns about particular diseases, problems with water, quality and quantity of available food, the high cost of living and the difficulty of paying children's school fees, the prohibitive cost of medical care, the pain and struggle of daily living, and above all disappointment with the state for not living up to widespread expectations about its responsibility to engage with the populace and to be sensitive to its needs. This is clear evidence of the political nature of health and well-being.

A first and most obvious area of concern was the diseases that continue to affect the health of the people of Luozi and the Manianga. Malaria, the major disease that afflicts nearly everyone and is the leading cause of death in the region, was mentioned by only one respondent. This suggests that it is regarded as a normal or unavoidable condition. Respondents were more concerned about, or at least more inclined to mention, other diseases. Bilharzia, onchocerciasis (river blindness), and filariasis were mentioned by village cultivators and fishers whose main water source was streams or rivers, and who did not have access to a good source of pure water.

- *Numanisa malaria tueti lomba kua beno bisi mputu mutu vana lusadusu*—To combat malaria we ask you of the North to give us help (both cultivators).
- *Nous cherchons comment s'en sortir contre l'epidemie de la bilharziose*—We are looking for a way to end this epidemic of bilharzia (fisher, cultivator).
- *Mpasi zeto i maza matueti nianga ka mena ma mbote ko . . . Tueti lomba mpasi leta evo zi organisme international za mavimpi mu kuiza kutu kuludila mpasi zo, Bilarziose. Kadi nkangu weti mena beba. Fisidi ko nga mavata 10 tunuanga maza ma bilharziose*—Our problem is that our water is not good. We ask for help from the state or international health organizations to deal with this bilharzia. Perhaps ten villages are using water so infested (carpenter, cultivator).
- *Nous cherchons la contribution ou participation du gouvernement de pouvoir nous proteger contre l'oncheroiseuse ou filariose*—We ask for the government to be able to protect us from onchocerciasis (river blindness) or filariasis (fisher, and cultivator).
- *Si nous pouvons avoir des gens qui peuvent nous aider a trouver des solutions sur les maladies que nous trouvons etrange: ex-l'AVC, la tension, la diabete*—If we could have experts to help us find solutions for strange diseases: ex-AVC, hypertension, diabetes (teacher, cultivator).

Clean water is a major preoccupation in the health consciousness of people because it is the means by which to eliminate of all sorts of waterborne diseases, such as diarrhea, typhus, dysentery, and even cholera. Some of the respondents requested maintenance or improvement of existing clean-water installations—for example, ensuring that the Luozi system did not have disruptions, or that it reached the higher-altitude households, or that springs once enclosed be maintained or repaired. Some were simply asking for improved water provided by a pump and well.

- *Amelioration et fonctionement de la REGISIDO: pas d'interruptions; fournir les parcels élévés*—Improve the functioning of the Regie des Eaux to eliminate interruptions and furnish water to the most elevated parcels (retired administrator, assistant territorial administrator).
- *Mpasi tueti mona mu sungula ko maza ma ndua Tueti lomba kua luyalu katu banzila mu kutu sukudila minlangu*—We have difficulty with our drinking water; we ask the government to clean our stream (tailor, cultivator).

- *Maza matunuanga meti kutulukisila bimbevo vo bulendakana mu kuiza kutu tudila bipompi aspirante va buala*—The water we drink makes us sick; may someone come to install a pump and well in our village (both cultivators).
- *Renforcer l'état de nos sources, car ils ne sont plus en bonne état*—Improve the quality of our springs; they are not in a good state (pastor and head of church post, retired nurse).
- *La source n'est pas amelioré; manque d'eau potable*—The spring is not encased; we lack clean drinking water (hospital chaplain, cultivator).

Food and nutrition are a further focus of the comments. Some lamented the simple lack of adequate food. Others complained of the bad quality of available food. A number asserted the principle that health depends on a good diet, and where this exists, diseases will be at a minimum. Others linked particular dietary weaknesses to specific diseases, such as hypertension.

- *Ndiuwulu vo y ena ya mbote, buna bimbevo kabidilendi kala ko*—If the diet is good, then there can be no illness (tailor, cultivator).
- *la consummation des aliments et autres chairs non-appropries pour la consommation. Ici l'état doit interdir l'importation de certains produits impropre, a la consommation*—Consumption of inappropriate foods and other meats; the state should forbid the importation of certain inappropriate products (city mayor, homemaker).
- *Malnutrition; pas de nourriture suffisant*—Malnutrition; insufficient food (university student, seamstress).
- *Ndiwulu yena ya mpasi beni i diadio dieti kuamisa zi nitu*—[Lack of] food gives us great pain, which is why our bodies suffer (mason, cultivator).
- *Parce que la population n'est pas bien nourri, elle devienne de plus en plus pauvre et malade*—Because the population is not well nourished, it becomes increasingly poor and sick (radio journalist, cultivator).
- *Ndiwulu yaka ya mbi*—Our food is bad (carpenter, cultivator).
- *Manque de proteine de la viande; on ne mange que plus de legume, c'est pourquoi il y a beaucoup de cas de l'exces de sang*—Lack of meat protein; people only eat legumes, which is why there are many cases of high blood pressure (pastor, nurse).

The maintenance of a clean house and yard was mentioned in a number of comments as contributing to good health. A few extended the importance of this practice to public spaces and streets as well.

- *Faire la sarclage tout autour de la maison*—Sweep around the house (chauffer, seamstress).

- *[On] doit se proteger contre la salette, se controler avant de manger*—One should protect oneself against being dirty, clean oneself before eating (merchant, seamstress).
- *Mvindu ya kinzungidila*—Removing filth in our surroundings (mechanic-chauffer, merchant).
- *L'insalubrite au niveau des avenues et aux entourages*—Filth in the streets and in the environment (NGO project director, teacher).

Many comments in this section connect shortcomings of health and lack of access to health care, narrowly defined, to shortcomings in the economy. A major source of the pain in daily life was the shortage of money, plain and simple. This economic failure or shortcoming extended to the lack of hospitals and health centers, the failure to properly maintain roads, the collapse of thriving markets that could bring good food and other goods, the absence of clean water wells, and the inability to afford school fees to properly educate children. These are the laments of living in a neoliberal and globalized economy in which everything is commoditized. What you have to sell brings low prices, and what you must buy is high.

- *Nsi eto ka yena ya mbote ko mu zingisa bantu. Mpasi za mbongo mu futa ku hopitila ye biskulu mpasi beni mu manisa bana mu skulu*—Our land does not do well at helping people live. It is difficult to pay hospital costs, and fees to get children through school (both cultivators).
- *Tueti mona mpasi mu luzingu*—We are suffering in our life (photographer, cultivator).
- *Nzingulu yaku RDC yena ya mpasi beni*—Living in the DRC is a struggle (blacksmith, cultivator).
- *Scolarisation des enfants est trop exorbitant*—Children's education fees are exorbitant (teacher, seamstress).
- *Ka tu tudilema companie kadi kiese mpia, mbongo nkatu; ndiwulu ya mbi; hopital mbongo za saka*—We need employers, for there is no joy, no money; food is bad, hospital fees extreme (carpenter, cultivator).
- *On paie chere a l'hopital. La vie devien de plus en plus dure*—One pays dearly at the hospital; life is increasingly difficult (teacher).

The litany of woes that one heard regularly became a kind of ritualistic performance, summed up with the recurring comment that the people had lost hope. Conditions of health, of life itself, were difficult because the country was in a bad state economically. Many of the comments express the desire that someone, usually the government, but also international agencies or companies would come to aid them in improving the people's lot.

CONCLUSION

The popular formulations of what health is and the popular concerns with un-achieved health may be seen as the first dimension of the legitimacy of an enter-prise as important as public health and health care. The people's voices, both their ideas about health and their laments about their leaders and circumstances, set the stage for the final three chapters.

PART III

The Legitimation of Power and Knowledge

6

Dumuna

Creating Authority from Below

Nsi vo yitumona beto tuna zinga, kansi vo nsi kayeti toma ko, beto i mpila mpasi mu toma zinga [If the land thrives, we will live; but, if the land doesn't thrive, we will have difficulty improving our lives].

> —Mama Jacqueline, Janzen intensive sample interview, 2013

In the Congo, failure is not an option.

> —Professor Kimpianga Mahaniah, founder, Centre de Vulgarisation
> Agricole; rector, Free University of Luozi. Comment to Janzen

Political legitimacy is rooted in the ability to fuse power and right in the service of the common interest.

> —Herman H. H. van Erp, British philosopher (2000, 197)

The voices in the epigraphs above bring together several strands of conviction and action regarding the links between the health of a society and its people, the critical role of leaders' resolve to pursue initiatives that bring about a better state of affairs, and the Western scholarly definition of legitimacy of power.[1] The first voice is that of a matron who conveys the popular understanding that individual well-being is tied to social well-being; thus for individuals to be healthy, society—the land, the *nsi*—needs to thrive. This term combines the meanings of "earth" and "country." The second speaker is a prominent educator, founding president of a Congolese development NGO, and rector of a university that trains many health care technicians and caregivers. He strongly advocates resolve, not even considering wavering in the face of serious challenges. The third voice is that of a scholar who has reviewed multiple definitions of legitimacy and formulated his own understanding of the concept. Out of the diverse echoes of popular, elite, and scholarly voices we may fashion our analysis of the legitimacy of the institutions and practices that shape public health and health care in the Lower Congo.

Social Legitimation:
Western and Kongolese Theories

The legitimacy of institutions and their leadership has been an active concern in social science scholarship and writing for many years. Legitimation theory emerged to inquire into the ways in which power is accepted and thus legitimized in society. Different types of authority became standard vocabulary in scholarship as well as public discourse. In Max Weber's tripartite typology of authority (*Herrschaft*), traditional authority, as found in archaic and local societies, rested in the legitimacy of custom, the acceptance in a society of having always done something in a certain way, presided over by elders or priests. Charismatic authority, as found in religious and political movements, recognized the impact of a society's superheroes in offering justification for new ideas and constructions that entered into practice and norms. Many scholars, and possibly Weber himself, judged that charisma was not intrinsic but was found in the credence lent to a popular leader. Finally, rational-legal authority, as found in the bureaucracies of states and large institutions, represented the role of law, courts, and explicitly systematic procedures in the governing of a modern nation-state (Weber 1980).

Weber's foundational work came to be seen as increasingly problematic in late twentieth- and twenty-first-century scholarship (Hesse 1979) because of its exclusive focus on the state (Beetham 1991). Modern secular states, large corporate organizations, and global political movements and networks required other kinds of perspectives. The "crisis of legitimacy" exposed by Jürgen Habermas (1975), who is seen as a perpetuator of the Weberian paradigm (Isenboeck 2006; Schechter 2013), identifies modern secular society's difficulties in providing a sense of solidarity such as that offered by nationalism, ethnicity, and religion, by way of a "transcendent" quality or identity. Habermas questions whether a complex secular society and secular state are even capable of offering individuals any meaningful identity. He has written (and continues to write) critical views of the European Union, with regard to the reemergence of its subnationalities despite, and therefore in contradiction to, its economic sovereignty.

Alternatives to the Weber-Habermas state-centric understanding of social legitimacy look at more basic attributes of sociopolitical organization. David Beetham defines legitimacy as the conformity of power to established rules, its justifiability by reference to beliefs shared by both dominant and subordinate parties, and evidence of consent on the part of the subordinate party (Beetham 1991; Pierson 1992). This analysis is particularly useful to our examination of Equatorial Africa because he explores legitimacy in a number of settings outside of Western industrial democracies, including Islamic societies, nonlegitimate expressions of state power, and both legitimate and nonlegitimate power entirely outside of the state. What we need for the present project, however, are theoretical formulations of nonstate actors and institutions that take the place of the state by providing services formerly expected of the state.

The notion of governmentality has been put forward by a number of theorists to describe both state and nonstate agencies as "a range of forms of action and fields of practice aimed in a complex way at steering individuals and collectives," and allowing for "a plurality of governmental rationalities, . . . depending on assumptions about starting points, means and goals, criteria of legitimacy, and acceptability" (Brockman, Krassling, Lemke 2011). Governmentality by itself has been productively applied to situations with a range of nonstate players, such as international NGOS and private entities. Ronnie Lipschutz extends the notion to entities that are not strictly state entities, noting that they draw their legitimacy from global civil society networks and from the "capillaries of social power" (Lipschutz 2005). In other words, the combined presence of local jurisdictions, special-interest NGOs, and ad hoc initiatives constitute multiple legitimacies with a variety of bases. Such a diversity of governmentality is "associated with biopolitics, . . . which is concerned with matters of life and death, with birth and propagation, with health and illness, both physical and mental, and with the processes that sustain or retard the optimization of the life of a population" (Lipschutz 2005, 236).

Analysts Maria Rusca and Klaas Schwartz (2012) speak of the "divergent sources of legitimacy" that take the place of the "hollow state" in bringing international NGOs to deal with the all-important service of urban water provisioning. They point out that NGOs operating in many African settings have tended to seek legitimacy in the accomplishment of a given task, rather than formal, normative, or legal legitimacy—that is, recognition as legal within a host country's laws. This has often caused friction between project output and normative legitimacy in development settings.

In situations where government fails entirely or substantially, other agencies must be introduced or called to life to deliver urgent services. Joanne Macrae, who addresses the post-civil war situation, suggests that the most important feature of organizational or initiative legitimation is "finding a constitution for decision-making" (Macrae 1997). In conditions of crisis resulting from a power vacuum, finding a constitution means taking control of decision making about the use and distribution of internal or external resources, and determining whether that is agreed to by those most affected. Multilateral agencies can exert leverage in defining basic health planning, or a neutral party can mediate with local institutions. In the case of internal institutions such as those that emerged in the Congo to coordinate health care and public health after the collapse of the state and its ministries in the 1990s, the same qualifications for legitimacy will obtain—namely, do they represent a constitution for legitimate decision making over resources?

A further socially embedded understanding of the legitimation of power features the critical moment when dissatisfied citizens object to a loss of voice or to a situation that upsets them, or they find themselves in a conflict with authorities (Boltanski and Thévenot 1999). Debate, discussion, and the expression of grievances between the subjects and authorities, along with the invocation of a narrative rooted in former traditions or values, become a form of justification that yields a new legitimacy embraced by both parties to the dispute (1999, 360–61). In the Lower Congo such a critical moment would be citizens' all-too-frequent lament of the withering of the state, of their rulers' abdication of responsibility, and of the withdrawal of the state from its obligations.

The fragmentation of power in the Congo gives us pause, however. Is the Boltanski-Thévenot model of a critical moment that is followed by debate, leading to the imperative of justification, at all fitting for the failed-state situation in which there is no one with whom the citizens can debate? When there is no they there? The articulation of social theory around the absence or fragmentation of power needs to be carefully considered too. Kongo thought and political theory has much to offer in this common situation. We will move to that perspective via the central axiom of the Foucauldian paradigm: that the state shapes subjectivity, which internalizes biopower. Paul Geissler, Richard Rottenburg, and Julia Zenker (2012) warn against applying Foucault's framework reflexively and reductionistically simply because it has been so successful in other settings. This warning is especially valid where dysfunctional institutions and serious chronic diseases and poverty make an impact upon subjectivity, or where internalized power is not the biopower of a nineteenth-century total institution, but rather the abyss in the wake of the collapsed kingdom, chiefdom, or postcolonial state. Can we envision the subjectivity of such biopower? This absence of state biopower may be seen as yielding to the upsurge of the illegitimate, diffuse, and dangerous power that the people and scholars usually refer to as witchcraft or sorcery (Geschiere 1997; Schatzberg 2001; Ashworth 2005), as do Kongo theories of power and legitimation.

The scope of social legitimation ideas and idioms in Kongo conceptions of health and the practice of healing cover much the same ground as the social science ideas explicated above. This is particularly the case because we are looking at institutions that must operate without state sanction, or with a missing or toxic state. Furthermore, some of the impetus for the operation of these initiatives and institutions arises from the people's own convictions. In the absence of public financing or insurance coverage for health care, the question of who pays for medical services is of critical importance. A Kongo pattern of shared cost within the nuclear and extended family, or lineage, is supported by traditional convictions that such sharing is essential to the survival of the family line. In earlier work I identified this process as "therapy management," and the ad hoc but sanctioned set of individuals who came together to discern and accompany the sufferer through therapy as the "therapy managing group" (Janzen 1978, 1987, 2002). The creation and nurturing of alliances built on marriage are also seen as essential for survival in times of health crisis. Education, professionalization, and emigration to a land of greater opportunity become part of this moral framework of the family.

But in Kongo thought and tradition there is a sense of the essential connection between sickness and social chaos, as well as their converse, health and social order. In the admittedly haphazard record of evidence for this equation, very often the justification for recruitment of an individual to a position of authority—as a chief or healer—is the individual's sickness, which is considered to be a form of calling from the ancestor or spirit world. The initiation to such an office is a therapeutic ritual that culminates in the endorsement of the individual by a wide circle of supportive allies. The extent to which such a traditional order of both ideas and instituted roles or social arrangements exist today depends on particular circumstances.

Scholars have identified a wider Central African pattern of social roles that are the site of legitimate and illegitimate power. Michael Schatzberg, writing about power and authority in ten countries of "Middle Africa," sees the common structure as centered on a father figure (chief, president, or other leader), spirituality (whether traditional, ancestor-based, Christianity, or Islam), and sorcery (the other of enemies, illicit use of any means in opposition) (2001). Wyatt MacGaffey (1970b) has put forward a structure of authority that is identified with much of Central Africa, but especially Kongo society, based on four interrelated roles: the chief (*mfumu*), the prophet (*ngunza*), the priest or magician-healer (*nganga*), and the witch or sorcerer (*ndoki*). He refers to these social categories as "religious commissions" because they are all imbued with a transcendent aura.

Chiefship in Kongo thinking is associated with a strong hand, resolute decision-making, the wisdom to settle conflicts, and ultimately the will to use the sword—or poison or another method—in the interest of the public good. Modern chiefs are but a faint echo of the image of the powerful chiefs of old. Mercantile traders and the colonial government destroyed the big historic chiefs, who regularly had thieves executed and are even said to have sacrificed kinspeople in their inaugurations. Nevertheless, the image of the chief is that of someone who has the will to take life—literally or mystically—for the good of the community. A legitimate and powerful chief or authority is essential in creating a viable social order.

The witch, or sorcerer (*ndoki*), on the other hand, who also is associated with death and killing, uses power, including mystical means, for self-enrichment at the expense of the public good. In Kongo thinking about power, *kundu* is the visible physiological accumulation of life energy that the *bandoki* have taken from their victims. Detecting *kundu* was the one reason for performing autopsies on human cadavers in the premodern era. In more recent times *kundu* became a metaphor to describe the disintegrative effects of European colonial influence (for example, money, power, education, foreign knowledge) that caused people to envy one another. In the ideology of this *kundu* power, an effective chief or family head should be able to bring together assets—wealth, individual influence, knowledge—for the betterment of the community.

The role of the prophet (*ngunza*) is that of an unpredictable critic of established power, an outside innovator who has interests in the public good similar to those of the chief. The role of prophet, though not well documented, emerges no later than the eighteenth century with Kimpa Vita, also known as Dona Beatrice, a priestess/prophetess who sought to restore the Kongo kingdom, which had been paralyzed by a succession conflict. The current lines of prophets date back to Simon Kimbangu and others who in 1921, early in Belgian colonialism, sought to revitalize Kongo society. Kimbangu, his adherents, and other prophets were perceived as a direct threat to the colonial order and were mercilessly hunted down, imprisoned, exiled, and kept under close surveillance until the late 1950s, the eve of independence.

The herbalist-healer-magician (*nganga*) shares some of the outside-innovator power with the prophet, but in a more technical sense. These specialists, historically and today, are masters of medicines and other techniques that address both physical and mystical issues. They divine the causes of misfortune, find witches, neutralize evil medicines, and heal the sick.

MacGaffey expands his model of power in Kongo society to incorporate the work of Mary Douglas on the differences between legitimate and illegitimate power. This difference is mainly couched in the effect on and perception of those affected by a fraught relationship or situation. Individuals may be seen as expressing either legitimate or illegitimate action, depending on the context and outcome of their actions with regard to furthering the public good. This is why those who perform great technological feats are sometimes seen with ambivalence. Whether they are good *ndoki*—or have good *kindoki*—depends on whether their contribution achieves the public good or is seen as robbing from the public for personal enrichment.

Although old-style powerful chiefs have not been seen since early colonial days, the picture of society given here continues to operate in the minds of many and in institutions. The reintroduction of traditional chiefship by the postcolonial state reminds people of what chiefs once could do, although now they are on the lowest rung of an administrative chain of command. People still consult prophets and healers, who interpret misfortunes. If events in the lives of people are seen as caused by human ill will or social chaos, the prophet or healer may identify individual actors in order to neutralize them or to protect the victim from them. Although the accusation of sorcery is regarded legally as serious slander, sorcery identifications have occurred in recent years, with a few cases of mob killings, described in chapter 4, during the chaotic preelection year of 2008. In 2013 we were told of two cases of sudden deaths that friends and family members interpreted as a mystical taking of life for personal gain.

All four of the Kongo commissions are believed to possess transcendental power, which may be either positive or negative, depending on the context and who is using it for what purpose. According to both the ethnographic literature and contemporary informants, standing over against the force of *kundu* accumulation and *kiungu*, both negative qualities defined by "eating too much," is the innate power of *mayembo*, which enables the holder to locate hidden objects, discern the thoughts of others, diagnose a disease, or find or identify a thief (Laman 1923, 26). *Mayembo* is a quality of spirit indicated by cramps or trembling of the body. It manifests itself in several modes: controlled expression, ecstatic outbursts of an unconscious nature, and that which comes suddenly with external stimulation, such as seeing something turning, hearing a steady rhythm, or clapping on water. For many people *mayembo* induces crying, trembling, and rolling on the ground. *Mayembo* is used to find sorcerers, to locate evil spirits that are attacking someone, and to interrogate spirits of the dead. Spirits of *minkisi* (or *bakisi*) manifest themselves in this way to come help the kin of the possessed. Drumming, dancing, hand clapping, or flapping a cloth can extend the ecstasy of *mayembo* to others, who then experience sympathetic ecstatic seizures. This technique is used to return the soul of a sick person to his or her body.

Contemporary prophets Tata Mayangi and Tata Luyobisa enhanced the foregoing portrayal from Laman's text of a century ago with several points, specifying that *mayembo* manifests itself in different places on the body: tingling in the hands that one feels before performing the rites of blessing, healing, and weighing of the spirit; twitching in the shoulders, which a hunter feels before success in hunting game, due to the way the hunter carries game home on the shoulders; twitching of the eyes before "seeing" spirits. Mayangi confirmed that this was how *bakisi* used to come to *banganga*, and how the Holy Spirit now comes to *bangunza*. This source of legitimation is signaled in the ritual of *dumuna* in healing, the blessing of interclan alliances, inauguration to chiefly office, and in the weighing-of-the-spirit rite of prophetic churches.

Mbuta Kusikila, the mayor of the commune of Kivunda in the north Manianga from 1960 to 1972, explained to me his understanding of Kongo social intricacies and values. His was the most sophisticated analysis I encountered among Kongo politicians and administrators. He not only gave me the standard explanations of events and issues; he had developed original theories that often reflected his wide reading. But most of all he was wise and could theorize his experience. I found his views on power most intriguing because he tied them to *kindoki* (what people called witchcraft) on the one hand, and to sickness and healing on the other. He understood *kindoki* to be the ability of a person to influence and affect others, for good or for ill. This is close to the classical meaning of the proto-Bantu term *loka*, the root of *kindoki*, the power of words. Chiefs, elected mayors, and presidents possessed legitimate *kindoki* and needed it to govern, whereas what most people called witches, sorcerers, or *bandoki* were those who used *loka* in an antisocial, illegitimate manner. The latter was what people feared. People who had grown up in colonialism did not know what legitimate power was or what it looked like. But in Kusikila's understanding it was made up of persons like himself, duly elected, exercising power for the good of society (figures 6.1 and 6.2).

The importance of the will of leaders or persons in positions of authority to assert themselves in the enactment of health and well-being is evident in cases Kusikila related to me in which he had exercised his authority in communities where dissent and chaos reigned, and where people were sick. In one such situation he had ordered the community to clean up their houses and streets by his deadline, or else he would imprison them. Their complaints stopped, as did their sickness. They became his strong supporters. He had used his positive *kindoki* for the well-being of this community.

Kusikila systematized his insights on power and legitimacy in the booklet *Lufwa evo Kimongi e?* (Death or Pestilence, 1966). *Lufwa* is the straightforward Kikongo term for death. *Kimongi*, on the other hand, is translated as pestilence, or foreign or strange death. The two words represent the two opposing poles of the

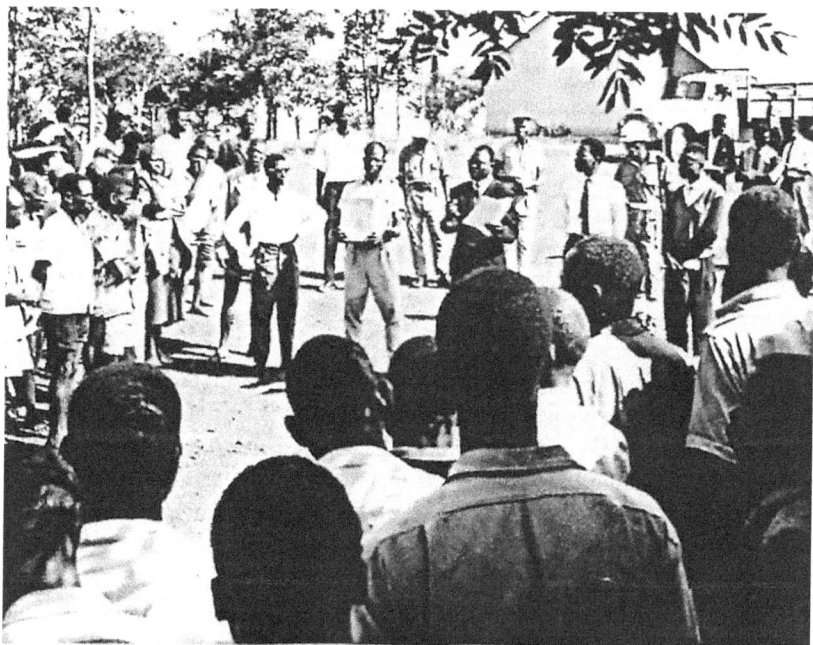

FIGURE 6.1. Yoswa Kusikila as communal mayor, explaining the balloting in the general elections while potential voters and police officers listen attentively. Photo: John M. Janzen, 1965.

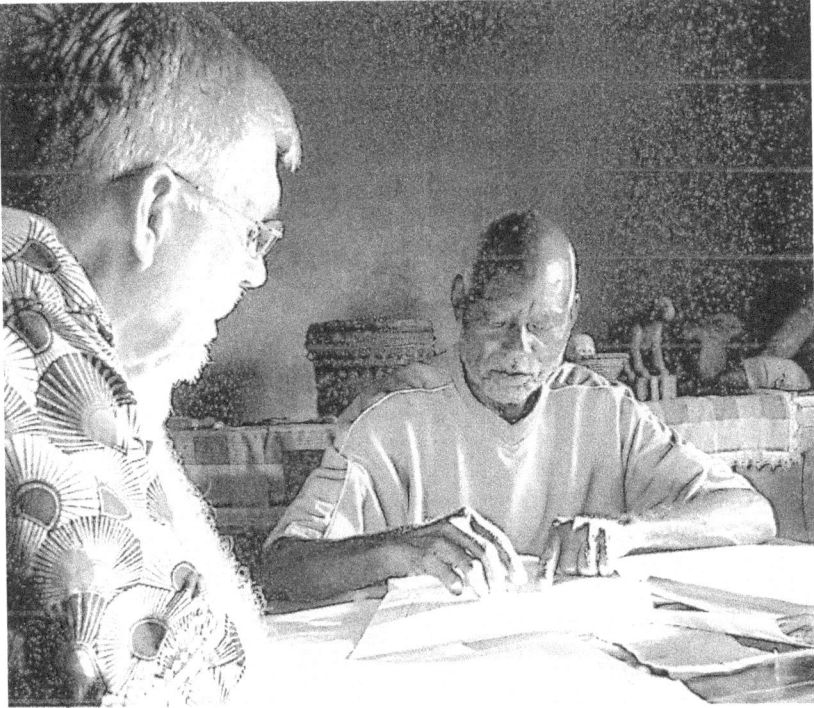

FIGURE 6.2. Conversation with Kusikila, at his home in Tadi (Kivunda). Kusikila is the author of *Lufwa evo Kimongi?* (Death or Pestilence?), an essay on political authority and legitimacy produced in the 1960s while he was an active leader and judge in Kivunda. It remains one of the most thorough articulations of the nature of power by a Kongo practitioner. Photo: Reinhild Janzen, March 2013.

diviner's dichotomy: a death can be straightforward, "of God" (*lufwa*), or it can be "of man" (*kimongi*). However, the framework is broader than that employed by most diviners.

Kusikila describes the causes of *kimongi*, the strange, unnatural death. Adultery leads to broken homes, sexually transmitted diseases, infertility, and a declining birth rate; parental ignorance leads to sick children; malice leads to diseases that cannot be treated by medicines. Although there are literal poisons that kill people, metaphorical poisons are more pervasive and injurious (for example, wrong instructions in school, certain kinds of study abroad that alienate the youth from their home country and traditions, the shunning of agriculture, wanting to be like Europeans, and abandonment of one's language). Breaking oaths leads to loss of trust in institutions like courts, economic contracts, and civil service. Reliance on magic (from Europe) or the lust after easy riches and theft, instead of work, leads to a kind of craziness. Slavery and colonial forced labor led to a distaste for work. Finally Kusikila comes to witchcraft, where he develops his theory of legitimate and illegitimate power. A country must develop in the vision of its true nature to prosper. Each country has its roots where it must find its future. He closes with a call to enlightenment, a challenge to build on science and leadership and to escape the reign of pestilence.

Academic legitimation theory and Kongo thought and ritual share several common features. Power may be legitimate or illegitimate. The former is used for the common good, the latter for personal gain at the expense of the common good. The common good in both traditions reflects the consent of the weakest members of society to actions taken by the most powerful, usually on their behalf. This is possible where there are laws or procedures, summarized in a set of principles like a constitution that everyone agrees on and that is grounded in commonly held precepts. In some of the academic theories and emphatically in Kongo thought, all power, legitimate and illegitimate alike, is anchored in transcendent reality. In Kongo theory, the legitimate common good is a form of public health of the polity; by contrast, its absence is considered a form of public sickness.

I discussed, debated, and mulled over these formulations of the legitimation of power with a number of individuals in various combinations and settings during my time in the Lower Congo (figures 6.3 and 6.4). Considerations of the legitimation of power in social order and social healing provide analytical avenues for understanding the divergent legitimations currently structuring and carrying out health and health care in the Manianga.

Dumuna—Creating and Restoring Legitimate Power

The evocative ritual of *dumuna* offers a touchstone to the deeper current of innovation, renewal, and assertion of legitimate authority in Kongo history. *Dumuna* is the outward manifestation of transcendence, or contact with the spirit world. Anyone who has seen or experienced this ritual remembers it forever: a vigorous set of three leaping, jumping handshakes or other physical contact between the one being jumped and the one administering the jumping. Although *dumuna* is nowadays known as a ritual practiced by prophet churches in the Lower Congo, it has a broader and much older history that a few informants suggest dates back to eighteenth-century prophetess Kimpa Vita, or Dona Beatrice, if not to the counselors of the earliest kings in the Kongo kingdom. I am using instances of the ritual *dumuna* here as a kind of canary in the coal mine to identify situations and developments in social relations that were deemed in need of recharging, or recentering. The photographs and ethnographic accounts and my personal observations of the rite offer a few of its applications that illustrate its likely purpose or consequence in a variety of domestic and public settings (figures 6.5 to 6.8).

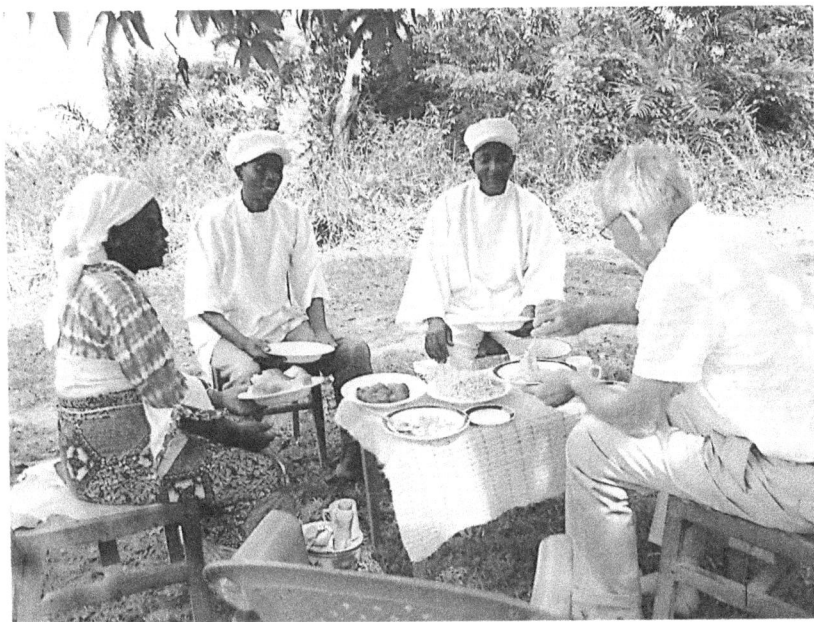

FIGURE 6.3. Conversation with (*left to right*) Mama Bakima, Tata Mayangi, and Tata Luyobisa, over breakfast under the trees at Nzieta. The occasion was the fiftieth anniversary celebration of the postcolonial founding of the Church of the Holy Spirit in Africa. The church was formally founded a few years after the leaders and many members returned from internal exile. Mayangi's father, Masamba Esaie, longtime head of the church, was regarded by Belgian colonial authorities as a particularly dangerous radical in the Ngunzist prophetic movement. Mayangi was born and experienced boyhood with his parents at the Oshwe Labor Camp in Bandundu, a common place of exile for Lower Congo colonial-era detainees. Photo: Reinhild Janzen, 2013.

When I shared with my Kongo friends and interlocutors my intention to use *dumuna* to illustrate the moments and circumstances of renewal of authority and legitimacy, they suggested that I knew what I was speaking about. But they cautioned me with the warning that the youth would not understand it. Nevertheless, based on my long acquaintance with North Kongo society, a number of instances of *dumuna* in widely varying situations demonstrate it as an apt and deeply held behavioral icon of social healing and relegitimation: for resolving family conflict, reestablishing social control, inaugurating leaders to new offices of authority, testing spiritual wholeness, and creating appropriate new techniques and institutions in a time of special need. These examples all illustrate the place of transcendence in connection with the work of the healer, family head, chief, and prophet-in-the-making in repairing social legitimacy in North Kongo society.

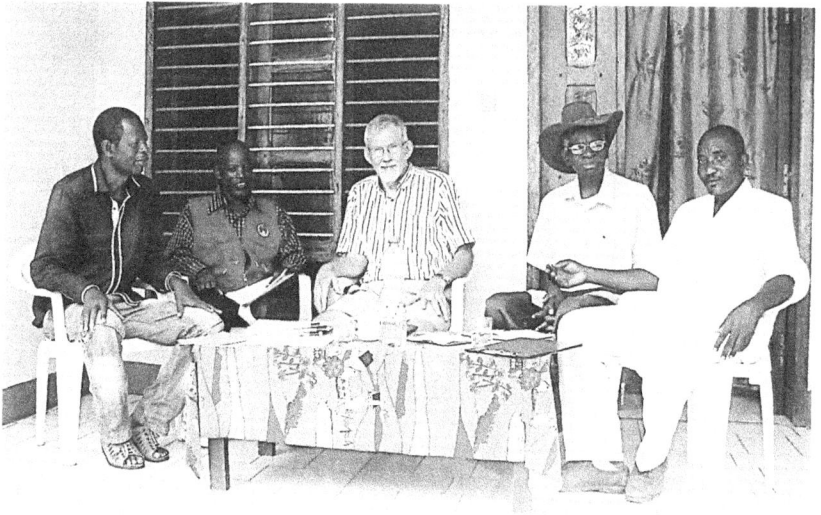

FIGURE 6.4. Conversation with the Luozi Brain Trust. An impromptu seminar occurred frequently on our veranda in Luozi. *Left to right*: Mbuta Kisolokele Thomas, retired sector chief and administrator and consultant for the Centre de Vulgarisation Agricole; Tata Célestin Lusiama, director of Radio Ntomosono ("Development") of the Université Libre de Luozi; the author; Tata Kimuengi Masamba Ronsard, Luozi merchant; and Tata Luyobisa Jackson, pastor of a prophetic church. Photo: Reinhild Janzen, 2013.

In the Healing Work of the *Nganga*

Healers put their subjects, or patients, through a *dumuna* ritual during or after treatment to indicate the conclusion of a successful treatment. In 1969, Kongo doctor/*nganga* Nzoamambu (figure 6.6) had a woman patient pass thrice between his spread legs following a hot-iron relaxation of her lower-back muscle cramp. Following that, he led her three times in a small jumping handshake. The kink in her lower back clearly loosened, and she went off happily to her day in the field. Although this short and direct physical treatment did not demonstrate dimensions of transcendence, it did suggest the transformative healing hand of the expert.

A far more dramatic *dumuna* leap was depicted in the 1920s by Swedish photographer Josef Öhrneman. The *nganga* is making an "ecstatic leap" with his *mfunka* whisk in his left hand as he is "seized by the spirit of an *nkisi*" (figure 6.5), while the participants accompany his dance-leap with song and rattles. The ethnographer-photographer does not identify the particular *nkisi*, but could it be *nkisi* Dumuna (Laman 1936, 134)?

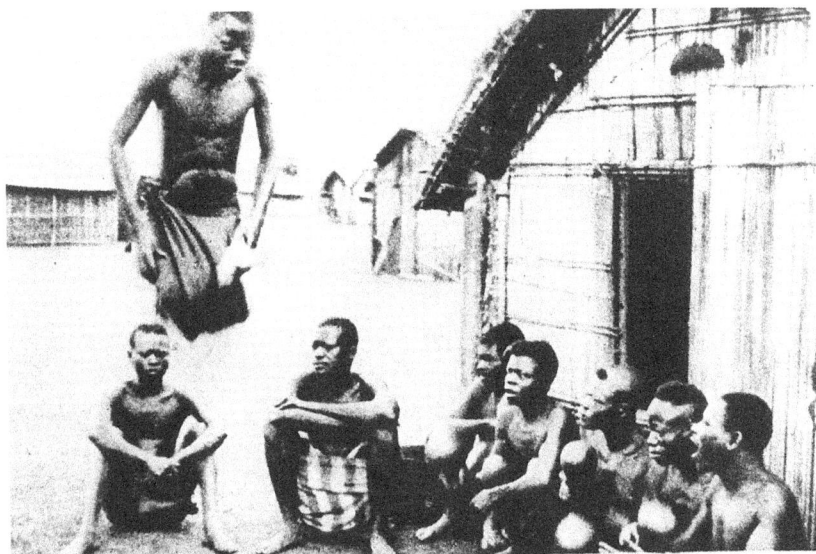

FIGURE 6.5. "The *nganga* leaps in the ecstatic moment he has come in contact with the *nkisi* spirit. In his hand he holds a *funka* (fly whisk). The men to the right accompany him with rattles." Bemba people in Kolo, Republic of Congo. Photo from a film by Josef Öhrneman, 1927. Published as picture 135 in Ernst Manker, *Bland Kristralbergens folk* (Stockholm: Albert Bonniers Förlag, 1929), 164–65. Reprinted by permission of Ethnographic Museum, Gotenburg, Sweden; museum database licensed through Carlotta system, CC-BY-NC-ND for free access and use.

In Blessings of Alliances

The soundness of alliances between exogamous clans is considered in Kongo society to be so essential for the ongoing life of the community that when the nodes of such alliances, particularly marriages, are troubled, it is imperative to resolve the problem. Misunderstandings and lingering hostilities between clans may jeopardize the reproductive capacity of women, and therefore the very survival of the community. In the case presented here to illustrate the place of *dumuna* blessing in restoring such an alliance, we see these axioms in action.

A judge in the government court of Matadi sent his wife home to the clan of her fathers to seek their blessing—or *dumuna*. The precipitating cause of this action was the death of her fourth child. The second and the fourth had been delivered by cesarean section. Her husband, the judge, suspected that the difficulties in both births might be caused by a conflict between her parent clans. The woman was a member of the Mpanga (Kingoyi) clan of Kumbi; her husband of the Kimbanga clan of Nsundi Mongo. Her fathers (*mase*) are the Kikwimba of Kisiasia, of which a portion remained at Kisiasia where they had once been slaves

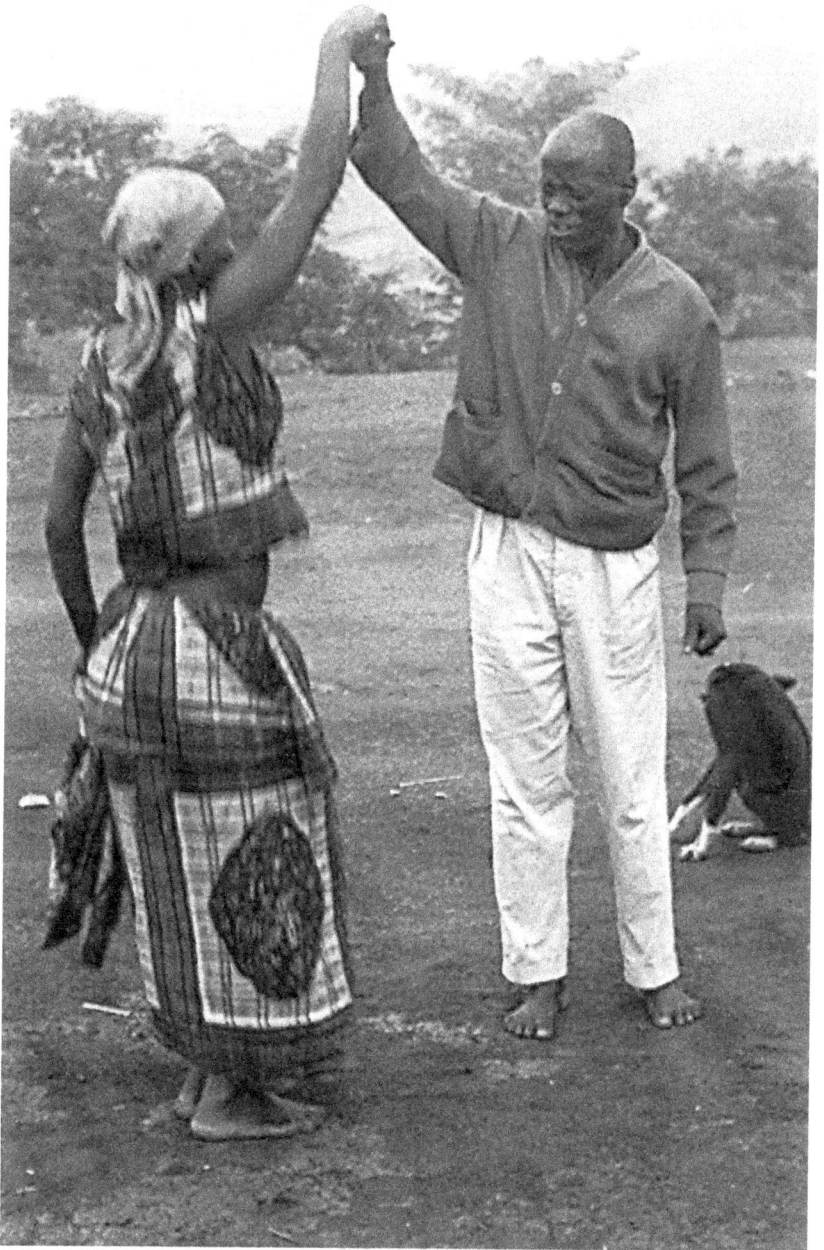

FIGURE 6.6. Nganga Nzoamambu of Mbanza Mwembe doing *dumuna* following treatment for "stitch in the side." Photo: John M. Janzen, 1969.

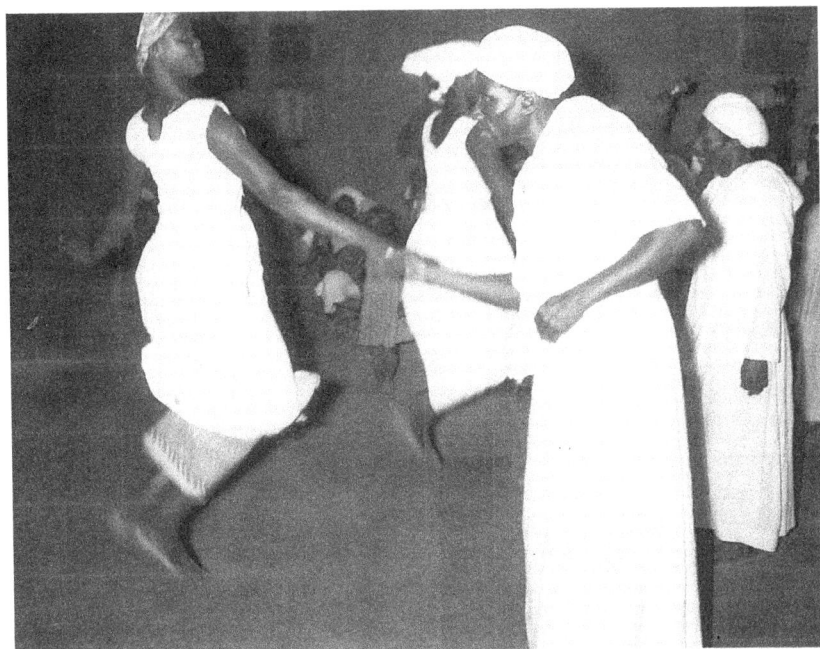

FIGURE 6.7. Weighing-the-spirit *dumuna*, Church of the Holy Spirit in Africa, Nzieta. Photo: John M. Janzen, 1969.

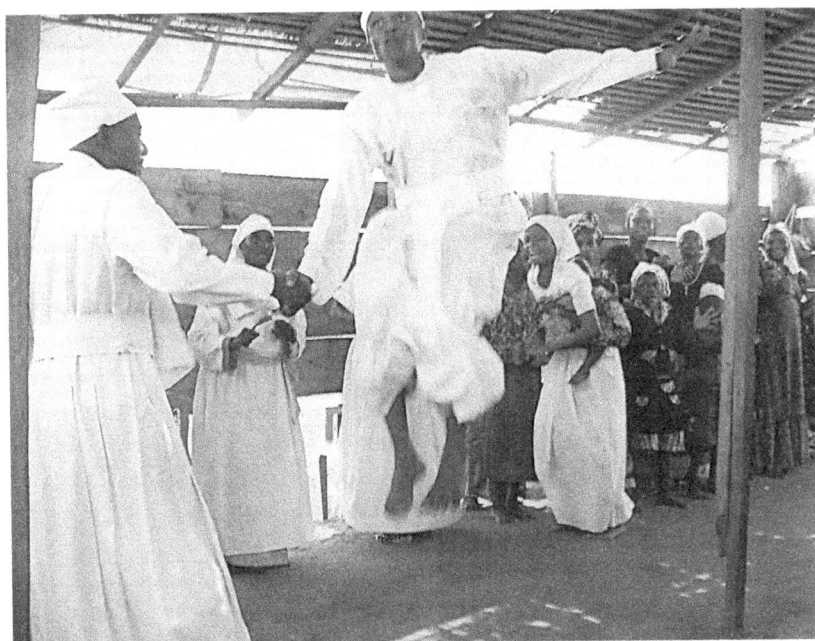

FIGURE 6.8. Inauguration-of-healer *dumuna*, Church of the Holy Spirit in Africa, Boma. Photo: John M. Janzen, 2013.

of the dominant Nsundi. Upon buying their freedom the majority had returned to Balari, their ancestral territory.

The misunderstanding between the clans that threatened the woman's reproductive career was explained to me as being due to the original bride price not having been properly divided between the bride's father's clan and her mother's clan, which was also her own. The marriage had taken place during colonial times when there had been a ceiling on bride price. The bride's maternal family was accused of having "eaten" the entire sum, or a great share of it, thus causing the paternal side's discontent. Now, although both sides had given the couple their blessing, there was reason to suspect and that it was no longer valid, and that the father's clan was to blame for having "tied up the woman's womb" (*kangidi kolo*). The woman wanted the blessing of her fathers, but the hang-up was that her father's clan, in their turn, were asking for a supplement to their share of the bride price. Thus the dispute had simmered since the marriage.

All of this was discussed around a circle as the affair opened on a November day in 1965, in Kisiasia village of Kivunda commune, where I observed the deliberations and the follow-through with the *dumuna* blessing. The woman's paternal side, the Kikwimba, represented by their speaker (*nzonzi*), opened by rhetorically asking that the marriage be annulled if the maternal clan wouldn't turn over some of the bride payment. After having minimized the gravity of the whole affair, and having laid the blame for the father's lack of money on the father's clan, the woman's maternal uncles—*bangudi nkazi*—withdrew *ku nenga* to deliberate. At this point the uncles were faced with two alternatives: refuse to pay the additional bride price to the Kikwimba, the father's clan, into which their own sister had married, thus running the risk that they would destroy the marriage by their continued disgust; or pay the father's clan the agreed-on, bargained-for sum—in a sense buying the blessing for their *mwana nkazi* and assuring her every chance of having healthy children again.

After multiple trips by the *nzonzi* between the two groups, it was settled that the woman's matrilineal uncles, the *bangudi-nkazi*, would hand across an additional 2,000 francs of *makwela*, or marriage money, plus *malafu* wine worth 320 francs, and 140 francs as *ndombulu a lusakumunu kwa mase mankento*, or request for the woman's paternal blessing. A member of the Kikwimba clan suggested to me that the maternal clan of the woman agreed to hand over 2,000 francs of additional *makwela* to the fathers only after the husband had agreed to pay them the sum, which would have been his obligation originally.

The blessing is not just the conveying of parents' consent; it is a well-prescribed societal rite, one of the old customs that everyone knows about but most can't do very well. There was a lot of discussion about how it was to be done and who should do it. The *nzonzi* came to the rescue and showed them what to do. The woman was brought to the center of the circle before the man who represented her fathers. The maternal uncles spoke, imploring the *mase*/fathers, who had allegedly been defrauded, to bless her and open her womb. Then they addressed the woman as their only hope: "If you are barren, we will die." The *malafu* wine for the blessing was put beside her, another portion of the 90 francs of *malafu mayuma* ("dry wine") was placed before the chair, and the oldest of the grandmothers from the *mase* fathers came and stood facing the woman. She put her hands, palms up, over the outspread palms of the woman (*mwana*) and pronounced a long blessing to the effect of "May you go in peace, have lots of children; may those who are behind you not bother you." She closed with the words of a Protestant prayer: "in the name of the father, the son, and *mwanda velela*." Then the grandmother put her hands under the armpits of the woman, and the woman likewise put her hands under the grandma's armpits, and they jumped (*dumuna*) together three times.

This procedure was done by two more women of the Kikwimba clan, and then finally by a father. The rite was carried out in absolute silence. To close, the deaconess led everyone in a hymn:[2]

Bizitu biabio tuna tuala,	All troubles we will bring
Kwa Yisu unatanga bio	to Jesus who will carry them
Zingolo zazo zena Yandi	He possesses all strengths
Mu Yandi tusiamuswanga.	In him we will be welcomed.
Ref. I munkisi wena ye ndwenga	Oh the nkisi has intelligence
Mu dedisa mambu mamo,	To unscramble all issues.
Kadi Yesu ulenda sala	But Jesus can act
Monso mena mampasi kwa nge.	To relieve all your pains.

The closing prayer was of the same order, proclaiming that Jesus knows everything, that he is intelligent; that God undergirds our lives, that he directs all.

People may also seek the blessing of the maternal side in order to be successful in family, in work, and in other undertakings. The harmony of the relationship is the most important factor, especially where the bride price is involved. Yet the relationship between the father (*se*) and the child (*mwana*) is the link in the chain that over time ensures the alliance between lineages in the wider society. Disharmony between two families is reflected or taken out on the offspring. One family can accuse the other of having caused misfortune; if any incident or past situation is not quite resolved, the families will fixate on it as the root cause of the trouble.

Creating Authority from Below in the Landed Domain

In earlier times Henry Stanley and other agents of the Congo Free State were obligated to negotiate for legitimate use of the Kilemba overlook after they had seized it by force and experienced several natural disasters. Later, in postcolonial Congo, newly arrived residents and developers rented, purchased, or paid use-right gifts to the land chiefs of Luozi. Now, in the twenty-first century, town officials are in the process of annexing the land and villages to an urbanizing Luozi. These landed estates, or local domains, are the *nsi*, the most widespread Western Bantu political institution that has endured for centuries (MacGaffey 1970a, 202–3; Vansina 1973, 313; 1990, 81–83; Janzen 1982a, 44).

In Kongo society, the *nsi* usually is organized through at least two allied but exogamous houses. The clan (*luvila*) is a category of descent from a putatively common ancestor, legitimized by genealogies and migratory stories. In the region of the old Kongo kingdom, narratives of clans such as Mpanzu, Mbenza, Kinsaku, Kindamba, Nsundi, Bwende, Kingoyi, and Mazinga invariably lead back to ancestry at the capital of the kingdom and migration to the present locale. The local house (*nzo, dikanda*) consists of locally related individuals with common descent from putative ancestors. Adoptions, replacements of kin groups without descendants, and outright takeovers by subordinates are known, so it is clear that we are dealing here with an ideology of consanguinity and alliances as the basis of political formation.

The making and unmaking of authority in Kongo history is a hornet's nest of claims and counterclaims at local and regional levels. The aim of this section is to sketch the process by which offices of authority in the Manianga were maintained and sometimes newly created, and to describe the ideology that characterized the fragmentation of authority as a social affliction, and the restoration of authority as social healing.[3] This is important for our understanding of the legitimacy of institutions in the region because the process underlies all authority, like the foundation for local and regional government, and the validity of purchases of land from land chiefs for private initiatives—or for urban development, as in the town of Luozi.

The authority of land chiefs in the local domain, the *nsi*, needs to be understood in relation to the historic kingdoms that emerged in the whole Lower Congo area from the twelfth century on: the Kongo kingdom founded around 1200 at its capital in northern Angola; a series of smaller, older, and as durable kingdoms, such as Nsundi, Loango, Ngoyo, and Kakongo; and many smaller scattered chiefdoms. These states evolved a set of similar institutions, titles, and structures that for some centuries dominated the political culture of the region. For example, in the Kongo kingdom sacerdotal authority was vested in the autochthonous Nsaku ne Vunda clan, whose ancestors were associated with the Earth. The monarchy was held by a conquering clan. This complementarity was mirrored in many later local arrangements. In Loango governors rotated to the four provinces in a particular order before acceding to the kingship. In other coastal kingdoms, the office of the priest of the Earth, who inaugurated the king, held authority separate from the kingship. According to the ideology of this tradition of authority, one did not inaugurate oneself. Rather, another kind of power bestowed authority on the line or individual holding office.

Records from the northern reaches of the Nsundi kingdom (the northern province of the Kongo kingdom) indicate that this form of authority was formalized in the kingdom structure (Luozi Territorial Archives, Dossier 129, 1916).[4] The *mpu* title was extended by the *ntotila* king of Nsundi in recognition of the payment of tribute. These titles were usually symbolized by shrine boxes that contained either bits of bone or mementos of former office holders, a whisk of buffalo or elephant hair, a leopard skin, a bracelet, and a hat or crown. The insignia of some of the chiefships north of the Congo River included old European swords obtained in trade or ancient battles.[5]

But in many regions the most common and widespread office to combine principles of wider authority with the *nsi* landed domain was the *kimfumu mpu*, sometimes also called the *kimfumu nsi*, chiefship of the land (Mertens 1942; Van Wing 1959; Doutreloux 1967; Thornton 1983; De Heusch 2000; MacGaffey 2000). Beyond the boundaries of the historic kingdoms, the *kimfumu mpu* was constituted from below by kinsmen, affines, and loose political allies. The *mpu*'s ideology of consanguinity with a sense of place tied to land generally focused on the claim to a legitimate cemetery, evidence of lengthy occupancy in the locality. The *nsi* domain was thus the basis of the claim to the right to own an *mpu*. In practice, the chiefship tended to be identified with a local clan section with one cemetery, at that point in its genealogical reckoning where several—often three, senior, middle, and junior—local lineages of the same house (*mielo nzo*, doors of the house) extended from a common source.

Other complementary arrangements included local clan and village organizations and market systems, which are organized either locally around the four-day market week, or as part of long-distance trading networks, ultimately connecting with the coastal international trade handled since the fifteenth century by Portuguese, Dutch, British, French, and other merchants. There were shrine and cult hierarchies and networks, related either to local landed estates or to functional specialties around misfortune, including problems with reproduction. By the seventeenth century the centralized polities that had existed earlier were destroyed and replaced by mercantile networks, which were in turn ceremonialized through such *nkisi* cult orders as Lemba (Janzen 1982a).

The North Manianga region never was brought into the centralized tribute, title, or authority sphere of any of the area's kingdoms or chiefdoms, so it was essentially an acephalous society at the beginning of, and in many ways during, the rule of the Congo Free State beginning in the 1870s. The mode of political action and judicial intervention tended to center on a council rather than the office of a political leader and the leader's court. Congo Free State agents, and after 1908 agents of the Belgian Congo, had considerable trouble dealing with these councils, which they considered to represent a kind of anarchy. They sought repeatedly to impose or to tease into being what they considered proper centralized chiefship.

In the absence of a higher regent to issue the *mpu* title over an *nsi* domain, this authority could be created de novo, from below. A combination of types of nominations was used: consensus among the *nkazi*-elders and, as important, determination of election by the spiritual world—the candidate was "elected," *tumbwa*, through ancestral call,[6] as evidenced by the individual's ecstatic seizure or trembling.[7] The judgment of an outside diviner-expert was often an important source of legitimation of the candidature. Following the diagnosis by a diviner of misfortune in the clan, or that of an individual who was afflicted, and pronouncement that the only hope for the health or well-being of the community lay in the candidate's investiture to the chiefship (Mertens 1942, 48; MacGaffey 1970a, 235–56), the elaborate process of organizing a healing-inauguration would begin.

Sickness is here defined to include both the physical symptoms and signs of the afflicted individual, and the social and political chaos that was suspected to have caused them. Healing was intended to establish or reestablish authoritative rule or consensus, as well as the consequent disappearance of the symptoms and signs of sickness. Structurally, the *mpu* was held in a free clan with clear title or claim to a permanent clan cemetery. It was often held in the junior house (*belo*) of the clan.

Legitimating Authority in the Face of Colonial Chiefship

The Kingoyi clan, dominant in the region north of the Congo River, was one of the clans that had received the *mpu* from the *ntotila* king of Nsundi, itself once a province of the Kongo kingdom. By the twentieth century, the ultimate *mpu* giver clan, Nsaku na Vunda, autochthonous of the Kongo capital in the thirteenth century, was represented in two sections in the Manianga.[8] Evidence of their clan and place name, Kinsaku of Kivunda, suggests that they may have been part of the vanguard of the eighteenth-century Kongo migration north across the Congo River— possibly to control trade routes or copper mines. In typical conquest voice, their origin narrative told of how the first man, Mwene Vunda, had come from the Kongo capital, Kongo dia Ntotila, to Kivunda Muyenze, with his sisters Makulu Makaku, Makulu Masengele, and Bubu of the land at Kivunda. According to the local narrative, Kinsaku and Mpanga were the only free clans; Kingoyi and the other clans were their slaves. But Kingoyi were present in all villages, and was thus the most populous, whereas Kikwimba, Kimpanga, Kindamba, Kinkumba, Kimbanga, and Nsundi were present in fewer settlements. Nsundi and Nsaku were present in only one settlement of the sector of Kivunda.[9]

Kingoyi's narrative was that they, together with the Kimpanga, also originated from Kongo dia Ntotila. The land was empty when they arrived. Claiming affiliation with another Kingoyi clan of south of the river, they dispersed at Zimba (from *zimbalala*, "to disperse") near Kimbanza, a district of Nsundi near the old Manianga market.

When Belgian colonial agents established the Kimata chiefship in 1916, they seem to have been clear in their minds that Kingoyi should have the medallion chiefship. Territorial agent O. Vercraeye believed that this clan's origins were similar to those of the royal Kinsaku. When the third holder of the colonial medallioned chiefship of Kimata, Mabaya-Luzunia, was diagnosed in 1933 by a prominent diviner to require investiture to the *mpu* because "he was sick," Vercraeye studied the process carefully to understand indigenous authority. He wished to avoid the mistakes made by earlier colonial agents during the Free State, of appointing slaves or commoners as chiefs whose true chiefs were boycotting and sabotaging the government.

It was common in the precolonial and colonial Lower Congo for individuals to accumulate several titles. But the particular conjuncture of the *mpu* and the colonial medallion chiefship was filled with contradictions. The *mpu*, in the several other settings related earlier, reflected recognition of marginality that was transformed into religious power, as in a cult of affliction, through an appeal to the ancestors. The colonial medallion chiefship was intended as an administrative role to facilitate the recruitment of workers, the construction and maintenance of roads, and the collection of taxes. Combining the two was a significant challenge. Yet the attempt to do so reveals the rapidly changing nature of public authority in the region.

Vercraeye was seeking a legitimate candidate for colonial chiefship, one who would be recognized and accepted by the community. Typical among Belgian colonial officials, he suggested in his notes on Mabaya's recruitment and inauguration that a royalist model would best fit the Kimata group, in which only one *belo* line would hold power. However, evidence shows that the people in these sister *bibelo* communities wished to share power as a commission, with each *belo* holding office in succession.

It is difficult to know how powerful or substantive the Kimata chiefship may have been before the Belgian colonial government recognized it and endowed it with its own title. The region was located within several hours walk from the Manianga market, which was situated along the main trade routes between Mpumbu market at Malebo Pool and the ports of Loango, Kakongo, and Ngoyo at the Atlantic Coast. Local memory and names give evidence of wealth in cloth, guns, and slaves. The memory of the trade remained in their clan epithet which alluded to "our mother, the palm sapling, which brought European cloth, guns and iron upriver from the coast."[10] In any case, the junior line was recommended for the *mpu*, through the divination on Mabaya.

Calming the Land: The *Mpu* Investiture as Healing Rite

This account of Mabaya's therapeutic investiture draws from Vercraeye's extensive notes.[11] Mabaya, sick for a long time, was told by the *nganga ngombo* diviner Babahoka of Mpete village, Kimbimbi region, that he would be healed only if he were invested to the *mpu*. On Konso day all the children born of fathers in the Kingoyi clan of Kimata (thus patrifilial children), were called together to give their father Mabaya the *mpu* so he might be healed. Konso is the most auspicious of the traditional four Kongo market week days, often associated with sacred rites, events, or sites. Here it was the time of purification.

The patrifilial children of Kingoyi-Kimata came, drank wine, and got to work cleaning the path to the cemetery. The ceremony was not, however, held in the cemetery because of Mabaya's ill health. Rather, they brought him out of his house, leading him by hand to a mat near the *mbazi*, the courtyard where conflicts are resolved. There he sat down cross-legged, and one of the patrifilial children, calling for silence, announced:

Mwana	Assistant
Bimbi, Nsungu, Bayaya.	*Bayaya.*
Nguba ngiene	*Ngiene*
I have groundnuts	
Makaya ngiene	*Ngiene*
I have greens	
Sudia ngiene	*Ngiene*
I have pepper	
Nsusu ngiene	*Ngiene*
I have a chicken	
Ngulu ngiene	*Ngiene*
I have a pig	
Mbwa ngiene	*Ngiene*
I have a dog	
Malafu ngiene	*Ngiene*
I have wine	
Bima nyonso ngiene	*Ngiene*
I have all things	

The assistant repeated the *Ngiene* call three times and sat down cross-legged *funda kata* as the chief. This position denotes, in Kongo thinking, a particular stance of authority, sometimes emulated in sculptured figures. A priest from among the patri-filial children took the ceremonial opening medicine (*mabonzo*) of *malemba-lemba*, *mumpoko*, and roots of *ntondo* and the palm, in which a bit of *mpemba* white earth and *kala* charcoal had been mixed. Dipping this in water, he approached the chief and sprinkled him.

These colors, white and black, and plants, reveal the Kongo theory behind every consecrated medicine or ritual inauguration. The ingredients are together often called *nkisi*, which means the composition and application of knowledge in the creation of a chemistry of efficacious material or human wisdom. *Mpemba*, or *luvemba*, drawn from white chalk from the riverbed, represents the hallowedness of ancestral presence. Charcoal, *kala*, represents the confusion of the human world, which stands in contrast to *mpemba*. The plants for the asperges have to do with the mediation of these two realms. Lemba-lemba, which is planted at the entrances to villages, tranquilizes and calms (*lemba*); *mumpoko*, a wild plant, mediates the domestic and the wild; *ntondo* and *diba* are parts of the palm tree, a plant of ancient uses and meanings connecting the two realms. In application to the purification of the *mpu* chief, they signify the chief's preparation to become a vessel of the beyond in the world of the living. The chief literally becomes an *nkisi*.

Turning toward the candidate, the assistant repeated "*Bimbi, Nsungu, Bayaya, nguba ngiene*." The priest, among the patrifilial children, then cleared his throat to make himself important and all repeated this. Pouring wine and water on the *mabonzo* for the asperges, he placed a hand on the head of the chief, pushed him back slightly, and with the other hand squeezed several drops into the chief's mouth while he incanted:

Nganga	Assistant
E tata, tata	
Oh father, father	
Mpemba nkuluntu	*Mpemba nkuluntu*
Sacred elder of the "white"	Elder of the "white"
Mpemba nkuluntu	*Mpemba nkuluntu*
E tata, tata	

Then followed the ceremony of *ntoba*. The earth was brought from the cemetery of the clan ancestors and mixed with palm wine and water. Taking this mixture, the *nganga* incanted:

Tusa mamba
We pour water
Tusa malafu
We pour wine
Ntsi ma muene tulemba
The domain of the lord, we calm it.

The forehead, the temples, and the entire body of the chief were anointed with *ntoba* cemetery earth. When this was finished, the *nganga* cleared his throat, and all present imitated him. Then the drums sounded, guns fired *bizongo* salvos to honor the candidate, and the children rejoiced with wine and food offered them by their father.

The purification of the candidate and the earthly domain, the *nsi*, had been completed. Water, palm wine, and cemetery earth from the Kingoyi ancestors fully integrated the ancestral and human realms. It also opened the human community to the power of the Earth and prepared the way for the final stage of the investiture of the chief at a later date. In other accounts of the *mpu* investiture, the candidate spends up to a month in isolation before the closing event.

Two days later, on Mpika, another of the four market days, the ceremonies of *sunga* (armband), *lunga* (bracelet) and *mpu* (crown) were observed. Again the chief was brought out of his house by the patrifilial children to the mat in the *mbazi* courtyard. Mpika is the antipode to Konso. The priest opened the rite with:

Bimbi, Nsungu, bayaya

and sprinkled the chief. Making a sign to the patrifilial children, he announced:

Tata Mbanda
Father Mbanda
Tata Mbanda
Father Mbanda
A wele kobila.
He goes to bathe.

This was repeated by the chorus of those present. Several patrifilial children picked up the chief and carried him to three successive crossroads of the village. At each one they stopped and the nganga repeated:

"Mbimbi, Nsungu, Ba Yaya"

Then they returned and placed him on a leopard skin that had been put on the mat where he had sat before. Just as the temporal cycle brought the ancestral white space into the midst of the human community, now the circular course of the sacralized chief past the village entrances brought the power of the leopard skin into the conventional courtyard, in an amplification of authority. Then the priest, with armband, bracelet, and crown in hand, advanced, jumped toward the chief. Balancing the three insignia he announced:

E kamba a gangu
Speak about it
nza watambula wau
Come fetch [insignia]
E wa wawa!

The priest returned in his tracks and repeated the procedure. He then attached the armband to the left arm of the chief. Again he returned, chanting the same words, and put the bracelet on the left wrist of the chief. Finally, in the same way, he put the *mpu* hat on the head of the chief.

Now there remained only the naming of the chief. This exchange was central to this part of the rite:

Nganga	Assistant
Bimbi, Nsungu, ba yaya	
Yandi luzebi nkumbu?	*Aha aha!*
Do you know his name?	
Yandi luzebi nkumbu?	*Aha aha!*
Do you know his name?	
Yandi Manswame?	*Aha aha!*
Is he Manswame?	
Yandi Maweza?	*Aha aha!*
Is he Maweza?	
Ta Mbanda, Ta Mbanda	He he he!
He's called Mbanda	
Ta Mbanda.	Heeeee.

And again gun salvos were fired. When all was quiet, an old patrifilial child arose and pronounced the following *mwina*, or *longo*, interdictions on the new chief.

Now that you are chief
That you have put on the *mpu*
You will not cultivate the earth
You will not dig up peanuts
You will not draw palm wine
You will not carry palm wine
You will not harvest mushrooms
You will not eat bloody meat of an animal killed that day
You will not eat leopard
You will not eat *kinkanda* monkey
You will not lead pigs to market
You will not plant banana trees
You will not eat palm nuts
You will not eat palm almonds
You will not break palm nuts
You will not carry anything on your head.

After these interdictions were pronounced, the same patrifilial child announced:

Tata wayenda
Father is going
Naku nanguna?
Who will raise him?

The head patrifilial child moved, jumping, toward the chief and took the chief's little finger of the right hand, and while he rose the two together they raised both hands into the air. The patrifilial child cried out, and those present replied:

ana simu	*tela*
children of the other shore	arise
lubulubu	*lubu*
lubulubu	*lubu*
ana simu	*tela.*

At that moment the chief jumped up, feet together, leaving the leopard skin. The ceremony was finished. This jumping was a sign of contact with the white of spiritual power. The "children of the other shore" are probably the onlookers, the patrifilial children, who are invited to behold this display of ancestral energy before them. Simu Nzadi, the shore of the great Nzadi River, is an analogy of the cosmic river, and the sight across this river of one who has passed over.[12]

The creation of the *mpu* chief entailed sustained obligations for the patrifilial children. They must pay a tribute called *budi dia mfumu*, a part of each harvest and of the animals killed in the hunt. They must carry for him everything he needs on his travels. They must build and keep trimmed his *lumbu* enclosure and build his house therein. The entrance to the *lumbu* of Mabaya was forbidden to all adult freemen (*mfumu kanda*) of the Kingoyi clan. Patrifilial children were on hand as courtiers, *nkengi a lumbu*, to watch over the chief, *kenga mfumu mpu*.

This healing-inauguration had included the use of signs of sickness to recruit to a position of authority, the transformation of the identity of the sufferer to that of ruler or priest, the healing of the community and its alliances as the sufferer was invested to an office of authority, and the empowerment of a junior or marginal segment of the community by renewal of an alternative office of authority. In the elaborate ceremony the transformation of the individual chief was like that of creating an *nkisi*, sacred medicinal agency, defined as rooted in the other world of the white (*nza mpemba*), hedged in on all sides with elaborate rules and prohibitions, and possessing otherworldly power, all for the good of the community. *Dumuna* is the final signature act that establishes sacred legitimate power.

The Ngunzist Appropriation of *Dumuna*

This final scene of the sacralized chief is reminiscent of the rites of purification, of healing, and of the weighing of the spirit among Manianga prophets. These performers of the spirit compare the tension between the sacred and the profane to electricity that is so powerful that one who has it can hardly be touched. The appropriate posture in approaching contact with such an empowered one is this jumping described here, *dumuna*.

About half of the fifteen churches in Luozi derive from the early twentieth-century prophetic movement known as Ngunzism, after *ngunza*, prophet or seer. Simon Kimbangu is usually regarded as the first of the twentieth-century prophets, and the largest independent African church that was organized after his followers returned from exile is the Église de Jésus Christ sur la terre par le prophète Simon Kimbangu (EJCSK), whose schools, dispensaries, and sanctuaries are found in Luozi and the countryside. But in the Manianga and cities of the region one also finds independent churches among followers of Mbumba Filipo, a contemporary of Kimbangu, of the western region of Kinkenge, and Samuel Kitoko, of the Sundi Mamba region, bearing names such as Dibundu dia Mpeve a Nlongo en Afrika (DMNA, Church of the Holy Spirit), Église du Saint Esprit, Église du Saint Esprit en Afrique (ESEA), Communauté du Saint Esprit en Afrique (CSEA), Église Prophetique Liberale, and Nsimba Yenge (Embrace Joy) (Mahaniah 2009).

The Church of the Holy Spirit in Africa, one of many independent Christian churches in the Lower Congo, has incorporated the *dumuna* rite as a climactic finale to its worship services. In addition to the blessing, the healing, and general singing-dancing and scripture reading, the jumping, dancing, hand-shaking *dumuna* is at the heart of the weighing of the spirit. Each of these rites has incorporated elements of traditional rituals into its liturgical repertoire. The blessing was first used by Masamba Esaie when he was taken into exile. He was permitted to bless his followers who remained behind. The *dumuna*, or weighing of the spirit, was first done in the church context by Mbumba Filipo in the 1920s in the Kinkenge region (Basolwa 1983). In this rite a ranking prophet stands with hands trembling in the spirit. Another adherent, whose spirit will be weighed—evaluated or measured—dances out before the officiant. The weighee extends a hand to the weigher. If the hand is not grasped, that is if the spirit is not adequate for them to connect, the weighee must confess before the weigher. If the weighee measures up, the hands connect, and the weigher propels the weighee into three leaping handshakes. Three times this routine is repeated, each time the jump more spectacular than the one preceding it. So prominent is this rite that the hilltop center of the Church of the Holy Spirit, at Nzieta, was nicknamed Sala Duma, the place where they do *dumuna*.

Prophetic Insights

Mayangi Charles is the son of famed colonial era Manianga prophet Masamba Esaie and spiritual leader of one of the branches of the Communauté du Saint Esprit en Afrique (formerly DMNA). In February 2013 we joined him and several others at Nzieta for the anniversary of the founding of their church. Mayangi explained the nature of *kingunza* as an independent line of visionary spirituality going back throughout Kongo history and expressing *mayembo* outside the institutionalized channels of chiefship, *kinganga*, or *kindoki*. It was present with twentieth-century prophet Kimbangu and the eighteenth-century prophetess Kimpa Vita, or Dona Beatrice, and even alongside the royal figures of the ancient Kongo kingdom.

Mayangi was a child of colonial exile, having been born in Bandundu Province where his father and other Manianga Ngunzists were in colonial labor camps around Oshwe and Boko from 1952 until 1960. This group, including Masamba, who was categorized as one of the most dangerous, was required to report daily to the police. They did very difficult forced labor, although they were allowed to grow their own food and live in their own houses. *Bangunza* and other dissidents considered dangerous to the colonial order were all over the Belgian Congo.[13]

Allowed to go home only at the time of independence in 1960, they gathered close to but not in their clan villages. The new settlement of Nzieta, which I first visited in 1965, was masterminded by Masamba as a collective settlement where everyone worked together and shared many resources. The founders of this particular group of prophets, including Kitoko and Masamba, were members of the Kindamba clan of Nsundi-Kibonga. There were others earlier; Kimbangu (whose family he said was from the Manianga, and sought land across the river in Ngombe), and Mbumba Filipo of Kinkenge were the most noteworthy.

Prior to 1952 the Masamba and Kitoko group met in a forest near Nzieta that they referred to as a forest of birds to hide its prophetic associations from the government. This is where Masamba and others met, along with Nzimbi Nsadisi, the son of a Portuguese merchant and a Congolese woman. This whole group was in Protestant schools and the Protestant church while they continued their informal meetings, rituals, drumming and singing, and expressions of *mayembo*. After they were arrested in the 1950s they were no longer able to meet or worship together. This is why, upon their release, the settlement at Nzieta became so special to them. Also, after independence the Protestant church authorities refused to allow them to remain a part of their church. So they formally founded their own organization.

Mayangi describes his father as a genius who had little education. As a young man he was very restless and went to various cities to find employment, always for short periods of time. He is also said to be athletically skilled and to have miraculously cured a leg fracture in a soccer game. His decision to marry was also unique:

he selected a young woman with a chronic festering foot sore, which his kin advised against. He paid the bride price, they married, he nursed her back to health, and they had six children. His wife supported the high value he placed on cleanliness and order, even at Nzieta. This settlement of returned exiles was organized as a communal society, with heads of particular areas of activity such as the fields, the worship place, and the pigeon farms kept behind the twelve residences. Mayangi was not sure where his father had gotten the idea for a communal settlement, but he had very clear ideas of how it should be run. In the end, after his father's death, it was unsustainable, even though it had represented their highest values.

He mentioned values in our conversation about what the prophetic church held in highest esteem from the Kongo tradition and the teachings of the missionaries. Mayangi stressed that the ancestors before missionaries had had a relationship with God, Mpungu Tulendo, Mentete (First One), or Nzambi, especially in times of crisis, such as the sickness of a child. A sick child would be taken to a stream, bathed, and laid in the sun, where the light of Mpungu, or Mentete, was held to have worked. *Banganga* said in connection with their work that they healed the outside, God the inside. But the *bangunza* are special in that they exist outside normal roles because of their *mayembo*. *Mayembo* is associated with trance. It comes to individuals with no training and overwhelms them, making them say and do almost crazy things. They have visions and dream all kinds of things; they can see the future.

Mayangi noted that the Kongo of the Manianga were able to select the values that were good from the tradition and blend them with missionary teachings. *Minkisi* had been used mainly for protection, but the missionaries and the Bible brought the Holy Spirit, which could replace the *minkisi*. Jesus the teacher was also made central to Kongo spirituality. But much that existed in earlier Kongo life and thought was also good. This the *bangunza* protected. Masamba's values brought the two worlds together. Before 1952 he had concurrently been a student catechist at the mission and a follower or novice of Samuel Kitoko in *kingunza*. This process of selecting the Kongo prophetic voice of God or truth, Mayangi emphasized in our conversation, "was not syncretism."

Dumuna as Initiation to Spiritual Healing

A national evangelist visiting the Boma congregation had said he would need to spend a night with the novice—a young chauffeur and mechanic—to question him and examine the strength and consistency of his vision. He had begun this work the morning after his arrival in Boma and continued the next day, a Saturday, before the Sunday service. In conversations Saturday we learned that the candidate was faring well in his evaluation and that there would indeed be an initiation on Sunday.

Sunday we were fetched around 10:30 a.m. by our chauffeur at our hotel and driven up a hill overlooking the city and Congo River. We walked up higher along a footpath through tall grass to the very top of the hill to a makeshift shelter of poles, boards on the sides, canvas, and a cloth roof. This was the site where a permanent structure would be built. The service was already in process. We placed our shoes outside the respective male and female doors and were ushered to our plastic chairs at the front on the male side. The national evangelist, the deacon, and several other prophets were seated at the table, Bibles and hymnals open. The song leader was directing a song, while a male worship animator was dancing opposite a young woman with a child strapped on her back. The evangelist translated much of the service—scripture reading, meditation—into French, and sometimes into Lingala. The parishioners, we were told, did not all know KiKongo very well. He translated my short words of greeting into Lingala.

The evangelist preached an Easter sermon, stressing the redeeming power of the resurrection. He also named the day Women's Recognition Day, noting that it had been women who at every step of the story of salvation—the Fall, the birth of Christ, the resurrection—had led the way, had recognized the significance of the moment.

Then came the initiation, ritually staged within the frame of the *dumuna*. The novice was positioned beside the evangelist as is the case when the weighing of the spirit is done. To strong polyrhythmic drumming and singing, the novice danced out to do the *dumuna*. Approaching the evangelist, he stopped and was motioned to kneel. The novice spiritual healer on this day, in *dumuna* terms, had three chances to succeed. If his hand failed to connect with his weighing prophet a third time, the ritual would end then and there, as a sign of his lack of readiness. But on the second try he succeeded in grasping the weigher's hand and did three, even four, tremendous leaps to finish the routine. Next, still in *dumuna* mode, he approached the evangelist and knelt again for counsel and scripture reading. Then the evangelist handed him the *kidimbu* sign of his office,[14] his own white towel. The novice healer then knelt between four senior prophets standing around him in a cross-like pattern. The evangelist read a scripture passage while he laid a trembling hand on the novice's head as a blessing. Then the presiding prophet-evangelist performed healing on him, the towel wrapped closely about his head. Then the prophet-evangelist waved the towel before him to create *mupepe*, or *mpeve*—wind. With this the novice had become a fully authorized healer in the Communauté du Saint Esprit en Afrique.

Conclusion

The most pivotal meaning that *dumuna*, the verbal concept and ritual action, has received in its long and complex history is its use to clarify relationships and to create or renew public authority. In both applications the condition that is being overcome is considered a kind of sickness, and the anticipated condition is defined as healthful. Along the way *dumuna* and related verbal concepts express the concentration of spiritual energy toward a particular insight, solution, or cure. Thus *dumuna* expresses the power of some *minkisi* that brought together the elements of nature, society, human will, and the technical methods needed to resolve the problem at hand. This was most evident in the *nkisi* called Dumuna, although we do not know the nature of the particular problem that it addressed.

Dumuna was used by some *banganga*, like Nzoamambu Oscar of Mbanza Mwembe earlier in the twentieth century, to mark the successful closure of his therapeutic interventions. *Dumuna* as a ritual also expressed the transparency of a paternal blessing to resolve a problematic, unfinished alliance between two clans, as well as, according to Thomas Kisolekele, any blessing an elder bestowed on a junior in the face of mysterious affliction.[15] In a similar vein, *dumuna* in chiefly inauguration represented the legitimation of a candidate by the patrifilial children— that is, the children of the men of a matrilineage, comprising the natural kin-based allies living as adults in their own matrilineal homes or elsewhere in the region or the world at large. The creation of legitimate authority out of sickness and disintegration reflects the general Central African premise that society may require a social healing that involves empowering its marginal elements.

This entire ideology of mystical power continues to engage the imaginations of the people of the Lower Congo, and no doubt more widely. There are those who suggest that this ideology is a form of debilitating collectivism that paralyzes efforts at social and economic development. But the realpolitik of many people leads them to seek to solve serious social problems, among the chief ones being those related to health and, beneath them, the issues of political economy. These initiatives need more than just a plan, a collective effort, or individual initiative; they need the embrace of social legitimacy to succeed.

7

Science, Sorcery, and Spirit

A nursing student at the Free University of Luozi wrote in her master's thesis, titled "Evaluation of Care in Gastro-Enteritis Fever in Children from 0-5 Years: Case Study in the Catholic Hospital of Luozi": "'The Lord is my light and my salvation; whom should I fear? The Lord is the refuge of my life; of whom then should I go in dread?' (Psalm 27:1). Take life as it comes, without regret, nor surprise, nor being upset, for the essential thing is that which remains for you to do." The thesis was dedicated "to the Eternal, my God, the Almighty who protected me and upheld me during all the years of my studies until today."

Eddy Makiedi Mambu's research thesis at the Free University of Luozi, Faculty of Health Sciences, on "The Evaluation of the Nurse's Contribution in the Care of a Case of Microscopic Positive Pulmonary Tuberculosis: Case Study at the State Hospital Centre of Kisenso" carries the epigraph "'In thee, O Lord, I have taken refuge; never let me be put to shame. As thou art righteous rescue me and save my life; hear me and set me free . . .' (Psalm 71:1–2). Holy Father, bless me in my life so that I will acknowledge my father, my mother, and all those who have helped me surmount the many obstacles encountered during the three years of study at the Free University of Luozi."

Mamy Nzumba Mbundu's thesis on "The Contribution of the Nurse in the Care of Infected Operating Wounds," at the Catholic Health Center of Luozi in 2005, was inscribed: "Blessed be the Eternal, for He hears my voice, my supplications and He lends his ear toward me during the period of my studies; may my cry reach thee, O Eternal; give me the intelligence and the wisdom according to your promise; may my supplication reach Thee; deliver me according to your promise. May each work with his hands to have something to give he who is in need (Saint Paul)."

Situating Science

The theses quoted above are three of the many at the Free University of Luozi that situate the student's first original research project in the context of a sacred space, often defined by a scripture passage and an invocation or wish. Many students express gratitude to parents, siblings, other kinfolk, elders, and ancestors for their support and for having modeled the wisdom and intelligence needed to complete a course of study. Some observers of this pattern might explain it as a manifestation of youthful enthusiasm, perhaps an attempt to impress the examiners with their diligence and piety. But these verses and invocations that festoon the title page of every thesis at the university follow the common practice in Kongo of invoking transcendent reality to order the world, especially where specialized techniques or knowledge are involved. This was also true of the consecrated medicines of old, the *minkisi*.

Legitimation of expert knowledge within a transcendent framework also means that there is a less clear-cut distinction between what we in the West call science and what we call religion. How they are integrated varies from era to era and from case to case. But such integration of divergent kinds of knowledge into one framework seems to be a fairly widespread historic and contemporary African phenomenon, found in such realms as metallurgy, agriculture, warfare, political office, family relations, and especially approaches to sickness and healing (Feierman and Janzen 2011). Although there would seem to be a realm in which technical knowledge is regarded as natural, crises such as sickness, accidents, brushes with death, and sociopolitical chaos transform the situation into a moral issue (Janzen 2015b, 2017). Steven Feierman and I suggest (2011, 248) that "the moral and humanistic envelope of knowledge that integrates science and religion may well be a unique contribution of African tradition to the world community."

This chapter examines a number of dimensions of this integration of science and religion within the distinctly North Kongo setting, both among professional elites and in expressions of popular sentiment. A review of the rapid development of the fields of medical anthropology, the history of science and medicine, and applied areas of public health provides a broader intellectual backdrop for this discussion.[1]

In the early postcolonial 1960s, most Western scholarship adhered to the sharp contrast between the objective knowledge of science and the backdrop of biomedicine, and the rest of human thought, which was characterized either as superstition or, most generously, folk knowledge. The traditions of objective knowledge were said to be the result of centuries of unilineal scientific progress that had produced the wonders of the Enlightenment, the Industrial Revolution, modern medicine, and other scientific achievements. However, like slowly trickling drops of water on stone, other thoughts were beginning to percolate that would challenge the received wisdom on knowledge. African Studies and other disciplines, such as history of science and philosophy, were confronted with the ramifications of E. E. Evans-Pritchard's seminal work (1937) on the thought world of the Azande people of Northeast Congo and Southern Sudan. Evans-Pritchard had argued that Azande thought, epitomized by Azande beliefs in witchcraft as an explanation for misfortune, was rational, even though it was based on assumptions that were different from those of Western science.

Generations of philosophers and anthropologists puzzled over this challenging evidence. Robin Horton's writing on Western science versus "African thought" (1967) had a very long life, as these stereotypic constructs, which were asymmetrical in the extreme, were endlessly compared with ever more local studies to argue one or another perspective. Others framed their studies, policy recommendations, and proposals for research in terms of modern medicine versus traditional medicine (Foster and Anderson 1978) or of modernization in contrast to primitive or traditional society. The comparative study of medical systems, launched first by scholars of Asian medicine, yielded the notions of medical pluralism (Leslie 1976) and epistemological pluralism, invoked for the serious consideration of alternative ways of seeing the world—Western scientific, Asian, and African. Some medical anthropologists insisted on seeing the field of all therapies in a given location as "medical culture" (Last 1992), thereby encouraging the possibility of commensurability between diverging logics and types of knowledge.

A radical shift in perspective on the nature of the relationship between culture and science emerged in American anthropology and the history of science and medicine as scholars asserted that science itself is culturally constructed. Thus one could examine the culture of biomedicine—the values and structures of thought that expert and instrumental knowledge illustrated (Hahn and Gaines 1985; Lock and Nguyen 2010). From this point in the 1980s and 1990s, the field of medical anthropology evolved rapidly, with an understanding of the biosciences that was much different from what had reigned in the 1960s era of science as objective-empirical knowledge. The undoing of some universalist models of disease (for example, depression [Kleinman and Good 1985], Alzheimer's [Cohen 1998], and menopause [Lock 1995]) in favor of culturally or nationally distinctive syndromes opened the way to visualizing conditions more commonly dealt with in African settings in terms of cultural variability and culturally specific constructions.

The reading of diseases in Africa in terms of their cultural construction was slow to occur, however, especially in tropical Africa where diseases such as malaria, cholera, HIV/AIDS, and Ebola raged. But researchers of the colonial history of science in Africa noted the African setting's transforming effect on science. The unique situations faced by colonial scientists in fields such as agriculture, environment, medicine, and public health created a new and distinctive local cast to the results, with far-reaching consequences (Tilley 2011). Phrases such as *endogenous knowledge, vernacular science,* and *competing epistemologies* now characterize this growing attention to variability and adaptation in science (314–28). Distinctive understanding of the cultural, social, and political contexts of health conditions in African settings appeared in due course with regard to the cultural and moral dimensions of disability (Ingstad and Whyte 1995; Livingston 2005), the moral and emotional-humanizing consequences of HIV/AIDS (Dilger and Luig 2010), and the broader consequences of living with malaria (Fulwilley 2011) and other conditions. Within medical anthropology an entire subfield emerged in the study of science, where one leading scholar refined the concept of "epistemic cultures" arising out of PTSD (Duclos 2009) to deal with the continuities and discontinuities in specialized knowledge. Without totally relativizing science, it is possible to see variability in knowledge and truth that is shaped by environment and culture and is open to creative applications that arise in the face of unique needs and urgencies.

An all-inclusive formulation of the relationship of knowledge to its sociocultural setting is proposed by the science and technology studies under the heading of coproduction. The coproduction of natural and social orders is how we know and represent the world. The ways in which we know and represent the world is inseparable from the ways in which we choose to live in it (Jasanoff 2004, 2). "Knowledge and its material embodiments are at once products of social work and constitutive of forms of social life; society cannot function without knowledge any more than knowledge can exist without social supports. Scientific knowledge, in particular, is not a detached mirror of reality. It both embeds and is embedded in social practices, identities, norms, conventions, discourses, instruments, and institutions" (2–3).

The global reach of public health has created another perspective on science in and about health in Africa, one that P. Wenzel Geissler and his associates portray as an archipelago-like network of institutes, centers, research projects, donor-run patient support centers, experimental huts and villages, demographic surveillance systems, specialized labs, and clinical research centers. Although this network of sites of science may resemble earlier scientific institutions, as well as training programs within public universities, referral hospitals, and national ministries, they are part of an asymmetrical empire of knowledge generation and legitimation that favors the northern institutions and funding sources (Geissler 2015). Data and body materials—blood, genetic samples, lab data on diseases—are extracted from local sites, but the value-added analysis and publications are conducted in the North, with results being shared with local and regional centers only after the fact. The archipelago of science described by Geissler parallels the neoliberal economy of resource extraction and consumer consumption of world products at global prices.

Whether this model of global health science fits the Lower Congo is debatable. In my research I found no examples of ongoing research or training programs conducted by northern institutions. No doubt the officials in charge of hospitals, clinics, and universities would have been very pleased to have had such partners. The suggestion that African science sites are isolated, underfunded, and therefore unable to connect with the powerful centers in the North is closer to the truth. The bare-bones operation of the Congolese health zones, which lack even computers, and their linkage with the World Health Organization (WHO) resonate with Geissler's portrayal. But a more accurate picture of science in the Manianga region of the Lower Congo is that of courageous independent scholars, researchers, and practitioners applying their insights directly to onerous health problems and reporting their findings to local, regional, and national audiences and colleagues as best they can.

Santé Rurale du Congo (SANRU), the major broker of global funds for public health initiatives in the Congo, has established a research department office that is focused on the "implementation and operational researches to (1) evaluate and document its past projects, (2) study areas that may improve the performance of its current or future projects; and (3) study areas to improve the performance of health systems."[2] Across the country many research initiatives are underway that resemble those in the Manianga, including some that reflect a keen interest in local herbaria and healers. Local research centers are working to find medicines to treat common communicable and noncommunicable diseases, and their efforts have led the Ministry of Health to create a subdivision on traditional medicine. The danger that these local, or even national, research agencies may merely serve as handmaiden project implementers of well-funded northern research centers is offset by the vigorous fund-raising efforts of SANRU and its success in the 2010s at becoming the principal recipient of funds for major public health research that is supported by international financiers such as the Global Fund, Global Alliance for Vaccines and Immunization (GAVI), and the Centers for Disease Control and Prevention (CDC) for projects in the Congo.[3]

This chapter continues with a closer examination of malaria's impact on people's lives and thoughts in the Manianga, and the related effect of sickle cell anemia, which results in multiple deaths of children. How are these illnesses understood and dealt with? What is the impact of medical knowledge, especially about modern genetics, on the people and families who have to contend with the sickle cell. These scenes from the world of health and healing in Western Equatorial Africa raise important issues having to do with science, medicine, and religion. How is authoritative knowledge produced? How is it legitimated, circulated, shared, and applied? Particularly, how are the sometimes competing claims of spiritual and scientific modes of knowing reconciled, interdigitated, or fused?

Malaria, Sickle Cell Anemia, and the Salience of Evolutionary Biology

The prevalence of malaria and its complications in the Manianga, the overall educational level of the population, and the focus on education that is relevant to basic health problems have resulted in a fairly high degree of consciousness of the scientific knowledge about the disease. This includes an understanding of evolutionary adaptive processes in determining who is affected and how, and what should be done to ameliorate conditions.

Given the historical absence of knowledge that malaria is a vector-spread infectious disease—on the part of both the Congolese and the colonial powers—the common practice of locating human settlements atop the many high hills that dot the region could be seen as an adaptive response to the relative danger of the lowlands. Conversations about the prevalence of historical settlements atop these high hills evoked comments about refreshing breezes, the smaller number of insects, and the overall more favorable conditions in the higher settlements. A similar sentiment about the common practice of keeping the yards around houses free of grass and the bare earth swept naked suggests that the main reason for these practices is insect and snake control. Of course, there is also an aesthetic consideration to a cleanly swept yard.

In order to facilitate administrative control of the population, the colonial government forced hilltop settlements to move into valleys, nearer to roads, and often alongside forested streams. The result was an increase of malaria. Colonial labor and tax policies also contributed very negatively to the health of the resident Congolese population. Flight from labor recruiters and tax collectors, not to mention punitive expeditions to control recalcitrant communities, meant that entire villages fled to the protection of lowland forests along streams, and directly into the ecological zones most heavily infested with tsetse flies and *Anopheles* mosquitoes. As a consequence, the Congo Free State period was deadly for those regions most closely involved with Europeans. Conditions were not much improved with more systematic colonial administration. Villages were forced to settle alongside new roads, where population control—sometimes justified in the name of public health—became a common feature of administration.

Public awareness of the nature of malaria infection and contagion has kept up with medical science advances. Knowledge of the role of mosquitoes in malaria is universal. Yet generally, despite an awareness of the role of commercial prophylaxes, Congolese people do not take them. Quinine continues to be a regular treatment, but it does not confer immunity, and if taken in too large doses for too long, it causes ringing in the ears and may result in temporary mental dissociation. Generations of other drugs have come and gone, with some degree of efficacy and usually with side effects if taken for long periods of time. Maniangans use a range of traditional local products and methods to deter malaria. Some people rub themselves with a poultice of several plants—one called *latta* is a favorite—before they go off into the bush, or they chew the leaves and swallow the juice. They say that the aroma of the plant repels mosquitoes. About a third of the households in our survey mentioned keeping the yard around the house free of grass and sweeping it daily to keep mosquitoes and other insects away; indeed, these households reported fewer incidents of malaria than those not mentioning this technique. The WHO's campaign to distribute medicated mosquito nets to all households through the health zone was accepted with anticipation. And all people with whom I spoke said they used them.

Despite the availability of drugs to calm bouts of malaria, medicated bed nets to prevent nighttime bites, and popular prophylactic poultices to repel mosquitoes during daytime work in fields and forests, most Maniangans accept occasional malaria infection, with weeks of being feverish and sick, as a normal feature of their lives. The outside observer would conclude that the cultural absorption of scientific knowledge about malaria contributes to a certain tolerance of the disease, but ready referral to medical specialists or medicines when the disease becomes life-threatening.

Both the medical community and much of the populace have become aware of the tendency of the spirochete *Plasmodium falciparum* as well as the *Anopheles* mosquito to develop resistance to chemicals used to eradicate them. Two further areas of knowledge of malaria have increased both medical experts' and some of the populace's knowledge of evolutionary processes at work in malaria and its effects. First, there has been a growing appreciation of the importance of using multiple medicines—commercial or herbal—to combat malaria, with the understanding that single, simple chemicals are more likely to result in resistance than complex or varying plants or chemicals. Second, a growing awareness within the medical community of the nature of gene frequencies, transmission of genetic material from generation to generation, and adaptation has contributed to distinctive approaches to dealing with the differential consequences of malaria in the community. In particular, the differential manifestations of sickle cell anemia within the community and families has prompted a better understanding of evolutionary biology in general.

Currently there is experimentation with medicines and protection methods that take into account the evolutionary proclivities of the target. The medicated mosquito nets that everyone in our survey used, courtesy of WHO, the Ministry of Health, and the health zone, has reportedly reduced malaria incidents somewhat. But many people are still bitten in early twilight or in the morning before mosquitoes withdraw for the hot sunlight hours. Pharmaceutical experimenters have discovered that synthetic drugs designed around a single chemical property or process are more easily resisted than chemicals with complex structures, such as natural products like quinine. Manianga pharmacist and drug manufacturer Batangu Mpesa, founder of the Centre de Recherche Pharmaceutique de Luozi, has conducted extensive experiments with about a hundred medicinal plants known to have been used by healers as antimalaria medication. Out of these he has identified a dozen or so that when used alternately and in combination produce a treatment that thus far has not produced resistance. His company currently serves about a million clients annually with Manadiar, a prophylaxis, and Manalaria, a treatment especially for infants that relieves the fever and calms the diarrhea that often accompany malaria outbreaks (Batangu-Mpesa 2009).

The manner in which Batangu legitimizes his research on malaria is illuminating. In a 2009 lecture to a national colloquium on scientific research on malaria in the Democratic Republic of Congo (DRC), he situated his work within the overall program and priorities of WHO. This includes taking note of WHO's recommendation that medicines be combined into cocktails—as is Coarsucam, which is made up of Artesunate and Amodiaquine—to stand a better chance of resisting resistance on the part of *Plasmodium falciparum*, the leading variant of malaria spirochete in tropical Africa (Batangu-Mpesa 2009, 12). Noting the lack of research on new malaria drugs in relation to the overall global output of drugs, Batangu lays out WHO's program for research into new medicines, primarily from the existing work of herbalist-healers. Such healers use materials of plant, animal, or mineral substances and practice manual techniques and therapies of spiritual healing. The researcher's goals are to identify and extract the active principles of these substances; to study their toxicity on experimental animals; to stage clinical trials of medicines that show promise, with an ethical review framework; to request market authorization; and then to make the new drugs available. Earlier efforts to successfully commercialize herbalists' medicines have often proved chimerical because of the high costs of drug experimentation and the doubtful future of a new drug. As well, the history of relatively quick biological resistance to new drugs has made pharmaceutical companies reluctant to invest large sums in uncertain outcomes (Janzen 2012, 115–37).

Despite such cautions, Batangu presses on with his own research and development program. Malaria is a crisis. It is the leading cause of morbidity and mortality across the DRC, especially in poor sectors of the population. He explains that his own motivation for his thirty-year research program rests on his care for himself, his family, his immediate community, and others. With his track record clear for all to see, he has obviously not poisoned his family or others who benefit from his medicine, including the some million households per year who buy Manalaria (2009, 31–32). This is an intriguing comment and postulate that reflects the fear in the community of exactly such a possibility, and the relative absence of the rule of law that would deal with powerful, unethical persons with drugs. Then follows the passage where Batangu lays out the moral foundations of his project (2009, 32).

- I am a native of the Luozi region;
- I am a pharmacist-analyst;
- I am a political person;
- I believe in God.

These four anchors assert identification with the region and offer evidence of scientific expertise, political acumen reflected in his days as a national parliamentarian, and finally, invocation of the supreme being. These claims encourage everyone to identify with Batangu as a researcher, citizen, leader, and believer. They encourage trust in his skill as a pharmacist, and confidence that he will take care of people as a former national deputy. Finally, that he is in touch with the true source of power and the natural world.

This cosmological manifesto is presented in visual form on a large mural extending across an entire wall of a large plant-drying shed and theater in Batangu's Luozi compound, not far from a plantation of medicinal herbs. The landscape scene, reminiscent of the Manianga with the Congo River flowing through it, features heroic male and female figures engaged in productive activity characteristic of their gender roles. The male figure is hauling in fish with a net, and a severely wounded crocodile has just been attacked by the fisher. The woman holds a hoe in her raised hand, ready to cultivate the garden plot before her. The title above this scene in French and KiKongo admonishes: "Work makes free and powerful." Smaller scenes in the landscape depict industrial and communications technology, while a dove hovers above, suggesting peace. Two biblical references offer further detail to anchor this social-realist depiction of the Kongo world of tomorrow to spiritual roots. In big letters beneath the male figure is Genesis 1:26–30, the passage in which God declares the creation good and gives Adam and Eve dominion over it. Beneath the female figure is John 15:5, the passage in which Jesus declares himself the vine and his disciples the branches: with him they will be fruitful.

Sickle cell anemia, or drépanocytose in French, affects many people in the Congo and in Western Equatorial Africa generally. It is a hereditary condition given by the heterozygous gene-carrying father and mother to some of their children. Statistically each child born to such parents has a 25 percent chance of not carrying the gene, a 50 percent chance of carrying the gene and having a sickling condition that gives some immunity against malaria, and a 25 percent chance of having full-blown sickle cell disease. Children in the latter group are susceptible to anemia and other health crises, and usually to early death if their condition is not carefully managed. No cure is available. In the DRC fully 30 percent of the population are carriers of the gene (Mbaku n.d.).

Joswe Mbaku, a professor of psychology at the Free University of Luozi, specializes in raising public health awareness about sickle cell anemia. In a pamphlet that he distributes to everyone in his entourage and classes (Mbaku n.d.), he explains the symptoms and life chances of those affected: The first signs of the sickness may manifest themselves as early as six months, in swelling of the feet and hands, in bone or head deformities, and in yellowing of the whites of the eye. Often severe physical pain accompanies the condition, due to deformation of red blood cells, which clog blood vessels, prevent good circulation and oxygenation. Anemia and infections follow. The immune system is weakened, and the child becomes prone to all kinds of medical ailments: malaria, retarding of growth, cerebro-vascular conditions, and so on. Sickling cannot be cured. It may be treated and, better, attacks may be avoided. But without care and attention, early death is very common.

With regard to treatment, Mbaku's tract recommends diminishing the pain of attacks by staying in well-ventilated areas with a stable temperature, frequently drinking water, eating a good and varied diet, and avoiding strenuous exercise. Medical treatments include very expensive drugs; blood transfusions may be necessary in certain cases.

The tract concludes by emphasizing that a long life is possible for children with sickle cell anemia, so their parents should be encouraged to put and keep them in school. They have a future in occupations that do not require strenuous physical activity, including some professions. Psychological counseling and moral support are very important elements of helping a person who is affected to live a reasonably normal life.

An analysis of the intensive sample in my 2013 study reveals a number of household couples who report as many or more deceased than living children. In the cohort of women in their fifties and sixties who have completed their reproductive cycles, four of twenty-two had lost at least half of their offspring; thus, they had probably parented children with sickle cell disease (table 7.1). One had borne eight children, of whom six had died; another had borne nine, of whom six had died; a third had borne six children, of whom five had died. This pattern of child loss produces an enormous burden especially for the woman, who is expected to bear children and is blamed for the string of child deaths. In the first-mentioned case, the woman was divorced by her first husband and remarried. Her second husband divorced her after the deaths of several more children. Her third husband had died. When interviewed she was living in a modest house in Luozi with her fourth husband. Both of them had been widowed. She said of him that "he agreed to take care of me, so we married" and he, a healer, seemed to favor this opportunity. The woman's only daughter, in her twenties, lived with them and was pursuing university studies.

Several of our acquaintances with whom I discussed sickle cell anemia said that before there was any consciousness of it as a hereditary condition, the children's deaths were usually thought to be caused by an unfinished, inadequately paid-up bride price. The importance of the alliance bond between families was so great that failure to establish it adequately brought to the fore undercurrents of miserliness and jealousy that could cause sterility or child death. Deaths of children were usually diagnosed as "deaths caused by man" (*lufwa kia muuntu*) as opposed to natural "deaths of God" (*lufwa kia Nzambi*). As awareness grew of the nature of the condition through public health education, it took the form of a vague sense that something was amiss in the biological makeup of the parents. But without an adequate understanding of genetics, this awareness was limited to identifying certain families or kin groups as somehow flawed, with the result that their children died. Manianga historian Kimpianga Mahaniah (2001, 54–56) has written a history of a lineage, his own, with such heavy sickle cell frequency that the family was formerly accused of harboring witchcraft in its midst, which occasioned anger, estrangement, and poison ordeals. In an entire chapter devoted to this he explains the genetics of sickling to a KiKongo readership.

With more schooling, especially in the biological sciences, and with the training of many lab technicians and the advent of numerous Congolese medical doctors and nurses, a fuller comprehension of sickle cell anemia has emerged in Manianga society, and in this wider region of Africa so heavily affected by malaria. Today genetic testing is becoming a prerequisite for marriage among educated young adults. If both are determined to be carriers or if one or both have somehow survived to marriageable age with sickle cell disease, medical counselors and psychologists routinely advise them to break off their engagement and find other partners.[4] This introduces a whole new source of tensions. Those who refuse to break off their engagement are asked to sign a document informing them of the likely consequences and indicating that they fully understand what they are confronting.

The emergence into public consciousness of a genetically transmitted condition as severe and life changing as the sickle cell gene, introduces new life choices, issues of identity, and moral considerations. Tampering with God-created nature or having to break off a cherished relationship may require a new kind of moral framework. Complicating matters even more, medical specialists suggest that there are multiple alleles in the genetic picture and that more refined testing can demonstrate gradations of severity in sickling. The consciousness of a sickling propensity introduces the kinds of ambiguities that have been confronted in genetic testing for fetal birth defects. Science and spirit are so intertwined here that a sophisticated moral and emotional compass is required at each stage of this complex condition.

This analysis of knowledge in the service of health and healing incorporates pharmacy, public health, medicine, and biology, including a keen grasp of the adaptive vigor of the malaria spirochete and the *Anopheles* mosquito in the human attempt to suppress or combat the carriers of the disease. In the understanding of such scholar-practitioner-politicians as Batangu, Mbaku, and Mahaniah, not only science but their own experiences and those of their clientele teach them the intricacies of the challenge of malaria. Their scientific knowledge is anchored in their learning and their experience, as well as in the global network of other researchers and practitioners. They also integrate the social, moral, and religious anchors of the context in which this science is applied.

For the educated citizenry of the Manianga, the knowledge they possess of malaria includes the scientific ideas, to the extent that they are grasped, as well as the tentacles of community pressure, including especially the widespread and deeply held idea that people can affect each other's health and well-being. Misfortunes such as children being chronically ill or dying of malaria introduces another logic

TABLE 7.1. Offspring of women in age group 50s–70s in intensive sample, by education and ratio of surviving to deceased children

HH#	Age	Years in school	Total births	Age of youngest	# deaths	# living
1	67	5	11	N/A	1	10
8	58	9	7	9	0	7
10	58	8	8	21	6	2
11	52	15	6	17	0	6
13	67	0	12	15	2	10
15	52	7	7	13	1	6
19	54	8	7	15	0	7
27	54	8	7	13	1	6
29	51	3	8	2	4	4
34	51	10	1	N/A	0	1
40	53	8	9	3	6	3
44	50	N/A	10	13	3	7
56	71	5	8	18	1	7
57	51	2	7	12	0	7
67	61	10	8	13	3	5
68	61	6	9	4	2	7
80	54	6	6	N/A	5	1
89	67	3	6	18	1	5
91	61	14	6	18	1	5
92	53	8	10	17	3	7
104	50	9	5	12	0	5
Total			158		40	118
Average		6.5	7.2			5.36

SOURCE: Intensive sample of 105 households, 2013.
Note: Reproduction figures of these women show ages, years of education, numbers of children born, those surviving and those who have died. Shaded cases are those whose offspring were most likely to have suffered sickle cell anemia.

into the etiological equation. Sickling, even where it is understood as a genetic pre-disposition or phenotypic cluster of syndromes, raises the question of community sanction, or of one's own inherent flaws that result in children's death. The truth of science does not erase the other logics of a social, moral, or religious nature. Although there would seem to be a realm in which knowledge and technique are regarded as conventional or natural, the advent of crises such as sicknesses, acci-dents, and brushes with death propel the situation into the moral universe.

Crocodiles and the Moral Universe

The contours of a Kongo moral universe that frames knowledge of the world extends beyond the individual body and diseases such as malaria to the natural landscape and the creatures that inhabit it. The power of this natural world along the banks of the mighty Congo River was brought home to me quite by accident one morning as we—Reinhild and I, with our chauffeur Pierre—sat in a thatch-roofed shelter near the ferry harbor, or beach as it is sometimes known. We had missed an earlier passage and had three hours to spend until the next embarkation. Our waiting companions were mostly young Congolese men, some drinking morn-ing cups of tea or coffee, or enjoying an early snack from a nearby "restaurant" cooking pot. Others chatted with friends and neighbors.

Small talk and polite greetings gave way to a focus on us as Americans. A bold young man asked: "Are there poor people in America?" "Yes," we answered, "it's a class-divided society." This was supplemented by a further question: "Are there mad people (*zoba*) in America?" "Yes, why not? People get sick, they become bur-dened by conflicts, they overextend themselves." Finally, the question that always comes up in circles like this, and had probably been on everyone's mind from the beginning: "Do you have sorcerers (*bandoki*) in America?" My answer to this difficult question was "Not really, at least not people who do what we hear sorcer-ers can do here in Kongo." But I added, "We have people who do bad things to each other. They are like your sorcerers." These three questions, it turned out, were a clue to how these interlocutors saw their own world, the contours of which they were projecting onto questions about America.

I decided to turn the conversation around into one where I, the anthropologist, would set the agenda. Half in playful repartee, half in curiosity before this ready audience, I redirected the conversation in our thatch shelter on the Congo river-bank from poverty, madness, and sorcery in America to that all-time favorite topic in Congolese gossip circles, the crocodiles in the Congo River, and asked an open question about the so-called Crocodile Problem. It appeared that the crocodiles on the Congo River and in streams that flow into it had, over the years, attacked men, women, and children who came to the river to draw water, to bathe, to wash clothes, or to fish. Crocodiles had also attacked fishing canoes, upsetting them and gobbling down the frightened fishers. A peak of crocodile attacks had occurred in

1987 when, in the sixty-three-kilometer stretch from the upriver rapids of Manianga and Mpioka to the downstream rapids of Isangila, twenty-three persons had been attacked, killed, and usually eaten by crocodiles (Mahaniah 1989). In 1988 and in the years following, the attacks had almost ceased.

I asked the eager conversationalists around me: "Why did the Congo River crocodiles stop grabbing and eating people in 1988 or thereabouts?" Typically, whenever this issue came up in conversations around town in the company I kept, some individuals would put forward the street opinion, and then offer that they might not believe it. Others might offer alternative explanations. On this morning, in this crowd, I was told that the reason for the cessation of crocodile attacks on the Congo River around Luozi was that the perpetrator of this activity, an *homme-croco* ("man-crocodile") had left town and returned to Europe. "Who was this person?" I asked. "It was the Catholic priest in Luozi. He had been taking lives and selling them in his coven to enrich himself."

Needless to say, I was amazed by this answer and probed further to determine how widely such a conviction was held. I asked our chauffeur, Pierre, if he believed this story. Pierre, a highly trained mechanic and chauffeur with some years' experience with the Iranian embassy in Kinshasa, and a self-identified Buddhist, said he believed the account. I then asked the entire circle seated under the thatch shelter to raise their hands if they believed this version of why crocodiles had attacked and eaten so many humans a few years earlier. Several raised their hands. The boldest of the young men volunteered for the others, "We all do." No one dissented. We wondered if possibly these young men with time on their hands might be playing a game with us, offering us tantalizing tales of an exotic Africa they may have thought we wanted to hear. The issue is complex.

Crocodiles are a part of the wide and awesomely powerful Congo River. People die regularly from drowning, having been caught in the middle of the two-kilometer-wide river during storms, and occasionally from crocodile attacks. The drownings are sometimes attributed to the mostly invisible but powerful and irritable *bisimbi* water spirits, which register their objections to some human endeavors having to do with the river. This was the local explanation of the drowning death of Henry Stanley's colleague Frank Pocock, whose canoe was destroyed in a descent of the rapids upriver from Manianga in the late nineteenth century. However, crocodiles are a presence in their own right. Their life cycle and character are known by every local inhabitant. Females lay eggs in the sand bars, in quiet banks, or in marshy areas. The young hatch out of these eggs and then fend for themselves. Sometimes the eggs or the young crocodiles are seized and eaten by large birds, but eventually the hardy survivors make their way into the water, where they live on fish they catch; some, in the younger stage, are eaten by large carnivorous fish. The river folklore includes a rich repertoire of stories about fishers and communities living on the banks of this mighty river with all its creatures and spirits.

One theme has to do with the relationship between crocodiles and humans, which can be either cooperative or predatory. Just as hunters have their dogs that go out before them to flush out the game, so fishers may have river dogs—crocodiles—to herd fish into their nets. The crocodiles do this by defecating in the water and then swimming toward the nets as the fish follow them eating the droppings. Just as hunters may develop a close, almost personal, relationship with their dogs, so some fishers have particular crocodiles with whom they cultivate a relationship of collaboration. Whether this in fact is possible or happens no one was able to tell me definitively, although some individuals who had grown up in riverside villages said they knew of cases where this was true. Thus some in this circle believed that with the right powers one could engage a crocodile to do one's work. On the other hand, they also believed that some fishers with crocodile helpers had offended their crocodiles, resulting in the crocodiles attacking their masters.

An *homme-croco* is another type of being altogether (figure 7.1). This is a human with magical powers who can take on the form of a crocodile in order to attack an enemy or rival in a way that resembles a crocodile attack. In popular thinking around Luozi, the twenty-three killings of 1987 were perpetrated not by regular crocodiles but by an *homme-croco*. As if to confirm this story's plausibility, rumors circulated about the capture of such a being on the Congo River some years ago in Lukungu, a fishing village upriver from Luozi. There was even a published newspaper article by a journalist who had gone to see the *homme-croco*'s corpse in a riverside village.

Although many folks with whom we discussed this matter of the crocodile attacks believed in the *homme-croco* or domesticated crocodiles, some doubted, or at least thought there were other explanations. The thinking on this matter among university-educated persons may be represented by that of Diallo Lukwamusu, project coordinator for the Free University of Luozi, who did not provide me with an outright negation of the popular version but answered my question as to why Congo River crocodiles had stopped attacking and eating people after 1987 with four hypotheses, each of which was plausible.

The first hypothesis was the popular version of the *homme-croco* who had left town and returned to Europe, or somewhere, around 1988. In the absence of such a person seeking many lives to achieve phenomenal powers, the ordinary crocodiles did not usually attack people.

A second hypothesis had to do with a night-time hunting expedition that had been organized by then-parliamentary deputy Batangu Mpesa, who had engaged a team of upriver hunters with high-powered rifles and spotlights to shoot and kill as many crocodiles as they could find. However, our chauffeur, Pierre, and many others, discounted this explanation, arguing that Batangu had produced only one dead crocodile as evidence. When later asked about this, Batangu had said that in

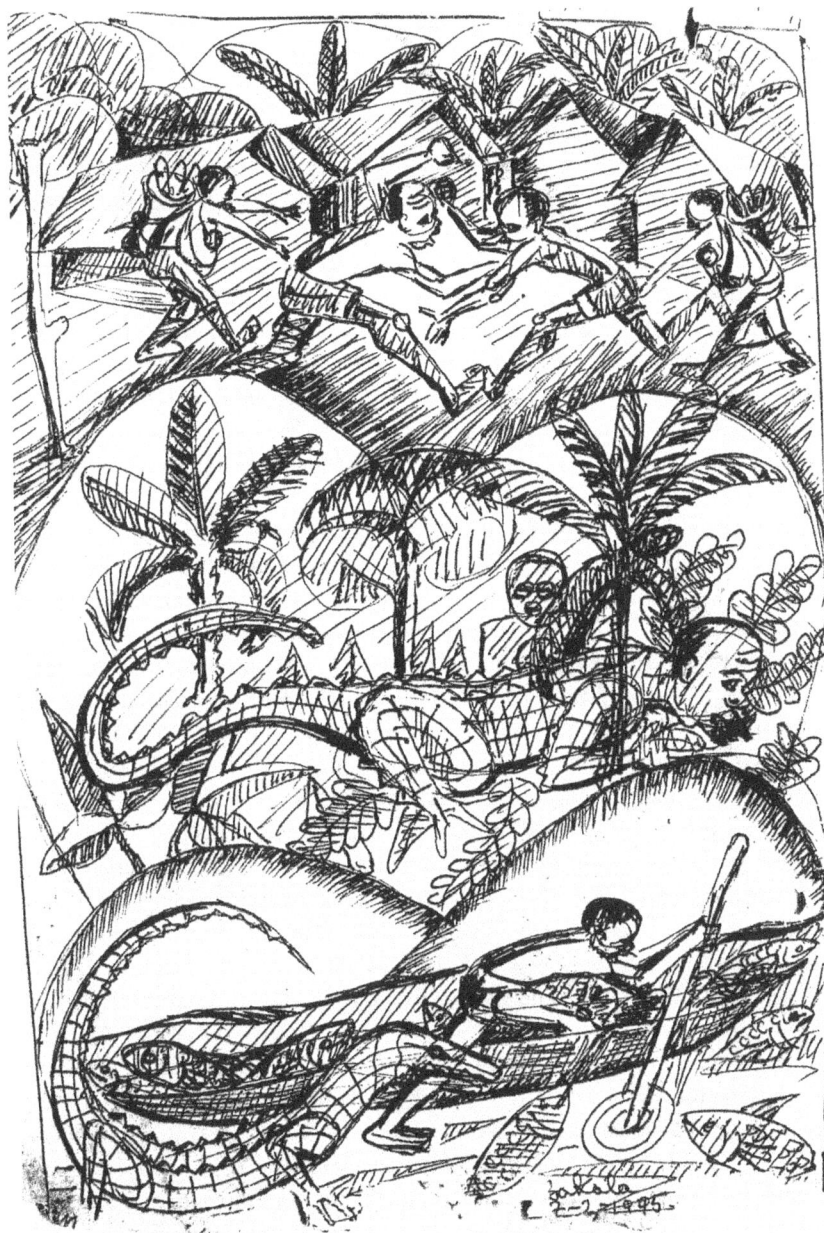

FIGURE 7.1. Crocodile man. Artist Bakala Daniel's sketch depicts the popular Manianga idea of a human transformed into a crocodile (*homme-croco*) to enact vengeance upon a human antagonist. The human crocodile specter hovers over a fisher who is in his canoe hauling in nets full of fish, while a flesh-and-blood crocodile attacks him. The source of the antagonism is a village conflict shown at the top of the tableau. Unbridled anger is believed to find expression—with or without human intention—in such mystically mediated attacks. Photo of sketch: John M. Janzen, 2013.

the all-night hunting expedition many crocodiles had been hit, but they had simply slid off their perches into the river, either escaping or, most likely, dying in the water to be eaten by other crocodiles. He had taken the one crocodile cadaver, which was retrieved for display in Luozi and then at his pharmacy in Kinshasa.

Lukwamusu's third hypothesis had more to do with accounting for the increase in crocodile attacks in the 1970s and 1980s than with the apparent end of the attacks. Among the Manianga elite in those decades, there emerged a rising awareness of the serious consequences of deforestation brought on by massive clear-cutting logging operations begun in the 1950s by outside companies. Entire forests were replaced with sisal, at the time a promising cash crop. The wood remaining after the logging operations was used in cooking fires and for the manufacture of charcoal for urban sale.

One of the most vigorous initiatives by the Centre de Vulgarisation Agricole over several decades has included an educational effort to raise consciousness about deforestation by spelling out the links between deforestation and declining agricultural productivity, as well as reforestation projects in Luozi and around the Manianga to create diverse secondary forests (Dianzungu dia Biniakunu 1987; Mahaniah 1989; Batukezanga 1998). These publications, especially Mahaniah's book, explained that the increase in crocodile attacks had resulted from an increase in the crocodile population, which in turn was due to a decline in the number, or even disappearance, of large carnivorous birds that used to prey on eggs and small crocodiles before they entered the water. Furthermore, overfishing had led to a decline in the number of carnivorous fish that eat small crocodiles in the river. An increasing population of hungry crocodiles led to their tendency to go after humans on the riverbanks. A simultaneously increasing human population on the river banks in towns like Luozi had also resulted in more women and children going to the river for water and washing at the same time as the crocodile population was increasing.

Lukwamusu's fourth hypothesis had to do with the installation of the Luozi water system in the early 1990s. Quite abruptly in 1993, the people of Luozi no longer needed to go to the river to bathe, wash clothes, or collect water for household uses. This, along with Batangu's hunt in 1987, had resulted in a dramatic decline in crocodile attacks. Among the small circle of university graduates, the combination of the latter three hypotheses, presented in scientific language, sufficed to account for not only the rise in crocodile attacks, but also their sudden ending. Yet the majority of Luozians and Maniangans apparently remained unconvinced, and continued to consider at least plausible the explanation that the rise in attacks had been due to the presence of an *homme croco*, or at least a sinister-minded individual with a domesticated crocodile, who preyed on innocent victims, especially women and children, to amass great power and wealth through mystical means.

Which brings us back to the questions asked at the river: in America are there poor people, mad people, and sorcerers? The first two groups have been marginalized in the realms of economy and sanity by the manipulations of the third group. If one sees this play of power as a zero-sum affair, then the ascent of the wealthy and the healthy has come at the expense of the impoverishment and the maddening of the many. The inquiries touched on the moral universe and questions of how power is handled, who gets pushed to the margins, who rises to the top and with what means, how evil is explained, and whether or how people can protect themselves. The Congolese moral universe has a logic to it that rests on the reciprocal exchange of gestures, acts of generosity, and intentions that should result in harmonious relations. If people share, help each other out, respect each other, and avoid antagonisms, the result should be a broader, more inclusive social circle and a moral society. One wonders if this is also how institutions are maintained, and whether the purpose of all the etiquette practiced by most Congolese is to check the fear of letting social exchange networks and relationships lapse or fall unattended, producing chaos and danger for all. To the outside Western observer, the juxtaposition of ecological analysis of multiple species interacting in an environmental niche on the one hand, and the mystical exploitation of natural creatures by sinister human agents is incongruous to say the least. Yet why should the multiple explanations—Lukwamusu's four hypotheses—not coexist within the same universe of thought?

Two further dimensions are at play in the moral universe seen here. One is the etiological pivot between "of God" and "of man" (human-caused) forces in accounting for misfortune, especially disease. The other is the shape of human personhood that is both more expansive than a typical Western, autonomous individual, and therefore more vulnerable to outside social forces and conditions.

To *Fiela* or Not to *Fiela*

The shift in causal logic during quests for healing from natural cause ("of God") to human cause ("of man") has been a common feature in Kongo and more widely in sub-Saharan African healing. Situations that may bring this shift about include lack of effective healing in a case that should have been resolved, a serious conflict of harsh or angry words that preceded or accompanied the misfortune or sickness, a sudden or surprising crisis that resulted in death or sickness, or the sentiment among family or colleagues of a sufferer that there is something else going on, more than meets the eye. In such cases the therapy managers of a case usually consult an expert, who examines the sufferer's relationships or recent life history, an action that is called *kufiela*, "to explore," or *kufimpa*, "to dig deep," terms that the anthropological literature would translate as "divination." It is important to recognize the process and results of divination as knowledge. A century of biomedicine in this part of Western Equatorial Africa has not dislodged sufferers' and their escorts' occasional need to know what else is going on. Why, when, and how such information is sought is at the heart of the legitimation of most knowledge in Kongo society.

Prior to 1921, the year that Kongo prophets after Kimbangu ordered the destruction of all *minkisi*, including those used for diagnosis and healing, diviners commonly investigated the causes of misfortune, illness, and death. With the *ngombo* basket, objects representing typical life situations were winnowed, and one or a cluster of these objects emerged to give the operator a clue, or a visual guide, for interpretation of the condition. Although the *ngombo* was abandoned, after 1921 this kind of investigative divination was taken over by a variety of people, including some *bangunza*-prophets and the remaining *banganga*, both of whom increasingly operated under the banner of Christianity. Christian missionaries vigorously resisted this practice because it presupposed the reality of sorcery, anger, and conflict in the cause of misfortune, disease, and death. Congolese people generally were more willing to accept such a reality, and often wanted to know who or what was causing their own or their close kin's misfortune. So *fiela* continued to be practiced by various personalities, usually by those who developed a knack for it, rather than being rigorously trained within the traditions of a particular *nkisi* like the *ngombo*.

In the 1950s and 1960s, Daniel Ndundu, a Protestant pastor and seminary professor, became an expert at *fiela* and had a widely respected tradition for practicing it with discretion. In the North Manianga, Marie Kukunda also had a favorable reputation and was able to *fiela* social cause and to mediate conflict situations without provoking political controversy (Janzen 1978, 2013a, 2013b). In 2013, at the time of our visit to Luozi and the wider Manianga, another independent *ngunza* enjoyed a good reputation for doing the work of *fiela*. Many pastors and prophets avoided the practice, however, because of the real potential that the identification of perpetrators of aggression would explode in their faces by provoking retaliatory lawsuits for slander, judicial action, or even extrajudicial violence.

Several instances of sorcery suspicion came to my attention. One case brought to the prophet whom we learned about in 2013 was that of a young mother who was told that she had experienced a curse—*envoûtement*—when she received a telephone call and heard a threatening voice that caused her to promptly faint. Her sister who was in the room sought their father. They managed to rouse her and bring her to the parents' house, where she was in shock. A prayer vigil and prophet-style healing-dancing were conducted, and she regained her composure. But the father sought out another prophet who examined the relationship in question. He determined that the threatening call had come from her husband's employer, who was trying to take her soul. Why her? Because her husband was too strong, so the employer had gone after the more vulnerable wife to fulfill his desires for power and life essence in his sorcery. The Communauté du Saint Esprit au Congo (CSEA) put the young woman through intensive therapy to return her soul to her and to protect her spiritually. Her husband resigned his position and moved to Kinshasa to find other work. In this case *mfiedulu* (the nominative of *fiela*) seems to have worked out because it was contained within a series of other rituals and supports that protected the targeted person.

I learned of open anger and continuing suspicion in the wake of misfortune in two further cases. In each one a high school student died rather suddenly—one from leukemia, the other from what appeared to be an aneurism. In both cases the deceased young person's friends or classmates came to the homes of the parents, where the wakes were being held. In both cases these gangs of youth, in their grief, attacked the parents, especially the fathers, accusing them of having taken the souls of their own children to gain power and wealth. In one case the teenagers assaulted the father with stones so forcefully that he and his family fled the scene to seek shelter.

Behind such actions was the idea that a death or misfortune, especially one that came as a surprise, had to have been caused by a malicious agent plotting to take the life. In the logic of such an hour it is always possible to find a personified other who connects society's members to each other, especially kinsfolk, in a malevolent tangle of evil intentions and selfish desires. The extensive literature on witchcraft and sorcery in Africa, beginning with Evans-Pritchard's work on the Azande, has tried to explain the assumptions in this logic. In this instance we need to fit it within the worldview of youth who are in school and studying science. We require contextual understanding of how one set of assumptions is applied at one point, and another set at another time, or of how the multiple logics operate concurrently in the same mind or social group.

These cases demonstrate the underlying connection between *mfiedulu* for "human cause" and public order, or the lack thereof. Jean Masamba ma Mpolo (1981), a leading analyst of African witchcraft and sorcery, suggests that the very act of an accusation of illicit power establishes more of a link between persons than uncertainty over whether there are any relationships. Deep-seated insecurity and fear are sentiments that propel a situation toward suspicion and accusation of another individual or group. The plethora of sentiments expressed by respondents in our intensive sample over the failure of the state to provide support and leadership confirms the problem. In the case of the Bundu dia Kongo in Luozi and the Manianga, the need to call in special troops to squelch a public outcry demonstrates the complete loss of legitimacy of the weak or failed state, despite the formalities of a bureaucracy and personnel in their offices.

PERSONHOOD AND RELATIONALITY IN
SICKNESS AND HEALING

A further reason for the etiological shift to human agency lies in the more inclusive, expansive sense of personhood that has been widely noted in Central Africa, including Kongo society. My scholarly interest in personhood in Kongo therapeutic logic was aroused when I tried to make sense of *nganga* Nzoamambu's medical cosmology (Janzen 1978). The diagnostic gloss *kimbevo kia muntu* (sickness of man, human agency-caused) corresponded in his dynamic scheme to a sequence of ever more severe reactions of the heart, the "chief of the person," to insult or injury. This sequence of signs began with mere heart palpitations, which progressed to the heart's "wild beating" and on to "fear in the heart," "madness," and ultimately death. Such signs in a sufferer, especially if demonstrated sequentially over time, were evidence of something else going on. This entire model I called Nzoamambu's "theory of the person" (Janzen 1978, 169). But as we have seen in several illness episodes reported above, this theory of the person is more widespread than the thought of one clever twentieth-century *nganga nkisi*. It resonates in more widespread writing and practice in Central Africa and beyond. MacGaffey has summed up his understanding of the power of historic Kongo *minkisi* embodied within "the personhood of objects" (1990; 2000, 78). The *nkisi* mirrors the entire scope of relations between the *nganga*, the client, and the "other" of threatened aggression. These relations combine metonymic and metaphoric allusions, as well as artistry in the harnessing of unique styles and methods of diagnosis and therapeutic intervention.

The contours of this unique Kongo, Western Equatorial African personhood include a number of aspects of identity, rights, and believed associations. There are the rights at birth to one's mother's lineage land and other privileges and obligations focused on the relationship to one's *nkazi*, maternal uncle, who holds proprietary rights over his nephews and nieces, his sister's children. An individual also is held to have deep ties to the father and the father's kin that are often associated with intellectual and spiritual powers. A kind of bilateral identity includes within it networks with other individuals and roles. Yet the individual is still in some sense original and autonomous. Naming, for example, is independent of these other lineage or clan associations. Individual names may be changed by life-course transitions or personal whim (Janzen 2002, 141). But it is this wider fan of kin that is usually invoked when suspicions of something else going on are raised in connection with sickness or other misfortune.

In the twenty-first-century Congo, the impact of the state and other public power relations also affect this wider, more inclusive personhood. Beyond kinship, modern individuals are members of churches, workers for employers, and neighbors in towns. They own businesses, sell in markets and wider commercial networks, and work as officials in government and operatives and bosses in political parties. They are subscribers to internet services and users of cellphones. Each of these arenas or networks becomes part of the persona of the individual. Because these arenas are not necessarily hierarchical, they proliferate as segmentation of the self or alternative dimensions of personhood. The weak state is there as a shadow presence, possibly more threatening because of its unpredictable character. Respondents in our intensive sample of households spoke of the state using terms such as *abandonment, betrayal, failure,* and *loss of hope.* Fear of chaos was the dominant sentiment about the state. This could be internalized as a threatening other, a sorcery attack (Geschiere 1997; Ashworth 2005).

The broader, more inclusive, more widely connected personhood of Kongo thought and society, in which etiological suppositions about the fates and fortunes that are "of God" and human-caused coexist, also explains the manner in which God, the ancestors, nature spirits, and other individuals taking the form of animals, may occupy the same universe as narrowly defined scientific theorems. Although scientific understanding shifts the focus of specific etiology of disease, it does not obviate the general breadth of personhood. In any event, in Kongo thinking and living the person is often more expansive and complex than the post-Enlightenment bounded, autonomous, Cartesian, Christian individual of current Western psychological and medical construction.[5] This expansive personhood is also more vulnerable to whims of aggression and recrimination, which accounts for the proliferation of protective rituals and measures.

SPIRITUAL HEALING AND BIOMEDICINE WITH DR. BAKIMA

The young doctor Bakima, who passed his medical school exams recently in Kinshasa, is an accomplished and dedicated *ngunza,* or prophet. We met him in Boma, and he gave us a tour of the Hôpital Général de Référence, where he was interning for a year, doing specializations in pediatrics, surgery, and internal medicine. On the table of the single room he shared with three other interns, there were several thick medical texts. On Sunday morning he was wearing another type of white, that of the CSEA, with its characteristic skull cap and long gown with a wide belt. Before him at the Sunday service were a KiKongo Bible and hymnbook. In the Bible were the notes of a course he had taken on traditional African healing.

I had suspected that Bakima was fully immersed in the two different healing traditions. Conversations with him indicated how he integrated the two in his thinking, his persona, and his career. Just as he was now a diploma-holding medical intern, so he was qualified to practice all the rites of the CSEA: the blessing, the healing, the *dumuna* weighing of the spirit. After completing secondary school on the scientific track, with a specialization in chemistry and biology, he had taken his medical training at the Faculty of Human Medicine at Simon Kimbangu University in Kinshasa. He completed his MD degree in June 2013. He had chosen this university not to learn about spiritual healing—which they did not teach, he said—but for its high-quality professors and well-equipped laboratories.

I engaged Bakima in a conversation to understand his simultaneous involvement in two such different healing traditions, biomedicine and faith healing. He explained that the two healing traditions fit together because of this great difference.

Biomedicine offers a narrow focus on a disease and its treatment and on the function of particular organs. Students learn the properties of medicines and how to apply them, as we saw that Sunday afternoon when he prescribed two antibiotics for Reinhild's incipient urinary tract infection. Spiritual healing addresses the whole person in context and offers assurance, contact with the Holy Spirit, protection, and harmony. There is a condition for its efficacy, however. One needs to believe in it. His training and practice was very much Christian, with reference to the life of Christ and the power of the Holy Spirit in healing. However, in his knowledge of African healing he also spoke of herbal and shamanic dimensions. He said that many of the CSEA rites and practices were distinctly Kongo in nature and were rooted in the work of prophets as early as Kimpa Vita Dona Beatrice in the eighteenth century, and of well-known later prophets.

Because they are so different, the two traditions are complementary. They fit together in Bakima's perspective and to a degree in his practice. Many patients he deals with expect treatment for the whole person, even if it is only a word of encouragement and hope for their suffering. When they are sick, they seek understanding of the source of the illness and they desire the hope of a counterforce to protect them. Bakima said that "we young physicians" are experimenting with ways to offer a more complete healing at our hospitals and clinics.

We discussed whether spiritual healing might lead to wrong ideas about the scientific knowledge of diseases. He discounted this possibility, pointing out that there is a big difference between spiritual healing and ignorance or lack of knowledge of diseases. We explored this with sickle cell anemia. Uneducated, uninformed people might interpret the multiple deaths of children of two parent carriers as being due to an incomplete bride price payment, or the witchcraft lust of one of the parents. Or there might be a vague understanding of something amiss in the biological heredity of the parents. But many educated young adults who seek marriage undergo genetic counseling, and if both are carriers or have the dominant strain of the disease, they are advised to break off their engagement.

Spiritual healing has nothing to do with bad information. It is all about the whole person's well-being in life's circumstances, and about receiving the benediction of a spirit-filled affirmation from the healer, one's family, and the community, he said. Because the CSEA practices healing, they claim that they remove the nefarious influence of bad spirits (when the healer circles the patient in a clockwise direction) and reinforcing good spirit (when the healer circles in a counterclockwise direction).

Bakima and I discussed the controversial practice of *fiela*, or *fimpa*, examination of relationships and the identification of individuals who might be the cause of a sickness through their ill will or malicious words. He stated that as a rule, and as a policy, the CSEA does not do this—at least not explicitly or publicly. In fact, one of their senior prophets told me that doing *fiela* is beyond the domain of religion. The healer has to know what is going on in the life of a sufferer but does not have to reveal it even to the patient.

However, other prophets in this tradition, and in the prophetic tradition in general, have practiced *fiela*, as the *banganga ngombo* used to do, and the few that are still around continue to do, and many people demand to know about. The process of *mfiedulu* presupposes the power of anger and ill will on the health of persons. So the CSEA allows for the reality of sorcery, anger, and other negative forces, and they heal and bless people so affected. But they do not dig around in such matters; nor do they help with the vengeance seeking that used to be done by *banganga nkisi* and may still occur. They call on the Holy Spirit to protect such people and to give them succor.

Finally, I asked Bakima if he could see himself opening a clinic with spirit healing and biomedicine as its announced practice. The main obstacle, he said, would be the licensing aspect, to get governmental acceptance. Some of his colleagues among the young doctors look askance at his dual interest, but there is at least one other young physician in the Congo who integrates his passions for both spiritual healing and biomedicine.

Conclusion

Science has become a pervasive dimension and vehicle of public health and medicine in the Manianga, and in the wider Western Equatorial African region. But the society's age-old structures and moral anchors remain strong. At the same time, the weakness of state power and the economic erosion many people have experienced have heightened anxieties and fueled paranoias. To address this condition, a range of knowledge types and therapeutic modalities have blossomed to provide substance and legitimation to the full gamut of anxieties and needs in a suffering population. Side by side, often in the same households, malaria attacks are treated with medications prescribed following examination of blood in a clinic, while fear about one's work situation or job insecurity arouses images of the use of illicit power, necessitating rituals of protection and restoration of the soul. Divination examinations thrive, and political opportunists take advantage of a fearful, desperate public.

The social and institutional settings in which these various modalities of knowledge are couched, and the extent to which they are legitimate and effective in coming to terms with the region's dominant diseases will be examined in the next, and final, chapter.

8

Legitimation and
Disease Control

Que le gouvernement puisse prendre en charge de sa population; et la population lui-
meme s'emprend en charge [Would that the government take charge of its
population, and that the population take charge of itself] (mechanic-chauffeur,
administrative assistant)

> —Intensive sample interview response, 2013

The people don't go to the clinic [I created at Kinsemi] to treat all the illnesses that
affect them. Can you find out the reason for this? Has it all been for naught?

> —Dr. Joseph Bila, Kinshasa, interview, 2013

The medical arrangement is unstable. Any part can falter or fail, impairing the
whole.

> —Dr. Alfred Monameso, MD, MPH, Head, Protestant Department
> of Medicine and Luozi Health Zone, *Vision 2017—Plan Strategique*
> *2013–2017*

In this chapter, ideas and illustrations of social legitimation introduced thus far
will be applied to interpret the structures, practices, and personalities behind the
public health, health care, and healing practices in the Manianga. Specifically, they
will be used to test this work's proposition that institutional and initiative legitimacy shapes the efficacy of a given program, course of action, therapeutic intervention, or public health policy. The same rubrics may be used to account for
and interpret both impressive successes in disease eradication and reduction (as in
the cases of polio, trypanosomiasis, smallpox, and leprosy) and the failures and
shortcoming (as with malaria, severe diarrhea, schistosomiasis, and the annual flu).

There is a hint of the issues in play in the comments of participants in our
intensive sample and in observations by administrators and professionals in public

health and medical institutions. The gap between satisfaction with services (presumably reflecting the full legitimacy and efficacy of institutions) and what the people perceive to be shortcomings (indicating inadequate legitimacy and ineffectual services) is glaring. Questions abound: How will the authorities deal with the absence of pure water sources in villages along the river? When will remote villages get health posts? Why is the quality of food in markets so bad? Why is entire infrastructure, including roads, schools, and the economy, so shaky? And the new faith-based public health and medical authorities ponder how to make the people aware of what they are doing to provide health care. Joseph Bila, famed for his early work on HIV/AIDS in Kinshasa, wonders why so few people frequent the clinic he has created in his own home village. These questions and observations reflect the objective indicators of statistical frequencies of diseases. And there are more. How can required health initiatives and the budgets of public health measures gain the backing of the public? What experiments or campaigns have been successful? Why have others failed? How is authority—consensual power—established or reestablished in social relationships, particularly kin relations, which often become tangled and contradictory? How is authority created in modern society? These questions culminate in a public cry for help: Why is the state so insensitive to its citizens?

DIVERSE DISEASES, DIVERGENT LEGITIMATIONS

In order to clearly consider the impact of institutional legitimacy on efficacy in dealing with diseases, it is useful to review the main lines of evidence and argument around three themes: first, a recognition of the distinctive characteristics of the diseases that make up the health challenge, and features they may have in common as targets of public health and medical attention; second, the institutional reconfiguration that occurred in the late 1980s and 1990s during the collapse of the state; and third, the threads of reasoning that produced an alternative picture of legitimation, one that recognized "divergent legitimations"[1] instead of a central state the source of all authority. Each of these topics receives brief attention here, then I assess the institutions that engage clusters of diseases.

I evaluate the nine principal diseases tracked by the Luozi Health Zone in terms of the legitimacy and efficacy of the institutions that are mainly responsible for dealing with them. Although each of these diseases has its own dynamics—bodily area or organ infected, bacterial or viral cause, nature of vector, environmental host, and so on—this analysis organizes them into six categories, with most conditions falling into more than one category (table 8.1).

Illnesses in the first category, water- and sewage-borne diseases, often lead to intestinal tract conditions like severe diarrhea, typhoid, dysentery, or cholera. The second category comprises diseases and conditions relating to maternal and child health, where control is considered critical for transforming the overall health of

TABLE 8.1. Categories of diseases in the Manianga region

	Categories of diseases					
	water- or sewage-borne	*maternal & children's*	*eradicated or declining in incidence*	*dangerous*	*steady-state*	*new or rising in incidence*
Principal diseases						
malaria					X	
severe diarrhea	X	X			X	
severe respiratory infection		X			X	
protein malnutrition		X	X			
seasonal flu / *grippe*						X
schistosomiasis	X				X	
tuberculosis				X	X	
typhoid fever	X			X	X	
HIV/AIDS				X	X	
Other diseases						
polio			X	X		
diabetes						X
Ebola				X		
cardiovascular disease						X
trypanosomiasis			X	X		

SOURCE: Luozi Health Zone records, 2012–13; intensive sample; Janzen fieldwork.
NOTE: The nine principal diseases tracked by the Luozi Health Zone and five additional diseases are cross-listed with six categories indicating how they are regarded by health and health care authorities.

society. Diseases here include severe diarrhea, especially among children, and protein malnutrition. In the third category are diseases that have been eradicated regionally and nearly so globally (such as polio and trypanosomiasis) and those that were in decline in the decade tracked (as is protein malnutrition).

Illnesses in the fourth category are regarded as dangerous by both the local and the international public health communities and therefore attract experts from afar to curtail such scourges. These conditions include HIV/AIDS, cholera, polio, tuberculosis (especially drug-resistant varieties), sleeping sickness, and, seen elsewhere in the region, Ebola. Diseases that have remained constant in their incidence constitute the fifth category. They do not receive the same attention from the international public health community as those in the first, second, and fourth categories, possibly because they represent no threat to the international order. The populace accepts them as normal, although they can be debilitating. Illnesses in this category include schistosomiasis (bilharzia), typhoid fever, respiratory diseases, and, above all, malaria. Finally, diseases in the sixth category are increasing in incidence. Manianga is seeing a slight increase in cases of severe diarrhea, and a more serious and dramatic rise in the incidence of annual flu (la grippe) because of regular travel to centers like metropolitan Kinshasa, Matadi, and beyond. This category also includes diabetes and cardiovascular conditions, new diseases that affect especially the nonagricultural class.

The institutional reconfiguration of the 1980s and 1990s turned the preexisting state-centric system on its head. The clinical- and hospital-centered medicine of earlier eras was reconfigured according to or became subservient to the health zones. Prioritization of curative medicine gave way to an emphasis on preventive medicine, including children's inoculations and maternal and children's health. The coordination of this new public health approach, organized around the decentralized health zones, was gradually taken over by church-based agencies, in particular Santé Rurale du Congo (SANRU), with the consent of a greatly weakened national Ministry of Health. In time and through various transformations SANRU became a national NGO, operating in parallel to state structures of health. Health clinics and hospitals were inserted into this decentralized system of health zones. A variety of private initiatives and organizations and global health NGOs—foremost among them the World Health Organization (WHO)—formed additional parts of this institutional configuration. The institutional upheaval and innovation complemented the continuing role of local government (including landed domains, villages, clans, sectors, and communes) in their responsibilities of overseeing water sources and sewage treatment (table 8.2).

The divergent legitimations of this new institutional configuration required us to find the most appropriate theoretical formulations that accommodated the nonstate players in this story—the NGOs, the civil society agencies and networks, and the churches. Such formulations as "capillaries of social power" (Lipshutz 2005) and finding the "constitutions for decision-making" (Macrae 1997) regarding the allocation of resources and the shaping of postconflict rehabilitation were put forward for this analysis. These ideas of social and institutional legitimacy joined Kongo thought with regard to the strategic transformations of creating vested social order out of chaos and illicit power. The literature on postconflict restoration of public services gave us the accurate description of divergent legitimation flowing from a number of sources of authority beyond the boundaries of a society. Our working definition of institutional legitimacy, fashioned out of this potpourri of concepts from varied traditions, may be summarized as follows.

Legitimate social and institutional authority presupposes the consent of the populace, the governed, the subordinate, and often in our focus, the sick and their

TABLE 8.2. Institutions and initiatives addressing categories of diseases

	Categories of diseases					
	water- or sewage-borne	*maternal & children's*	*eradicated or declining in incidence*	*dangerous*	*steady-state*	*new or rising in incidence*
local chiefs, clan heads, mayors	X					
health zones		X	X		X	
hospitals, health centers & posts		X	X		X	X
church medical ministries		X				
private clinics, pharmacies		X	X	X	X	X
ad hoc coalitions	X					
national NGOs: SANRU, REGIDESO	X	X		X		
international NGOs: WHO, CDC, GAVI	X	X		X		

SOURCE: Janzen fieldwork.

kin. Without this dimension few initiatives or institutional creations may be expected to be effective or long-lasting. Legitimate authority also requires the common good as a goal of powerful actors, because it is their influence and control of resources that makes possible effective action. Further legitimate authority must include a set of rules or laws that clearly enunciate procedures in terms of which actors and officials are held accountable, whether these rules emanate from national legal codes or international conventions and agreements. These rules or procedures must be coordinated with a constitution shared by the community being served. Such a constitution need not necessarily be a written document. The entire corpus of ideas about the society, its assumptions, and its normative codes makes decisions possible and morally binding, and thus real.[2]

Legitimate authority may emanate from the concerted engagement of recognized international bodies in the health affairs of a local society and in the application of outside funds and resources, such as medicines, experts, and medical practitioners. But the practitioners of such outside initiatives must take into account local authorities who may resist their action out of a sense of threat to their own authority. Also the failure to take into account local knowledge—the society's constitution—

in the introduction of outside techniques and resources may result in failure of the initiative when the outside networks and flows come to an end. Finally, legitimacy of health and healing institutions and initiatives usually involves some sort of transcendent anchoring in tradition or in religious or ancestral points of reference.

Water- and Sewage-Borne Diseases

The importance of pure water for drinking and relatively clean water for bathing is clearly at the forefront of Maniangan consciousness. Most people make the connection between pure water and the absence of gastrointestinal diseases like typhoid fever, severe diarrhea in children, and worse conditions, like cholera. In recent decades the idea of convenience, of proximity to the source of clean water, has been added to that of clean water's availability. The importance of pit latrines is also linked in many minds to healthful living and the avoidance of these and other serious diseases.

It has become abundantly clear that the legitimacy behind the clean water sources and pit latrines in the Manianga is the populace itself, as well as local government. There is no sharp division between populace and government at this level, where clan heads, village heads, land chiefs, and *groupement* and sector chiefs are all drawn from the local community by either election or appointment. A strong measure of self-serving preventive action is involved in digging a latrine pit or cementing in and pipe tapping a spring. In all jurisdictions of the region local officials are tasked with overseeing these health-enhancing measures and with sanctioning those who are lax in their attention to the expected measures. That these officials are supported in their oversight work provides a strong indication of consent of the governed. This legitimacy reaches far back into the precolonial past. Whatever reforms and refinements were made by the colonial government have been incorporated into the tradition of legitimate local government. Governmentality at this level enjoys a robust legitimacy in which self-serving self-help suffices to maintain a fairly high level of healthful living.

But there are shortcomings in the legitimacy of existing institutions with regard to water and sewage oversight and development. This is most evident from the outcries of those who lack these services, mainly among the villages of fishers along the Congo River. The near universal infestation of schistosomiasis-carrying and -transmitting snails in their water streams raised their ire, which they directed at the state. The legitimacy deficit voiced in this popular outcry was extended by the apparent absence of any health policies pertaining to dealing with the infestation or to providing an alternative source of water for drinking, cooking, and bathing. The fishing villages along the Congo River also demonstrated the legitimacy and efficacy deficit in that all respondents from these villages reported in the intensive sample survey that they dealt with their schistosomiasis symptoms through self-medication rather than visits to a health post or center. In other words, they appeared to have been abandoned in their plight with this pervasive disease.

Further legitimacy shortcomings are apparent in the maintenance of water provisioning infrastructure. Fully half of the village hand pumps that an NGO had installed with wells in the postcolonial era were nonfunctional.[3] The ones I asked about in villages I visited—including both wells in Kisiasia, North Manianga—were said to have stopped working some years ago. No one seemed to know what was wrong with them or who was responsible for repairing them. The territorial administrator's report recommended that this be investigated by the proper authorities but did not specify who those authorities were. Villagers in Kisiasia had returned to using the cemented-in springs that then-mayor Kusikila had installed back in the late 1950s with the help of former students. The only hardship with the use of these springs was that they were located at some distance from the village and required a steep walk uphill with a full container of water on one's head.

The same legitimacy deficiency is evident in the institutional administration of the Luozi waterworks. Coordination of fuel for the pump engines, parts for repair and upkeep, and overall management of the intricate system requires a much more complex level of specialized competence than single water pumps do. The institutional basis of the urban waterworks reached well beyond local government to the corporate public utility REGIDESO, an agency within the Department of Mines of the Democratic Republic of the Congo (DRC). It has its own cadre of engineers and company headquarters in Kinshasa that are, at least in theory, on call when things go wrong at the pumping station. Given its fee-for-service financial support from each and every user, paid monthly, it is designed to operate and support itself. Popular support and the strong desire to have clean water and to avoid trips to the polluted, crocodile infested, Congo River, make the legitimacy of the waterworks self-evident to everyone. Yet it is vulnerable to shortages of fuel and to delays in the availability of machine replacement parts. How the waterworks will fare as a privatized corporation remains to be seen.

Maternal and Child Health

Maternal and child health involves much more than combating diseases. It centrally entails the promotion of prenatal care and nutrition, safe birthing facilities and practices, and postnatal administration of vaccinations and supplements like Vitamin A. Luozi Health Zone reports for the 2003–12 decade indicate a slight decline in infant mortality rates, from eighty to sixty-six deaths per one thousand children under one year of age, continuing the significant decline from three hundred in 1935. The current infant mortality rate reflects the incidence of severe diarrhea and malaria. By contrast, the level of protein malnutrition fell steadily during the 2003–12 decade, no doubt due in part to the systematic distribution of Vitamin A supplements.

On the maternal health side of the equation, parents have strong concern for the well-being and education of their children, and the crucial place they see in this for family planning. The picture of maternal and child health is thus mixed, with a slight tilt toward improvement.

Maternal and child health is shaped by almost all the institutions listed in table 8.2. The first of these is the local community and government where the women and children reside, and where they benefit from whatever clean water and sewage treatment may be available, or suffer if it is not available. The services that are funneled through the health zone—inoculations, supplements, special campaigns—are directly beneficial to mothers and children. The health posts, clinics, and hospitals and their managing directorates provide care during emergencies and health crises. The gradual decline in protein malnutrition is a direct indicator of the legitimacy and efficacy of these institutions.

Yet there are legitimacy shortcomings in these institutions, too. Some followers of the nativist-nationalist Bundu dia Kongo movement harbor strong opposition to childhood vaccinations and dietary supplements. For them, a Christian church-managed medical institution obliging them to allow their children to be given foreign medicine is a gross violation of their convictions. The parental resistance to child vaccinations was one of the topics over which I had the most extended discussions with the staff of the health zone. They were greatly surprised to hear that such resistance, albeit for very different reasons, existed in the United States. In a setting where children still die from severe diarrhea, typhoid, malaria, and not so long ago polio, they could not fathom the antivaccination movement in the industrialized West.

Eradicated and Declining Diseases

Since the 2008 polio eradication campaign led by WHO, the Manianga has had no polio cases, and the disease has been dropped from the lists of principal and even occasional diseases. At the time of this writing, the WHO campaign is still working in a few pockets in a few countries. The only tangible evidence of the Luozi campaign is the hand-drawn map on the wall of the health zone headquarters.

A legitimacy analysis of the 2008 polio eradication campaign allows us to visualize the threads of support, endorsement, and resource flow, as well as resistance, through a number of institutions. The basic structure and staff of the campaign was the health zone. Because this was part of a global campaign, there was good publicity and advance knowledge about it. Financial resources as well as the vaccine were provided, along with expert technicians from WHO to ensure reasonable coverage. The pockets of resistance encountered did not, apparently, invalidate the campaign because there were no active infections in those enclaves at the time of the campaign. The polio eradication effort was not the first campaign on which WHO, the health zone, and SANRU or the Ministry of Health had collaborated;

therefore, public opinion was mostly in favor of the action. It was well organized at all levels of the chain of distribution and execution.

Largely the same story could be told about trypanosomiasis, with the difference lying in the more complex nature of the disease's transmission—human to vector, via other nonhuman carriers, to other humans. Furthermore, the disease may persist in mammals that are immune to it and may therefore transmit it to humans via tsetse fly vectors. The case of trypanosomiasis reported in chapter 2 reveals a gap in the institutional legitimacy of WHO campaigns, especially those that are localized and whose management depends on a team of strangers who come to a region for a few weeks, then disappear. This case raises the question of what is required to sustain the infrastructure and management of public health institutions and linkages for unspecified future outbreaks.

The third case of a disease on the decline with yet other implications for institutional legitimacy is that of protein malnutrition as tracked in the Luozi Health Zone. It declined from 553 cases in 2003 to 153 cases in 2012. Here the diligent work of the health zone staff, who regularly visited health posts and centers, ensuring that Vitamin A supplements were administered and other dietary rules were maintained, meant that most of the patients regained their health. But this disease is dependent on there being a reasonably sound economy and access to food by the poorest households. This requires not just WHO with its supplements, or even the presence of a distribution network in the health zone, but a viable local economy that includes even the poorest.

Dangerous Diseases

The category of diseases that are regarded as dangerous or highly contagious by international health agencies, and therefore a threat to the global community, is closely related to the foregoing category of eradicated diseases. However, eradicated diseases are part of history, part of the successful endeavor of global health institutions to eliminate major diseases, one after the other, from the face of the earth. Dangerous diseases are still active and must be vigilantly tracked and pursued. HIV/AIDS, polio, trypanosomiasis (sleeping sickness), and Ebola (which has appeared elsewhere in the DRC) have all received focused attention and campaign funding in recent years. Here the general demand or expectation of the populace has matched the NGO rationale for the advancement of global health.

Medications reported in the Luozi Health Zone or the intensive sample for these diseases were free to the patient, and the health zone has provided the format for carrying out these initiatives. Indeed, one can argue that the health zone infrastructure has been largely supported by the flow of international funds to deal with these dangerous diseases, to stop them at their source. But such initiatives have only gone partway in the creation of health-maintaining infrastructure and long-term institutional legitimacy.

Steady-State Diseases

Malaria remains the major chronic tropical disease in Western Equatorial Africa, and specifically in the region along the Congo River where Luozi, the territorial capital, is located. Institutions and initiatives that address this disease do not go beyond a general curative approach for each individual episode suffered. Fully a third of the populace is recorded to have visited a clinic for malaria each year in the decade from 2003 to 2012. Hospitals, health centers, health posts, and pharmacies all carry medications that bring down fever and help sufferers get through a specific episode. Infants suffering the dangerous combined effects of malaria infection—diarrhea, dehydration, and anemia—are regularly given blood transfusions, most often directly from a compatible kinsperson.

Malaria is considered a normal disease, and the populace mostly accepts it as a given. WHO-distributed medicated nets are enthusiastically welcomed. The nets may have somewhat lessened the infection rates, although the health zone statistics from 2003 to 2012 do not show it. They have in no way decreased the number of the mosquitoes that carry and spread malaria. Thus although the availability of cures offers medical institutions an aura of legitimacy in dealing with malaria, there is no engagement at the public level to change the status quo. This is evident in the malarial cures offered by private pharmacies and the absence of public campaigns to lessen malaria infection. Many households keep their yards free of grass and underbrush, and there is some awareness of the dangers of standing water pools. Yet there are no programs, nor even apparently consciousness of the need for elimination of such pools on the public streets and in ditches where mosquitoes breed.

The same conclusion might be drawn regarding seasonal upper respiratory infections and schistosomiasis, which is chronic among fishing communities along the rivers. The absence of a sustained public initiative on these major diseases is an indication of the lack of institutional legitimacy and the will to engage with these debilitating conditions. In both the malaria and schistosomiasis episodes in the intensive sample of our study, self-medication was high, suggesting that the populace either believes that it can take care of itself and that a visit to a clinic is time-consuming and expensive, or that it does not have high confidence in the institutions that might be expected to deal with these conditions.

Contagious diseases like typhoid fever, tuberculosis, and HIV/AIDS are present at a relatively low number of visits to health posts, health centers, and referral hospitals. Their treatment has been the focus of international NGOs that have usually supported tracking and medical treatment. Tuberculosis patients regularly receive antibiotics. Medical support in the form of the medication AZT is available for HIV/AIDS patients.

Schistosomiasis is a focus of WHO, although it is not clear what specifically is being done about the sites where snails are present. Malaria is also the focus of a number of international NGOs, although there was little evidence of this in the Manianga beyond the availability of medicated nets and of medications for infections on a case-by-case basis. Can the present level and nature of outside support to health zone and clinical care bring malaria infections down? This is unlikely because the program for intervention is largely individual and episode-specific rather than preventative.

In order for the malaria program to move to a different level of coverage, especially if it is to be preventive, the public sector of towns and cities, and the public places in them would need to be more fully engaged. Coordinating the elimination and prevention of water pools in street-side ditches and on roadways in towns and cities would require a new initiative through civic administrations that currently barely exist or are extremely understaffed. The case of Dar es Salaam, Tanzania, is instructive. There both individualized curative medicine and a rigorous program of filling pools and ditches or treating them with oils, and draining swamps and other *Anopheles* breeding grounds are in effect. The latter approach is more effective but requires extensive public authority to enact (Kelly 2012). Could international NGO involvement provide an avenue for this level of coverage and prevention? The Gates Foundation's malaria eradication program features research initiatives in genetic alteration of mosquitoes, as well as intensive tracking of cycles of infection in Rwanda and elsewhere. Although the Gates Foundation is a partner with SANRU, I heard nothing of these cutting-edge programs in Luozi. Until the public networks of the health zone are ramped up to far greater density and financing, it is unlikely that malaria incidence will decline much.

Is this an issue of legitimacy, of financing, or of both? The present structure of public health is underfunded for what it is trying to do, and it is also given very little structural legitimacy in the form of legal and constitutional cover. The health zone system did not receive a single mention in the intensive sample survey. Although it is seen as a critical program nationally and internationally, it has not been given serious legitimacy in a public sense.

New Diseases and Diseases with Increasing Incidence

The seasonal flu, known as *la grippe*, showed a dramatic increase in incidence across the Luozi Health Zone from 2006 to 2012, from zero to 3,158 cases seen by health posts, health centers, and the referral hospital. (Most likely it did not begin to be present in 2006 but began to be tracked in that year because of rising incidence.) Other than to relieve the fever with aspirin and other medications, there was no plan of an approach to the seasonal outbreak and global spread of the flu. Even if the knowledge of such a disease spreading globally had been known, and it may have been by some medical observers, there was no infrastructure in place to accommodate a massive campaign of flu vaccinations. This suggests that in the eyes of both the populace and health experts the flu is like malaria, a dimension of normal life with occasional sicknesses and unfortunate deaths.

A full range of legitimation anchors are needed if these services are to be effectively initiated and maintained, and if institutions are to have staying power beyond a crisis, epidemic, or infusion of outside funds on a one-time basis. Public demand and expressed need for services is but one aspect of the legitimation needed. The coordination of medical experts and institutional upkeep requires extensive legitimation of the kind that Max Weber (1980) called rational-legal authority and others refer to as adherence to a predictable legal code. Yet if the entire configuration of structures is not kept together by an overarching authority of the kind we usually associate with the state, can it be sustained? Although the churches of the Congo are clearly willing to carry out the extraordinary service of medical coordination, they do not find much satisfaction in doing the work of the state. They await fuller state partnership.

YEARNING FOR THE STATE

The appeal to the churches to take on the administration and coordination of the health zones in the early 1990s raises intriguing issues of legitimation. Clearly the will of the governed was engaged. The voices heard in the intensive sample suggest a groundswell of discontent, summed up in this comment: "The land is not thriving; there's great difficulty paying hospital and school fees. The government of the land should arrange matters to restore people's hope." Yet when the state fails, does the agency that comes forward to take its place find the legitimacy afforded a functional state, or even a state organized by patrimonial patronage ties? Alfred Monameso, head of the Protestant Department of Medicine (DOM), in both interview comments and in the Vision 2017 document (Communauté Evangélique du Congo 2012), voices serious doubts about the DOM's ability to meet expectations placed upon it. The funding base is insufficient to meet the need, and unstable. He voices the concern that many clientele do not appreciate what the DOM is doing, the sacrificial service it is providing. Several medical doctors expressed their concern over the fact that the populace does not avail itself of the medical services before it. They say that people instead run off to charlatan healers for panacea remedies instead of real medical care.

Vision 2017 suggests that an advertising campaign might be needed to promote the health zone and its medical institutions. But the long-range plan represented by Vision 2017 suggests that the heads of the DOM and the church elders see the present arrangement as temporary. Restoration of state support and coordination is the expected, hoped for goal. On the other hand, the churches do have the confidence of most citizens, and the church bureaucracies were the most durable corporate structures remaining after the collapse of the state in the early 1990s.

What more would they need to do to ramp up the work they are doing, in order to address new diseases and the significant increase in seasonal flu? If the global solution of annual flu vaccinations were to be adopted, such a move would require an initiative comparable to the polio vaccination campaign or the Vitamin A for children campaign, on an annual basis. In other words, an additional feature of public health coverage would be required. In the past, new rounds of medical procedures have been possible only with outside support. This is unlikely to occur until a new or rising disease is seen as a threat to global health.

The health zone framework itself is quite fragile in this entire scheme of divergent legitimations for public health and health care. Brought into existence in 1985, it is now the official structure within which to coordinate institutions, medical professionals, supplies, and services. The small team of an *animateur*, a nurse-*infirmier*, and a secretary is seriously challenged to visit all health posts on a regular basis. Locally, citizen teams are doing their best to encourage nurses and other medical practitioners to meet the needs of the people. Yet the Luozi Health Zone team lacked even a single computer to compile its results and had to rely instead on large paper sheets on the walls of its small offices to tabulate participation rates, medication records, and basic demographic and epidemiological information. The high expectations placed on these teams by the populace and by the agencies expecting good records (the shadow Ministry of Health and WHO, for example) gave them strong popular and outside NGO legitimacy, but this legitimacy was hardly matched by funds to carry out their multiple responsibilities. In sum, the health zone in Luozi and the Manianga is dependent on soft money—project-specific outside support—for its very existence. It lacks rational-legal authority or legitimacy.

Despite the success in bringing down protein malnutrition within a credible basic infrastructure of public health and special NGO attention to the condition, and financial support for stocks of vitamins, full legitimacy at multiple levels of coordination and resource availability is lacking for all the conditions in the health zone. The continuing chronic levels of diseases such as malaria, tuberculosis, schistosomiasis, and typhoid fever, as well as inattention to the rising rates of seasonal flu, can only be explained by the absence of overarching state power and legitimation, including especially the corresponding lack of funding. The infrastructure and funding created by a Geneva-based organization for vitamin A dietary supplements for children does not translate into malaria eradication.

This absence of overarching coordination and regular long-term financing is evident in some popular comments and in a round of voices from the intensive sample survey that leapt out of the data. These were in addition to pleas for economic revitalization and comments about specific diseases, particular water sources, and the quality of food. They addressed the elephant in the room: the leadership, the government, the state.

- *L'etat kaketi baka bantu en charge ko; makompani nkatu*—The state doesn't take charge of people; there are no companies (fisher, seamstress).
- *Tuetei sala mu ngolo mu ntoto kansi mbakulu yena mpasi. Tueti lomba kua zimfumu za luyalu batukubikila nsi*—We work hard in the soil but yield is meager; we pray the heads of government to put things in order (both cultivators).
- *Nsi ka yena ya dedama ko, mpasi mu futa mbongo ku hospital evo ku skulu. Luyalu lua nsi kakubika nsamu miami bima bantu balenda vuvama*—The land is not thriving; there's great difficulty paying hospital and school fees. The government of the land should arrange matters to restore people's hope (both cultivators).
- *Nga luyalu lenda sadisa kansi kaluena ko. Tueti nuana kaka mu beto kibeni*—Would that the government would help, but it doesn't; we are struggling on our own (both cultivators).
- *Vo tuena ye bisalu buna tulenda vuka. Idio vo luyalu lua nsi lulenda kutubanzila buna luvuvamu luna kala mu bantu*—If we had work, we would revive. Therefore if the government of the land would be able to think of us the people would again have hope (both cultivators).
- *Que le gouvernement puisse prendre en charge de sa population; et la population lui-meme s'emprend en charge*—Would that the government take charge of its population, and that the population take charge of itself (mechanic-chauffeur, administrative assistant).

CONCLUSION

These voices register the sentiment that divergent legitimation is not enough and is not coherent enough to meet the needs and longings for the people's health and health care. They suggest that the effort to create institutional alternatives to earlier state-based programs are not workable and not visible enough. The health zone system and its various NGO suppliers and brokers received no mention in the intensive sample survey. Can it really be the case that the health zone institutional structure is invisible to the respondents? Perhaps they do not differentiate between authorities in civic, religious, state, and NGO administrative hierarchies. For them, the coherence of leadership associated with a unitary state is the solution to all ills, especially those related to health care and economic well-being.

Perhaps there is hope again for fuller governmental involvement in public health and health care in the DRC. Despite the continuing news of conflict and deferred elections in the several years after this research in 2013, the DRC had, by early 2018, improved its standing on the Failed State Index, to seventh from its all-time worst position, of second from the bottom. This is in part due to the disintegration of other countries, like Syria and Yemen. Although the DRC's Ministry of

Health has few funds to distribute from the national treasury, it has reclaimed its role as a policy-setting agency that supports all the civic, international, and private initiatives in public health and health care.

SANRU has become a full-fledged, independent national NGO, with a secure niche as broker of funds and medical resources from a range of donors. At the time of this writing in early 2018, its financial contribution was on the order of $100 million annually, flowing in funds, services, and resources to most of the five hundred health zones across the country.[4] This agency, which had its origins in the distinctive Congolese decentralized health zone movement and was able to sustain the coordination and flow of resources throughout a dark and tumultuous period in the history of the DRC, holds a unique position in the annals of public health administration. SANRU is clearly given its power by outside funding agencies— USAID, the Gates Foundation, Global Alliance for Vaccines and Immunization (GAVI), the Centers for Disease Control, the United Nations Development Programme, and others—but it is now administered entirely by Congolese medical and public health professionals. This highlights its legitimacy from consent of the people. It is legally secured by the Congolese state as a national NGO and has a series of official partners, including its former parent, the national Protestant church council, Communauté Evangélique du Congo. It works alongside the Ministry of Health, from which it receives policy guidelines and program recommendations. The main shortcoming, in terms of the criteria of legitimation, is that its funding is from soft-money and project-specific sources, although some grants have gone to build up and restore health zones destroyed by war. SANRU exemplifies the best in public-private partnerships.

CONCLUSION

Two narratives have flowed through this work's chapters and pages. The first has been an epidemiological narrative about the incidence and nature of diseases that affect the human population. The second has been about the legitimacy of institutions, particularly those that attend to public health and health care in the Lower Congo and in the north bank Territory of Luozi. The chapters have progressively demonstrated that these two narratives, and their realms of discourse and reality, are profoundly intertwined. The double entendre of this book's title—*Health in a Fragile State*—is intended to capture this entanglement: the fragile state leads to fragile health. Conversely, institutional strength, as seen in full social legitimacy of institutions, empowers the public and those who work in such institutions to more efficaciously deal with diseases, yielding declining disease incidence and better health.

As I considered the many ways that health and society could be analyzed in the postcolonial Lower Congo, this approach rose to the top. First, I noticed the paradox of lingering levels of diseases for which there are full explanations and available treatments. Second, I had seen the seemingly arbitrary constellation of institutions that emerged to carry public health and health care when state-sponsored structures dissolved in the 1980s and 1990s. Third, I was able to see this institutional fluidity against the backdrop of many historical institutional dissolutions and re-creations—for example, the disintegration of the Kongo kingdom and other centralized polities, the emergence of cult-like trade-route networks like Lemba, and the arbitrary imposition of colonial chiefships, often bypassing established chiefs. The current institutional arrangement seemed merely the latest in a string of arbitrary orders. Surely the improvised and temporary quality of these arrangements have a profound impact on the way focused affairs like public health and health care must be organized to be effective.

The work investigates the layers of this topic in three parts and develops a cor-responding analysis. Part I, "A History of Population and Disease in the Lower Congo," shows the extent and locales of population displacement, disease, and mass death that resulted from forced labor policies and projects, especially in the Congo Free State period (1885-1907). The colonial government, in an effort to minimize the public relations disaster that was unfolding on the international front, made pro forma inquiries about the regions of depopulation and shrinking chiefdoms, and presented to the world a façade of reformed labor and governance policies that were considered good for the people and for the colony's productivity. Fortunately, foreign missions like the Svenska Missions Förbundet were there to model public health campaigns that eventually turned the catastrophe around. From 1930 on, the demographic evidence suggests a gradual decline in mortality rates and a rise in overall population. What makes this historical story relevant to the postcolonial story of health in a fragile state is its echoes in the memories of many people as they speak about their own health and living situation. The like-lihood of lingering unconscious memory around disease makes it worthwhile to revisit historical events in the Congo River region.

Part II, "The Social Reproduction of Health," presents the institutional here and now of the story: first, the domestic realm, where economic viability and shar-ing of risk occur at a most intimate level; second, the public institutions that do the work of public health and health care; and third, popular ideas and perspec-tives about what health is and means. The second of these presentations highlights the distinctive reconfiguration of loosely related institutions and initiatives that emerged during the 1980s and 1990s collapse of the Zairian state. Some of these, such as local government and the hospitals, were a continuation of what had been there before under state control and coordination. However, the centerpiece of the configuration, the health zone, was new. When the health zones became the backbone of national health care in the Congo, hospitals and clinics were to some extent placed on a back burner. Part II demonstrates that there is an ongoing and thriving, if fragile, public health and health care structure.

Part III, "The Legitimation of Power and Knowledge," focuses on the uses of authority and authoritative knowledge in health and healing. Institutional legiti-macy is difficult to measure, and even if it is identified by its attributes, it is difficult to apply as a causal explanation of the way things are. But authors and theorists can demonstrate the importance to overall social well-being of a relatively full contin-gent of legitimacy's features.

Definitions of and debates over legitimacy appear at several places in the vol-ume. A basic picture of the issues and a proposition about the relationship of institutions to disease appear in the introduction. Chapter 6, "*Dumuna*: Creat-ing Authority from Below," offers a more extensive discussion of legitimation theory and discusses which formulations are most appropriate for the reconfigured health and health care institutional setting after the collapse of the state. This presentation of theories of legitimation includes the tenets of an implicit philosophy of power in Kongo society as presented by several thoughtful and articulate spokespersons.

An ultimate formulation of the attributes of institutional legitimacy is presented in the opening of chapter 8. Its features are:

(1) the consent of the populace, the governed, the sick, and their kin;
(2) the common good as a goal of powerful actors;
(3) a set of rules or laws that enunciate procedures and regarding which there can be accountability;
(4) a written or implicit constitution shared by the community being served, which is referred to in decision-making over resources;
(5) allowance for the engagement of international bodies in the health affairs of the local society; and
(6) transcendent anchoring in religious or ancestral reference, or in tradition.

Chapter 8 also offers a nuanced picture of this entanglement of institutional legitimation and health. Six clusters of diseases, each with a different trajectory, is interpreted in relation to the institutions taking charge of its control. Diseases that are water- and sewage-borne are mainly addressed by local governments, which encourage the populace to keep their water sources clean and to build and maintain pit toilets. Those diseases that affect the health of women and children are addressed by a broad arc of public health and medical institutions. The eradication and declining incidence of certain diseases generally reflects the involvement of international agencies working through the new, nongovernmental institutions of public health, including the health zones, SANRU, and the Ministry of Health. Diseases considered dangerous are taken on by international experts, who work through health zones in order to control them at their source.

Diseases that demonstrate a steady state—a continuing level of infection and incidence—and those that are new or rising in incidence are of most concern to us, for they represent the ongoing state of affairs and evidence of new dangers. Three diseases are particularly noteworthy: malaria, schistosomiasis, and the annual flu. Malaria affects nearly everyone in the populace in a given year, and perhaps a third of the cases are serious enough for patients to find their way to institutional care. But this care, which is generally good, deals only with the specific episode and seeks only to get the individual sufferer through the episode. Little attention is paid to prophylaxis or environmental conditions that contribute to transmission, not to mention measures that would stop the cycle of transmission and thus lead to eradication of the disease. Schistosomiasis is similarly pervasive in riverside communities, particularly among fishers, who work in the water. Residents of these communities wish their drinking and bathing conditions could be improved, but no one takes them up on their pleas. The third disease, the global flu, is alarmingly on the rise. It is being tracked, but there appears to be no program for flu vaccines. Sufferers are on their own or can expect to receive only symptomatic care in the clinics.

If institutional legitimacy is the hallmark of effective disease control, what is missing here? If global health agencies were to take an interest in these diseases as they have in HIV/AIDS, Ebola, trypanosomiasis, and polio, and if they were to ship medicines and invest funds in treatment and prevention, no doubt change would happen. But it might last only as long as the funding and program assistance. Perhaps knowledge of disease control would find its way into the local repository of knowledge and stimulate responses such as Joswe Mbaku's program for assisting people with sickle cell anemia to create a meaningful life for themselves.

Health and healing knowledge exists in complex and intertwined formulations, characterized in this work as science and spirit. These types of knowledge are not the same as modern and traditional. Rather, science and spirit are complementary ways of articulating systematic connections between visible evidence and theoretical axioms. Science has to do with what we see under the microscope, in DNA, in the soil on the hillside, and in the automobile's engine, and can be understood with ideas taught in the university or by experts elsewhere in the world. Spirit has to do with the voice of and blessing by the spirits of nature, God, the ancestors, and the human community. In the minds of most Maniangans these two ways of knowing are intertwined; they can be marshalled together to bring about a coherent, collaborative approach to problem solving, to creating a better world.

If this complex knowledge is to become useful to individuals, families, the community, and the nation, it must be couched in and owned by a legitimate social body, whether that be the family, clan, school or university, the church, the state, or some institutional entity created by and responsible to the state. It is especially at the upper reaches of social order that the Lower Congo, indeed much of Western Central Africa, has seen so many and such pervasive political delegitimations over the past several centuries. The rise and destruction of successive political regimes, social orders, and cultural practices has created its own kind of traumatic collective amnesia that is expressed in fears of hidden illicit powers and suspicious forces, and spurious cures and panaceas to offset them.

Although the north bank of the Congo River was not significantly touched by the Kongo kingdom, the seventeenth-century defeat of the kingdom, followed by interregnum chaos, resulted in the heightened reliance on *minkisi* charms for the politics of social control. In the north bank societies, the rise of the coastal trade and the introduction of mercantile wealth and the slave trade from the sixteenth through the nineteenth centuries transformed the social compact within and between local communities. The end of this mercantile system, controlled by Congolese elites, came in the late nineteenth century with the introduction of the Congo Free State. Very quickly the new rulers shifted the centers of power and brought to an end long-standing chiefdoms and trade relations. Others were brought into being by the Free State's agents. Belgian colonialism solidified the Free State's structure of tribute-paying, forced-labor-recruiting colonial chiefs. This structure was overturned with independence and replaced by the even less predictable authorities of the postcolonial order. Although the Manianga region was not directly affected by Congo's postcolonial wars, the weakening of the Zairian state resulted in the evaporation of structures of service that had been developed in higher education, the postal service, roadways, railroads, and health care.

Despite major progress in the decline of mortality rates, especially infant mortality rates, major diseases whose treatments and cures are well known continue at unacceptable levels of infection. The worst of these, malaria, continues to infect and kill, despite the pervasive use of medicated mosquito nets and widespread knowledge and availability of prophylactics and cures. Bilharzia, sleeping sickness, and HIV/AIDS continue to make their appearance although in far diminished numbers compared to earlier times. Rising incidence of the annual flu challenges existing services. The availability of hospitals and clinics, trained personnel, and (usually) medicines drives citizens of Luozi and the hinterlands to dig very deeply into their pockets for emergency medical care. The high and rising cost of everything presses common folk to keep one foot in the subsistence economy to stave off destitution.

Living on the brink fuels paranoid worldviews and the embrace of panaceas. The moral universe that accompanies a neoliberal economy, in which everything can be bought and sold, frames who is marginalized, who is victimized, and who wins or holds power. Theories of illicitly gained power abound, as well as rituals of protection from the predators of souls and resources. *Sorcery* in the book's title reveals the space left by the absentee state and the failed or disrupted institution. This is Kusikila's *kimongi*, the unnatural death inflicted by uncaptured power that is loose in the land and in the perceptions of its people. It is there in the haunting, threatening, telephone call; the death of a fisher by crocodile on the river; the child's death from a malaria fever that the medical staff thought was manageable; the trusted elder's sudden and too-early death; the student's sudden death, for which his peers seek revenge on his parents. All these disconcerting events add to the paranoid fear of those who struggle to get by day to day. A leader like Muanda Nsemi can fan the flames of these fears and anxieties into the out-of-control brush fires of lynch mobs. The last vestiges of a fragile state, the military's special forces, kill several dozen protestors, and the tension and paranoia continue.

The legitimate integration of knowledge and power is pivotal to the achievement of effective disease control and enhancement of health in the Manianga region of the Lower Congo, and in many similar regions of the world. This work has focused on the way that multiple kinds of knowledge have been developed to heal the conditions that affect people in the region and the social and institutional structures in which this knowledge is couched. The study and its analysis may provide health planners and analysts, as well as independent scholars like anthropologists, with a perspective that accounts for successes and failures. Social legitimation—the public will, clear authority by duly elected or appointed officials, and experts with adequate resources at their disposal—are required in order to achieve popularly desired goals of health care and public health. Creative individuals will continue to launch special initiatives and to found institutions, but the burden of history suggests that effective action in any realm—transportation, education, scientific research and development, food production, and health and health care—requires long-term consistency that can best be provided by an enlightened democratic state based on a constitution that is accompanied by laws to guide it, and incorporating an adequate educational system to produce the needed health and health care experts. That is the social legitimacy that the people of the Lower Congo crave and deserve.

These people's voices are present throughout the work in the form of KiKongo and French citations of their responses in the intensive sample. Some of the statements are matter-of-fact replies to survey questions, whereas others are open-ended comments about the shortcomings of public health and health care, food, markets, the economy, and their leaders. Popular passion about their situation is evident. Like a chorus in a classical Greek drama, they are there, watching, acting, demanding, and waiting for appropriate and ample public health and health care.

NOTES

Introduction

1. Interview with Cyprien Opira, medical director at Lacor Hospital, Gulu, Uganda, November 2014.

2. Social anthropology seminar and interview with Norman Schräpel, University of Halle-Wittenberg, 2014.

3. Interview with Ngoyi Bukonda, professor of public health at Wichita State University, former student of Martin Ngwete, and adviser in the early administration of Zairian health zones; interviews conducted from 2012 to 2015.

4. Interviews with Pakisa Tshimika, who was instrumental in the creation and revitalization of the health zones in the Bandundu Province, whose capital is Kikwit; interviews conducted in 1991, 1995, and 2000.

5. Bukonda interview.

6. Ibid.

7. The use of the names "Congo" and "Kongo" is governed by the following scholarly and popular conventions. Congo refers to the modern states—the Democratic Republic of Congo (Kinshasa) and the Republic of Congo (Brazzaville)—the Congo river, and the entire Congo Basin. Kongo refers to the Kongo ethnic group and identity (Bakongo) resident in northern Angola, western DRC, and the Congo Republic as well as the historic Kongo kingdom, the KiKongo language, and as an adjective describing customary practices in these societies.

8. This figure is based on the average number of residents in an intensive sample: 579 individuals in 105 households equals 5.6 individuals per household. Thus 15,000 residents in Luozi divided by 5.6 equals approximately 2,678 households.

9. Interview and Luozi city tour with Henriette Kalusebolo Mattlola, secretary for civil affairs registration in the Luozi city office, 2013

10. Interviews and conversations with Thomas Kisolokele, former mayor and advisor of the Centre de Vulgarisation Agricole, 2013.

11. For a general overview of the movement Bundu dia Kongo and a summary of its teachings as contained in Nsemi's prolific writings, see Wamba-dia-Wamba (1999). For a

field study in Luozi that focuses on the choreography and body symbolism of the movement prior to the confrontation described here, see Covington-Ward (2016).

12. This seminar provided the case material and conceptual framework for *Quest*. The Quebec cases, assembled by Bates, as interesting as the Kongo ones, remain to be published.

CHAPTER 1. POPULATION DECLINE AND RISE

1. The phrase "longue durée" is from cultural historian Fernand Braudel (1979), who looked for trends that were outside of consciousness, shaped by a convergence of environmental, economic, sociopolitical, and ideational forces.

2. For another example of the links of memory between the atrocities of the Congo Free State a century ago, and twenty-first-century violence, see Nancy Rose Hunt (2008).

3. There were 531 births and 292 deaths in the five chiefdoms in 1938; the population thus grew by 239 persons, yielding a 1.31 percent growth rate (table 1.3).

4. Régistre d'Hygiène des Villages de la Chefferie de Kibunzi, Dr. Vilen, Kibunzi Hospital, 1936.

5. Ibid.

6. Conversation with Célestin Lusiama, head of Radio Ntomosono, voice of the Free University of Luozi, 2013.

7. Ibid.

8. Postcolonial acknowledgment of Stanley's role in founding the Congo's government is evident in the Luozi Territorial Zone's standard opening to recent annual reports: "Sous la dénomination de Manianga, la creation de Luozi en poste d'Etat de Mbula Matari par Henri Morton Stanley, explorateur Anglais, délegué du Roi Leopold II date du 1er Mai 1881." *Rapport Annuel du Territoire de Luozi, 2000.*

9. This allusion to "pain in the side" mirrors the syndrome *lubanzi* ("stitch in the side"), encountered in North Kongo research on healing. The condition is considered by patients and healers to be difficult or impossible for European biomedical doctors and nurses to treat successfully, because they did not understand its human cause, namely sorcery or ill will. The Luozi fisher's story that names Stanley's labor recruiter as "pain in the side" could be interpreted as a semiconscious or embodied traumatic memory of Congo Free State and early Belgian Congo colonial oppression of Congolese adult males. For a fuller view of *lubanzi*, see Janzen (1982b). For an original and poignant interpretation of the long-term impact of colonial forced labor and labor policy on Congolese male identity, see Gondola (2016). "Oppression, emasculation, and infantilization" are the words Ch. Didier Gondola uses (2016, 4) to characterize the practice and the policy. His analysis links this colonial policy of both the Free State and the Belgian Congo to the attractiveness of radically different liberating identities, such as the urban cowboys, the "Bills," named after Buffalo Bill of the Wild West, picked up in 1950s movies in Kinshasa.

10. The paysannat was a Belgian colonial initiative begun in the 1950s to stimulate agricultural production in regional economies. The initial Kundi project brought three hundred Congolese to settle eight-hectare plots. Under government supervision they were asked to cultivate Urena fibers as a cash crop along with subsistence food crops. The fiber plots were mechanically cultivated. The new community was organized into a cooperative (Nicolai 1961, 68–77). In 2013 the Kundi settlement continued, although fiber cash crops had been discontinued. A herd of beef cattle provided the regional economy with some good protein. A small medical center at Kundi was part of the health zone institutional system.

11. This scene is reminiscent of the Kuba experience during the same period, as reviewed by Vansina's exemplary investigation of the 50 percent decimation hypothesis (2010, 127–49). He is able to assess the numbers of fatalities involved in reported military attacks on the Kuba and in epidemics, as well as eyewitness accounts of villages or populations in a location (either in a settlement or in hiding). He concludes that the Kuba in Kasai Province were indeed reduced by 50 percent during the Congo Free State period.

12. Etat Indépendant du Congo, Dist. de Matadi, Poste de Luozi, Mod. B.I: *Rapports Politiques*, p. 3, "Rapport sur la reprise du Poste de Luozi," Luozi State Archives, 1909–1915.

13. Belgian Colonial Government, *Registre des Rapports sur l'Administration Générale*, Luozi Territorial Archives, 1916.

Chapter 2. Postcolonial Population and Disease Trends

1. Territoire de Luozi, *Rapport Annuel*, 1987, p. 11.

2. Territoire de Luozi, *Rapport Annuel*, 2000, 2002, 2010, 2011. Possibly some of the annual growth rate is absorbed in out migration.

3. See World Health Organization, "Smallpox," www.who.int/csr/disease/smallpox/en/.

4. See World Health Organization, "Human African Trypanosomiasis," www.who.int/trypanosomiasis_african/en/.

5. For more in-depth acquaintance with these diseases, the reader may consult the websites of the Centers for Disease Control (CDC), the World Health Organization (WHO), Santé Rurale du Congo (SANRU), and many other books and manuals on tropical diseases.

6. This obvious fact was noticed by Genevieve Riley, a student in my fall 2013 medical anthropology class. She suggested that these diseases' etiologies have in common a predominant feature of Manianga life: living and working outdoors and being vulnerable to the many diseases whose vectors also live outdoors.

Chapter 3. Health in Household, Family, and Clan

1. This section incorporates some of the ideas published in Janzen 2009.

2. Pierre Bourdieu's generalized economic, symbolic, and biological account of the Kabyle (of Algeria) lineage and how it maintained itself over time through strategies of resource control and marriage alliances was reformulated as the habitus, that social space within which all these resources converged to produce social and symbolic capital (Bourdieu 1977). Colin Murray examined Lesotho lineage societies caught up in labor migration to the mines and factories of South Africa, and the way that investments into local rituals kept home communities and identities alive (Murray 1981).

3. When Bourdieu turned more exclusively to the study of Western industrial society, social reproduction came to require its corollary, cultural reproduction: the way that education, media, the arts, religion, and communications ensure the perpetuation of society's structures, both those of the privileged and those of the marginalized (Bourdieu and Passeron 1977; Nash 1990).

4. Women weavers in Laos inspired Kristin Lundberg (2008) to adopt Bourdieu's habitus as a framework for the study of the social reproduction of health. Lundberg emphasizes the strategies of everyday life in the "identification and attainment of information, social relations, and material goods." Echoing Bourdieu's phenomenological perspective, she writes that "it is at the level of the lifeworld where practice exists and practical knowledge operates, that health comes to be, or is maintained and is reproduced."

5. Shawna Carroll (2008, 2012) studied determinants and consequences for insured and uninsured working women. Karen Stipp (2008) studied the conditions and consequences of lack of insurance for 9 million children in the United States. For both scholars the focus was on commoditized health care and health services, and society's commitment to social reproduction of health. Because health care has become so thoroughly commoditized in the United States, the evidence is strong that there is a social class hierarchy of differential access to that which enables health. Health insurance is not the end all of health; it is an indicator of society's deeper resource flows and structures of jural rights.

6. Carroll (2012) examines the effects of the variable of health insurance on women's cultural constructions of cardiovascular disease. Her hypothesis is that women who have insurance will use more of a biomedical model of risk in their understanding of cardiovascular disease, whereas those who lack insurance may use other models of the disease and the functioning of their bodies in relation to risky behaviors. Health insurance is hypothesized to play the role of a kind of self-fulfilling prophecy in the way women relate to their bodies and the ways they understand the risks of cardiovascular disease.

7. Stipp (2008) notes that children's health insurance accompanies the most important feature of having a "proximal care provider," someone who is regularly consulted by parents when the child becomes ill or there is a threat to health. And as a consequence, their health is better. The uninsured, by contrast, have no easy recourse to a proximal care provider. They thus tend to put off seeking care when children are ill, or they go to the emergency ward, where they encounter different caregivers who do not know them or their history. As a consequence, they are sick more often; have longer, more unnecessary episodes of ill health; and die more frequently. Stipp develops an ecology of health in her analysis that explores the stresses of disparity in health access on families. As a result of this pattern and the presence of a large number of uninsured children, the United States ranks rather low in health indicators among industrialized countries. The social reproduction of health reflects an exacerbated class division between rich and poor (Singer and Baer 2007, 151–80).

8. Jan Vansina's claim regarding the eighteenth-century invention of matrilineality in *Paths in the Rainforests* (1990) is critiqued by Wyatt MacGaffey (2013) for not explaining the connection of this social structural development to the rise of global commercial slavery. A matrilineal estate privileges accumulated capital in women, and their reproduction of labor power and slaves for commercial advantage. In addition, the export of male slaves outnumbered that of female slaves by three to one.

9. Filip De Boeck and Sammy Baloji (2016) feature the land chiefs in their recent anthropological and photographic study of Kinshasa. The search for land by developers, wealthy elites who wish to create their own peri-urban homes, and struggling squatters all provide the historic landowners a boom in rents, short-term use titles, and other arrangements. Technically, according to state and financial statutes, purchase and transfer of title is possible, but the uncertainties of Congolese governance means that the land chiefs are becoming wealthy and prominent in their own right within and on the outskirts of the city. See De Boeck and Baloji (2016), chapter 8, "Ngaliema's Revenge: Urban Expansion, Chiefs, and the Politics of Land," 257–94.

10. See Vansina (1990) and Janzen (1982a) for examples of such comparisons of value, particularly the changing price of a slave on the Atlantic market in the eighteenth and nineteenth centuries, in relation to cloth, livestock, and successive currencies of the region.

11. The set of malaria cures we purchased later to take with us to the United States, where we were advised that medical experts do not recognize malaria very well or know how to deal with it, cost 14,500 CF.

Chapter 4. Public Health and Health Care Institutions, Reconfigured

1. Kivunda Communal Records.

2. The prelude to the Rwandan genocide and war of 1994, and the ongoing low-grade civil war in Burundi offered several examples of local mayors or *bourgmestres* either being able to avert open conflict or seeing their locales break down in open conflict. See Janzen and Janzen (2000).

3. Territoire de Luozi, *Rapport Annuel*, 2008, p. 30.

4. Lettre # 090/BIS/CAB.GOUV/0682/ 2008 and Arret # 013/CAB.MIN/AFF.SAH .SN/08, respectively.

5. Territoire de Luozi, *Rapport Annuel*, 2008, pp. 30–33.

6. Territoire de Luozi, *Rapport Annuel*, 2011.

7. The national Ministry of Health operates as a policy clearing house but provides few funds to administrative units like the DOM of Luozi, according to Franklin Baer (personal communication, January 15, 2018).

Chapter 5. Rejoicing in Our Bodies

1. Interviews with Ngoyi Bukonda, professor of public health at Wichita State University, 2012-15.

Chapter 6. *Dumuna*

1. Parts of this chapter were presented in a lecture to the Center for Area Studies at the University of Leipzig, October 22, 2014, titled "Social Legitimation and Health in Lower Congo."

2. The song with which the ritual closed was hymn no. 527 from the then current Protestant hymnal, *Nkunga mia Kintwadi* (Svenska Missionsforbundet 1957).

3. These ideas were first broached in a 2004 lecture and a presentation on the panel "Voices from the Margins: Constructing Power and Authority," African Studies Association, New York, October 20, 2007.

4. Belgian Colonial Government, *Registre des Rapports sur l'Administration Générale*, Luozi Territorial Archives, Dossier 129, 1916.

5. The *nsengele wa mbele*, or *mbele a lulendo* (sword of power or authority; sword of status) is a vestige of the Christianized and Europeanized Kongo kingdom, widely represented in regalia and documents from historic Kongo. Cécile Fromont (2014) suggests that the *sangamento* dance or greeting by Kongo soldiers depicted in a number of historic drawings are the inspiration for the aggressive stance of nineteenth-century *nkisi Nkondi*. This nkisi was a statue bristling with wedges and nails, with raised arm holding a spear, and associated with magical vengeance. Clan origin legends at Kimbanza and Kimata along the Congo River near the old Manianga market refer to the historic loss of the sword in connection with the fragmentation of power and the dispersal of ancestors, and the consequent loss of clan lands (see Janzen and MacGaffey 1974, 93–94 and cover). Although I do not see any connection between the ways that *dumuna* is practiced and the *sangamento*, it is

possible that there is a continuity between the brandishing of the sword and *lusanga*, one of the names for the men's lodge, the place of political discourse and governance, as well as *nsanga zi Kongo*, a kind of scepter used in healing (Laman 1936, 756).

6. Interview with Bazola Samuel and his friend Jerome, Kintadi village, 1965.

7. Interview with Kintadi village elders, 1965.

8. E. O. Vercraeye, "Rapport de l'investiture *mpu* de Mabaya," AIMO/C2, P.V. #135, 20/8/33, Luozi Territorial Archives, 1933; interview with Kintadi village elders, 1965.

9. These comments on the origin of the Kongo kingdom and relations of regional clans to the kingdom's origins are based on local sources, either from colonial research early in the Belgian colonial era, as available in the Luozi Territorial Archives, or from informants in my own fieldwork. They are being used to illustrate the complexities of colonial administration in the Manianga and how the previously established authorities maneuvered to preserve their power in the face of the colonial state. This work is not the place to consider the numerous scholarly debates on Kongo kingship. But see Sahlins (2017) for a review of some of the literature on the origins of the Kongo kingdom, and Vos (2015) on late precolonial politics of the kingdom and its demise.

10. E. O. Vercraeye, "Rapport sur la chefferie Kimata," AIMO/C2, P.V. #135, 26/8/32, Luozi Territorial Archives, 1932.

11. E. O. Vercraeye, "Rapport de l'investiture *mpu* de Mabaya," AIMO/C2, P.V. #135, 20/8/33, Luozi Territorial Archives, 1933.

12. Kimpianga Mahaniah (2001, 16–20) provides a vivid account—in KiKongo—of the chiefly inauguration of his great grandfather in a chiefdom along the Congo River east of Luozi. The insignia are transferred from a predecessor in the Kindamba clan; the transfer of power closes with the *dumuna* rite.

13. Nancy Rose Hunt's study *A Nervous State: Violence, Remedies, and Reverie in Colonial Congo* (2016) includes a depiction of the zones of exile labor camps in upriver Equateur Province, where many Lower Congo prophets and their followers were sent. Hunt's work masterfully conveys the mental state of the colony, as well as of those who resisted it.

14. *Kidimbu, bidimbu* (pl.), marquee, signe, indication du grad. *Kidimbu kyandumunu*, signe en sautant (Laman, 1936, 119).

15. Interviews and conversations with Thomas Kisolokele, former mayor and advisor of the Centre de Vulgarisation Agricole, 2013.

Chapter 7. Science, Sorcery, and Spirit

1. The materials and issues covered in this chapter are taken in part from my earlier lectures and published work, including "Sickle Cell Anemia, Genetic Counselling, Marriage Planning, and Social Reproduction in Western Equatorial Africa," African Studies Seminar, Beyreuth University, October 28, 2014. The publishers of my following two works are hereby thanked for granting permission for reuse of this material: "Science and Spirit in Postcolonial North Kongo Health and Healing," *African Studies Quarterly* 15, no. 3 (2015): 47–63, and "Science in the Moral Space of Health and Healing Paradigms in Western Equatorial Africa," in *African Medical Pluralism*, edited by William C. Olsen and Carolyn Sargent (Bloomington: Indiana University Press, 2017), 90-109.

2. Mulamba Diese, personal communication, May 2018.

3. Franklin Baer, personal communication, 2018.

4. Jennifer Rosacker, an astute student of medical anthropology at the University of Kansas, on reading about this premarital test for the sickle cell gene, commented that it had become almost as integral a requirement as the bride price.

5. For other applications of the notion of personhood in Central Africa, see discussions of war trauma in Janzen and Janzen (2000, 203–7), and for further elaboration of the notion of personhood in the history of Western thought and medical anthropology, see Janzen 2002, 137–48, chapter 6, "Personhood, Liminality, and Identity."

CHAPTER 8. LEGITIMATION AND DISEASE CONTROL

1. An earlier version of this analysis was aired in my working paper "Divergent Legitimations" (2015a).

2. The reader may still wonder where this notion is grounded in practice or scholarship. In addition to Joanne Macrae's perspective on postconflict restoration and development, and the need for aid agencies to "find the constitution for decision-making" (1997), Kenneth Burke's (1962) understanding of the concept is also helpful: a constitution in its fullest sense is "the fundamental, organic law or principles of government of a nation, state, society, or other organized body . . . embodied in written documents, or implied in the institutions and usages of the country or society" (341). Elsewhere Burke refers to the "constitution behind the constitution" (362).

3. Territoire de Luozi, *Rapport Annuel*, 2012.

4. Franklin Baer, personal communication, 2017 and 2018.

BIBLIOGRAPHY

Antonelli, Richard C., and Donna M. Antonelli. 2004. "Providing a Medical Home: The Cost of Care Coordination Services in a Community-Based, General Pediatric Practice." *Pediatrics* 113 (5): 1522–28.

Ashworth, Adam. 2005. *Witchcraft, Violence, and Democracy in South Africa*. Chicago: University of Chicago Press.

Axelson, Sigbert. 1970. *Culture Confrontation in the Lower Congo*. Falköping, Sweden: Gummessons.

Baer, Franklin. 2007. "FBO Health Networks and Renewing Primary Health Care." Independent consultant report. www.sanru.org/reports/FBOs_and_Renewing_PHC.pdf.

Basolwa Kapita. 1983. *Mbumba Filipo et ses Adeptes au Manianga, 1921–1942*. Kinshasa: Centre de Vulgarisation Agricole.

Batangu-Mpesa, E. F. 2009. *Polyphytothérapie combinatoire et alternative du Paludisme*. Exposé aux 1eres Journées Scientifiques sur le Paludisme en RDC, sur le thème: Paludisme, Récherches et Perspectives en RDCongo. Faculté de Médécine, Université de Kinshasa, October 22-23.

Batukezanga, Zamenga. 1998. *Un Croco a Luozi*. 4th ed. Kinshasa: Mediaspaul.

Beetham, David. 1991. *The Legitimation of Power*. Atlantic Highlands, NJ: Humanities Press International.

Berman, Peter, Carl Kendall, and Karabi Bhattacharyya. 1989. "The Household Production of Health: Putting People at the Center of Health Improvement." In *Towards More Efficacy in Women's Health and Child Survival Strategies*, edited by Ismail Sirageldin et al., 113–29. Baltimore: Johns Hopkins University Press.

Berman, Peter, Carl Kendall, and Karabi Bhattacharyya. 1994. "The Household Production of Health: Integrating Social Science Perspectives on Micro-level Health Determinants." *Social Science and Medicine* 38:205–15.

Biershenk, Thomas, and Jean-Pierre Olivier de Sardan, eds. 2014. *States at Work: Dynamics of African Bureaucracies*. Leiden: Brill.

Bila, Joseph Kapita. 1988. *SIDA en Afrique: Maladie et phénomène social*. Luozi/Kinshasa: Centre de Vulgarisation Agricole.

Bilton, Tony, et al. 1996. *Introductory Sociology*. 3rd ed. London: Macmillan.

Boltanski, Luc, and Laurent Thévenot. 1999. "The Sociology of Critical Capacity." *European Journal of Social Theory* 2 (3): 359–77.

Boorse, Christopher. 1977. "Health as a Theoretical Concept." *Philosophy of Science* 44: 542–77.

Bourdieu, Pierre. 1977. *Outline to a Theory of Practice*. Cambridge: Cambridge University Press.

Bourdieu, Pierre, and J.-C. Passeron. 1977. *Reproduction in Education, Society, and Culture*. Beverly Hills: SAGE.

Braudel, Fernand. 1979. *Civilisation materielle, économie, et capitalisme, 14eme–19eme siécle*. Paris: Armand Colin.

Brausch, Georges. 1961. *Belgian Administration in the Congo*. London: Oxford University Press.

Brockman, Ulrich, Susanne Krassling, and Thomas Lemke. 2011. *Governmentality: Current Issues and Future Challenges*. New York: Routledge.

Burke, Kenneth. 1962. *A Grammar of Motives and a Rhetoric of Motives*. New York: Meridian.

Bush, Kenneth. 2000. "La poliomyelite entre la guerre et la paix." *Bulletin de l'OMS* 3:76–77.

Canguilhem, Georges. 1966. *Le normal et le pathologique*. Paris: Presses Universitaires de France.

Carroll, Shawna. 2008. "Cultural Construction of Disease Risk: A Measure for the Social Reproduction of Health." *Vienna Ethnomedicine Newsletter*, Summer.

Carroll, Shawna. 2012. "From Cultivation to Neglect: Women's Bodies in the Social Reproduction of Health." In *Bodies and Culture: Discourses, Communities, Representations, Performances*, edited by Damon Talbott, Marike Janzen, and Christopher E. Forth, 21-35. Newcastle on Tyne, UK: Cambridge Scholarly Publishing.

Chabal, Patrick, and Jean-Pascal Daloz. 1999. *Africa Works: Disorder as Political Instrument*. Bloomington: Indiana University Press.

Cohen, Lawrence. 1998. *No Aging in India: Alzheimer's, the Bad Family, and Other Modern Things*. Berkeley: University of California Press.

Communauté Evangélique du Congo. 2012. *Vision 2017—Plan Stratégique 2013–2017*. Département des Oeuvres Médicales, Luozi, Novembre.

Conrad, Joseph. 1965. *Heart of Darkness*. Englewood Cliffs, NJ: Prentice-Hall.

Cornet, René J. 1947. *La Bataille du Rail: La construction du chemin de fer de Matadi à Stanley Pool*. Brussels: Louis Cuypers.

Covington-Ward, Yolanda. 2016. *Gesture and Power: Religion, Nationalism, and Everyday Performance in Congo*. Durham, NC: Duke University Press.

De Boeck, Filip, and Sammy Baloji. 2016. *Suturing the City: Living Together in Congo's Urban Worlds*. London: Autograph ABP.

De Heusch, Luc. 2000. *Le roi de Kongo et les monstres sacrés*. Paris: Gallimard.

Dianzungu dia Biniakunu. 1987. *Nsi Yankatu Ngongo eto: Tuzolele Nsi yalubutu, yantoko ye Yicilumukanga Maza* [Our land, we resist: We desire a land that is fertile, beautiful, with sparkling clean water]. Luozi: Editions du CVA.

Dilger, Hansjorg and Ute Luig, eds. 2010. *Morality, Hope, and Grief: Anthropologies of AIDS in Africa*. Oxford: Berghahn.

Doutreloux, Albert. 1967. *L'ombre des fétiches: Société et Culture Yombe*. Louvain, Belgium: Editions Nauwelaerts.

Duclos, Vincent. 2009. "When Anthropology Meets Science: An Interview with Allan Young." *Altérités* 6 (1): 110–18.

Ekholm Friedman, Kajsa. 1991. *Catastrophe and Creation: The Transformation of an African Culture.* Chur, Switzerland: Harwood Academic.

Evans-Pritchard, E. E. 1937. *Witchcraft, Oracles, and Magic among the Azande.* Oxford: Oxford University Press.

Feierman, Steven, and John M. Janzen. 2011. "African Religions." In *Science and Religion around the World,* edited by John Hedley Brooke and Ronald L. Numbers, 229-51. Oxford: Oxford University Press.

Feierman, Steven, and John M. Janzen, eds. 1992. *The Social Basis of Health and Healing in Africa.* Berkeley: University of California Press.

Ferguson, James. 2006. *Global Shadows: Africa in the Neoliberal World Order.* Durham, NC: Duke University Press.

Fortes, Meyer. 1971. "Introduction." In *The Developmental Cycle in Domestic Groups,* edited by Jack Goody, 1-14. Cambridge, UK: Cambridge University Press.

Foster, George, and Barbara Anderson. 1978. *Medical Anthropology.* Hoboken, NJ: John Wiley and Sons.

Foster, Robert J. 1995. *Social Reproduction and History in Melanesia: Mortuary Ritual, Gift Exchange, and Custom in the Tanga Islands.* Cambridge: Cambridge University Press.

Fromont, Cécile. 2014. *The Art of Conversion: Christian Visual Culture in the Kingdom of Kongo.* Chapel Hill: University of North Carolina Press.

Fulwilley, Duana. 2011. *The Enculturated Gene: Sickle Cell Health Politics and Biological Difference in West Africa.* Princeton, NJ: Princeton University Press.

Fund for Peace. 2018. *Fragile States Index.* Washington, DC: The Fund for Peace. https://fragilestatesindex.org/.

Geissler, Paul W., Richard Rottenburg, and Julia Zenker, eds. 2012. *Rethinking Biomedicine and Governance in Africa: Contributions from Anthropology.* Bielefeld, Germany: Transcript Verlag.

Gerhart, Gail M. 1999. "Review of Chabal and Daloz, *Africa Works.*" *Foreign Affairs* (November/December).

Geschiere, Peter. 1997. *The Modernity of Witchcraft: Politics and the Occult in Postcolonial Africa.* Charlotte: University of Virginia Press.

Gondola, Ch. Didier. 2016. *Tropical Cowboys: Westerns, Violence, and Masculinity in Kinshasa.* Bloomington: Indiana University Press.

Goody, Jack. 1976. *Production and Reproduction: A Comparative Study of the Domestic Domain.* Cambridge, UK: Cambridge University Press.

Habermas, Jürgen. 1975. *Legitimation Crisis.* Boston: Beacon.

Hahn, Robert, and Atwood Gaines, eds. 1985. *Physicians of Western Medicine: Anthropological Approaches to Theory and Practice.* Boston: D. Reidel.

Hesse, Gunther. 1979. *Staatsaufgaben: Zur Theorie der Legitimations und Identifikation staatlicher Aufgaben.* Baden-Baden, Germany: Nomos Verlagsgesellschaft.

Hochschild, Adam. 1998. *King Leopold's Ghost: A Story of Greed, Terror, and Heroism in Colonial Africa.* Boston: Houghton Mifflin.

Horton, Robin. 1967. "African Traditional Thought and Western Science." *Africa* 37 (1): 50–72.

Hull, H. F. 1999. "Fighting Stops for Polio Immunization." *Mis à Jour,* December 14.

Hunt, Nancy Rose. 2008. "An Acoustic Register, Tenacious Images, and Congolese Scenes of Rape and Repetition." *Cultural Anthropology* 23 (2): 220–53.

Hunt, Nancy Rose. 2011. "Colonial Medical Anthropology and the Making of the Central African Infertility Belt." In *Ordering Africa: Anthropology, European Imperialism, and the Politics of Knowledge*, edited by Helen Tilley, with Robert J. Gordon. Manchester: Manchester University Press.

Hunt, Nancy Rose. 2016. *A Nervous State: Violence, Remedies, and Reverie in Colonial Congo.* Durham, NC: Duke University Press.

Ingstad, Benedicte, and Susan Reynolds Whyte, eds. 1995. *Disability and Culture.* Berkeley: University of California Press.

Isenboeck, Peter. 2006. "Verstehen und Werten: Max Weber und Jürgen Habermas über die transcendentalen Voraussetzungen Kulturwissenschaftlicher Erkentnisse." In *Aspekte des Weber-Paradigmas: Festschrift für Wolfgang Schluchter*, edited by Albert Gert. Wiesbaden: VS Verlag für Sozialwissenschaften.

Janzen, John M. 1977. "The Tradition of Renewal in Kongo Religion." In *African Religions: A Symposium*, edited by Newell Booth, 69–114. Lagos, Nigeria: Nok.

Janzen, John M. 1978. *The Quest for Therapy in Lower Zaire.* Berkeley: University of California Press.

Janzen, John M. 1982a. *Lemba 1650–1930: A Drum of Affliction in Africa and the New World.* New York: Garland.

Janzen, John M. 1982b. "Lubanzi: The History of a Kongo Disease." In *African Health and Healing*, edited by S. Yoder, 107-19. Los Angeles: Crossroads.

Janzen, John M. 1987 "Therapy Management: Concept, Reality, Process." *Medical Anthropology Quarterly* 1 (1): 68–84.

Janzen, John M. 1992. *Ngoma: Discourses of Healing in Central and Southern Africa.* Berkeley: University of California Press.

Janzen, John M. 2002. *The Social Fabric of Health: An Introduction to Medical Anthropology.* New York: McGraw-Hill.

Janzen, John M. 2009. "The Social Reproduction of Health." In *Essays in Medical Anthropology: Austrian Ethnomedical Society after Thirty Years*, edited by Ruth Kutalek and Armin Prinz, 91-109. Münster, Germany: LIT Verlag.

Janzen, John M. 2012. "Afri-global Medicine: New Perspectives on Epidemics, Drugs, Wars, Migrations, and Healing Rituals." In *Medicine, Mobility, and Power in Global Africa*, edited by Hansjorg Dilger, Abdoulaye Kane, and Stacey Langwick, 115-37. Bloomington: Indiana University Press.

Janzen, John M. 2013a. "*Minkisi* at the Articulations of Individual and Societal Stress Points." *Fragments of the Invisible: The René and Odette Delenne Collection of Congo Sculpture*, 46-53. Cleveland Museum of Art.

Janzen, John M. 2013b. "Renewal and Reinterpretation in Kongo Religion." In *Kongo across the Waters*, edited by Susan Cooksey, Robin Poynor, and Hein Vanhee, 132-42. Gainesville: University of Florida Press.

Janzen, John M. 2015a. "Divergent Legitimations of Post-State Health Institutions in Western Equatorial Africa." Working Paper Series 14, SPP 1448, Adaptation and Creativity in Africa. University of Halle-Wittenberg. http://www.spp1448.de/fileadmin/media/galleries/SPP_Administration/Working_Paper_Series/SPP1448_WP14_Janzen.pdf.

Janzen, John M. 2015b. "Science and Spirit in Postcolonial North Kongo Health and Healing." *African Studies Quarterly* 15 (3): 47–63.

Janzen, John M. 2017. "Science in the Moral Space of Health and Healing Paradigms in Western Equatorial Africa." In *African Medical Pluralism*, edited by William C. Olsen and Carolyn Sargent, 90-109. Bloomington: Indiana University Press.

Janzen, John M., and Reinhild Kauenhoven Janzen. 2000. *Do I Still Have a Life? Voices from the Aftermath of War in Rwanda and Burundi*. University of Kansas Publications in Anthropology 20. Lawrence: University of Kansas.

Janzen, John M., and Wyatt MacGaffey. 1974. *An Anthology of Kongo Religion: Primary Texts from Lower Zaire*. University of Kansas Publications in Anthropology 5. Lawrence: University of Kansas.

Janzen, John M., and Gwyn Prins, eds. 1981. "Causality and Classification in African Medicine and Health." Special issue, *Social Science and Medicine* 15B (3).

Jasanoff, Sheila, ed. 2004. *States of Knowledge: The Co-production of Science and Social Order*. London: Routledge.

Katz, Cindi. 2001. "Vagabond Capitalism and the Necessity of Social Reproduction." *Antipode* 33 (5): 708–27.

Kelly, Ann. 2012. "Serving the City: Community-Based Malaria Control in Dar es Salaam." In *Rethinking Biomedicine and Governance in Africa*, edited by Paul W. Geissler, Richard Rottenburg, and Julia Zenker, 161–76. Bielefeld, Germany: Transcript Verlag.

Kintaudi, Leon, Felix Minuku, and Franklin Baer. 2013. *A Short History of the ECC-DOM Faith-Based Health Network in DR Congo*. Kinshasa: SANRU.

Kleinman, Arthur, and Byron Good, eds. 1985. *Culture and Depression: Studies in the Anthropology and Cross-Cultural Psychiatry of Affect and Disorder*. Berkeley: University of California Press.

Kusikila kwa Kilombo, Yoswa. 1966. *Lufwa evo Kimongi e?* [Death or Pestilence?] Kumba: Academie Congolaise. Translated and published in John M. Janzen and Wyatt MacGaffey, *An Anthology of Kongo Religion: Primary Texts from Lower Zaire*, University of Kansas Publications in Anthropology 5 (Lawrence: University of Kansas, 1974).

Lachenal, Guillaume. 2017. *The Lomidine Files: The Untold Story of a Medical Disaster in Colonial Africa*. Baltimore, MD: Johns Hopkins University Press.

Laman, Karl. 1936. *Dictionnaire KiKongo-Francais*. Brussels: Institut Royal Colonial Belge. Reprint, Ridgewood, NJ: Gregg, 1964.

Laman, Karl. 2000. *Rayons de Vérité*. Stockholm: Svenska Missions Förbundet. Translation and reprint of *Sanningsstraelar: Animism och missionsmetodik bland primitive folk* (Stockholm: Svenska Missionsfoerbundets Foerlag, 1923).

Larson, Ulla. 2003. "Infertility in Central Africa." *Tropical Medicine and International Health* 8 (4): 354–67.

Last, Murray. 1992. "The Importance of Knowing about Not Knowing: Observations from Hausaland." In *The Social Basis of Health and Healing in Africa*, edited by Steven Feierman and John M. Janzen, 393-406. Berkeley: University of California Press.

Leslie, Charles, ed. 1976. *Asian Medical Systems*. Berkeley: University of California Press.

Lipschutz, Ronnie. 2005. "Global Civil Society and Global Governmentality; or, The Search for Politics and State amidst the Capillaries of Social Power." In *Power in Global Governance*, edited by Michael Barnett and Raymond Duvall, 229-48. Cambridge: Cambridge University Press.

Livingston, Julie. 2005 *Debility and the Moral Imagination in Botswana*. Bloomington: Indiana University Press.

Lock, Margaret. 1995. *Encounters with Aging: Mythologies of Menopause in Japan and North America*. Berkeley: University of California Press.

Lock, Margaret, and Vinh-Kim Nguyen. 2010. *An Anthropology of Biomedicine*. New York: Wiley.

Lundberg, Kristin. 2008. *Women Weaving Well-Being: The Social Reproduction of Health in Laos*. PhD diss., University of Kansas.

MacGaffey, Wyatt. 1970a. *Custom and Government in Lower Congo*. Berkeley: University of California Press.

MacGaffey, Wyatt. 1970b. "The Religious Commissions of the BaKongo." *Man* 5:27–38.

MacGaffey, Wyatt. 1990. "The Personhood of Ritual Objects: Kongo *Minkisi*." *Etnofoor* 3 (1): 45–61.

MacGaffey, Wyatt. 2000. *Kongo Political Culture: The Conceptual Challenge of the Particular*. Bloomington: Indiana University Press.

MacGaffey, Wyatt. 2013. "Notes on Vansina's Invention of Matrilinearity." *Journal of African History* 54 (2): 269–80.

Macrae, Joanne. 1997. "Dilemmas of Legitimacy, Sustainability, and Coherence: Rehabilitating the Health Sector." In *Rebuilding Societies after Civil War*, edited by Krishna Kumar, 183-201. Boulder, CO: Lynne Rienner.

Mahaniah, Kimpianga. 1981. "La structure multidimensionelle de guérison a Kinshasa, capital du Zaire." *Social Science and Medicine* 15B (3): 341–50.

Mahaniah, Kimpianga. 1989b. *La problematique crocodilienne a Luozi: Discours et moyens de lutte*. Luozi: Editions Centre de Vulgarisation Agricole.

Mahaniah, Kimpianga. 2001. *Kikulu kia chefferie Luangu*. Luozi: Presses de l'Université Libre de Luozi.

Mahaniah, Kimpianga. 2008. *Kikulu kia Bamanianga*. Luozi: Presses de l'Université Libre de Luozi.

Mahaniah, Kimpianga. 2009. *Carte postale du Territoire de Luozi*. Luozi: Presses de l'Université Libre de Luozi.

Mahaniah, Kimpianga. 2012. *Mon grandpère paternel: Souvenirs d'un notable congolais de Luozi*. Luozi: Presses de l'Université Libre de Luozi.

Manker, Ernst. 1929. *Bland Kristralbergens folk*. Stockholm: Albert Bonniers Förlag.

Masamba ma Mpolo, Jean. 1981. "Kindoki as Diagnosis and Therapy." *Social Science and Medicine* 15B (3): 405–14.

Mbaku, Joswe. n.d. [2013]. *Qu'est-ce-que la Drepanocytose?* Université Libre de Luozi, Psychology Department.

Meillassoux, Claude. 1964. *L'anthropologie économique des Gourou en Cote d'Ivoire*. Paris: Mouton.

Meillassoux, Claude. 1981. *Maidens, Meal, and Money: Capitalism and the Domestic Community*. Cambridge, UK: Cambridge University Press.

Mertens, J. 1942. *Les chefs couronnés chez les BaKongo Orientaux*. Brussels: Institut Royal Colonial Belge.

Miller, Joseph. 1988. *Way of Death: Merchant Capitalism and the Angolan Slave Trade, 1730–1830*. Madison: University of Wisconsin Press.

Mudimbe, V. Y. 1981. "Signes thérapeutiques et prose de la vie en Afrique noire." *Social Science and Medicine* 15B (3): 195-212.

Murray, Colin. 1981. "The Work of Men, Women, and the Ancestors: Social Reproduction in the Periphery of Southern Africa. In *The Social Anthropology of Work*, edited by Sandra Wallman, 337–63. New York: Academic Press.

Nash, Roy. 1990. "Bourdieu on Education, Social, and Cultural Reproduction." *British Journal of Sociology of Education* 114:531–47.

Nicolai, Henri. 1961. *Luozi: Géographie régionale d'un pays du Bas-Congo.* Brussels: Académie Royale des Sciences d'Outre-Mer.

Öhrneman, Josef. 1968. *Perspektiv från Kongo.* Stockholm: Gummerson.

Pfeiffer, James, and Rachel Chapman. 2010. "Anthropological Perspectives on Structural Adjustment and Public Health." *Annual Review of Anthropology* 39:149–65.

Pierson, Christopher. 1992. "Review of Beetham, *Legitimation of Power.*" *Sociology* 26 (3): 550.

Pirenne, J. H. 1959. "Les éléments fondamentaux de l'ancienne structure territorial et politique du Bas-Congo." *Académie Royale des Sciences d'Outre-Mer, Bull. des Séances* 3:557–77.

Richards, Audrey. 1930. *Hunger and Work in a Savage Tribe: A Functional Study of Nutrition among the Southern Bantu.* Reprint, New York: Routledge, 2004.

Rusca, Maria, and Klaas Schwartz. 2012. "Divergent Sources of Legitimacy: A Case Study of International NGOs in the Water Services Sector in Lilongwe and Maputo." *Journal of Southern African Studies* 39 (3): 681–97.

Sahlins, Marshall. 2017. "The Atemporal Dimension of History: In the Old Kongo Kingdom, For Example." In *On Kings*, by David Graeber and Marshall Sahlins, 139-222. Chicago: Hau Books.

Sanderson, Jean-Paul. 2000. "Le Congo Belge entre mythe et réalité: Une analyse du discours démographique colonial. *Population* 55 (2): 331–55.

Sautter, Gilles. 1966. *De l'Atlantique au fleuve Congo: Une géographie du sous-peuplement.* 2 vols. Paris: Mouton.

Schatzberg, Michael. 2001. *Political Legitimacy in Middle Africa: Father, Family, Food.* Bloomington: Indiana University Press.

Schechter, Darrow. 2013. *Die Kritik der instrumentallen Vernunft von Weber bis Habermas.* Baden-Baden, Germany: Nomos.

Silla, Eric. 1998. *People Are Not the Same: Leprosy and Identity in Twentieth-Century Mali.* Portsmouth, NH: Heinemann.

Singer, Merrill, and Hans Baer. 2007. *Introducing Medical Anthropology.* New York: Alta Mira.

Smith-Nonini, S. 2006. "Conceiving the Health commons: Operationalizing a 'Right' to Health." *Social Analysis* 50 (3): 233–45.

Sohier, A. 1954. *Traité élémentaire de droit coutumier du Congo Belge.* Brussels: Maison F. Larcier.

Soret, Marcel. 1959. *Les Kongo Nord-Occidentaux.* Paris: Presses Universitaires de France.

Stanley, Henry Morton. 1885. *The Congo and the Founding of Its Free State.* New York: Harper and Brothers.

Stipp, Karen. 2008. "Ecological Perspective on Inequality and the Social Reproduction of Ill Health." The University of Kansas School of Social Welfare, PhD diss.

Svenska Missionsförbundet. 1939. *L'oeuvre médicale de la SMF au Congo Belge. Rapport Annuel 1938.* Matadi, Congo: Svenska Missionsförbundet.

Svenska Missionsförbundet. 1957. *Nkunga mia Kintwadi.* Leopoldville: LECO.

Thornton, John. 1983. *The Kingdom of Kongo, 1641–1718.* Madison: University of Wisconsin Press.

Tilley, Helen. 2011. *Africa as a Living Laboratory: Empire, Development, and the Problem of Scientific Knowledge, 1870–1950.* Chicago: University of Chicago Press.

Trolli, Giovanni, and Lucien Louis Dupuy. 1934. *Contribution à l'étude de la démographie des Bakongo au Congo Belge 1933.* Bruxelles: Fonds Reine Elisabeth pour l'Assistance Médicale aux Indigènes du Congo Belge (FOREAMI).

van Erp, Herman H. H. 2000. *Political Reason and Interest: Philosophical Legitimation of the Political Order in a Pluralistic Society.* Aldershot, UK: Ashgate.

Vansina, Jan. 1973. *The Tio Kingdom of Middle Congo, 1880–1892.* London: Oxford.

Vansina, Jan. 1990. *Paths in the Rainforests: Toward a History of Political Tradition in Equatorial Africa.* Madison: University of Wisconsin Press.

Vansina, Jan. 2010. *Being Colonized: The Kuba Experience in Rural Congo, 1880–1960.* Madison: University of Wisconsin Press.

Van Wing, J. 1959. *Etudes BaKongo.* Brussels: Desclée de Brouwer.

Vos, Jelmer. 2015. *Kongo in the Age of Empire (1860–1913): The Breakdown of a Moral Order.* Madison: University of Wisconsin Press.

Wamba-dia-Wamba, Ernest. 1999. "Bundu dia Kongo: A Kongolese Fundamentalist Religious Movement." In *East African Expressions of Christianity*, edited by Thomas Spear and Isaria N. Kimambo, 213-28. Oxford: James Currey.

Weber, Max. 1980. *The Theory of Social and Economic Organization.* London: Collier Macmillan.

World Health Organization. 1978. *Primary Health Care* [The Alma-Ata Declaration]. Geneva: World Health Organization.

World Health Organization. 2000a. *L'annuaire statistique.* Geneva: World Health Organization.

World Health Organization. 2000b. *Rapport sur la Santé dans le Monde.* Geneva: World Health Organization.

World Health Organization. 2001. "WHO/UNICEF Joint Mission, DR Congo (18–29 Jun 2001)." World Health Organization, Kinshasa, June 29. https://reliefweb.int/report/democratic-republic-congo/whounicef-joint-mission-dr-congo-18-29-jun-2001.

World Health Organization. 2012. *Statistical Annual.* Geneva: World Health Organization.

Young, Crawford, and Thomas Turner. 1985. *The Rise and Decline of the Zairian State.* Madison: University of Wisconsin Press.

INDEX

postcolonial: health and healthcare transformations, 110–11; land access and ownership, 175; population and disease trends
of the, 65–86; reintroduction of chiefship, 164; scholarship in anthropology
on health, healing, and science, 191–94
power, 4, 8, 13, 24, 36–37, 89, 110, 112–13,
134, 144, 149, 159–60, 176, 182, 184, 188–
89, 198, 206, 226, 233; biopower, 162;
illicit or illegitimate, 4–5, 25, 163–64,
168, 213, 217, 233; legitimate, 36, 166,
168, 184. *See also* authority; legitimation;
sorcery; witch
primary health care (PHC), 10–12, 21, 44,
105, 119–26, 143–59. *See also* health;
health zones; public health; World
Health Organization
prophet (*ngunza*), prophetic, prophetism
(*kingunza*), 17–18, 42, 78, 102; appropri-
ation, and practice of *dumuna*, 168–70,
185; clandestine meeting, deportation,
or exile of, 186–87; divination by, 138;
healing the whole person, 36, 211–12;
role of, in Kongo religious commissions,
163–65. *See also* Dona Beatrice, Kimpa
Vita; Kimbangu, Simon; Kitoko,
Samuel; Masamba, Esaie; *ngunza*
protein malnutrition (*kwashiorkor*), 77–78,
263–65; 16, 220; as disease in decline,
222; as principal disease, 83–85
public health, 4, 13, 20, 23, 33, 44, 45, 49,
109–44, 190–91, 214–15; Belgian colonial, 60–61, 113; early launch, in Zaire/
DRC, 119–21, 195; intervention in sleeping sickness outbreak, 74–76; in relation
to sickle cell anemia, 198–99. *See also*
Baer, Franklin; Bukonda, Ngoyi; Fonds
Reine Elisabeth pour l'Assistance Medi-
cale aux Indigènes du Congo Belge;
health zones; Kintaudi, Leon; Minuku,
Felix; Ngwete, Martin; primary health
care; Santé Rural du Congo; Tshimika,
Pakisa

railroad: Matadi to Ango-Ango in Mayombe, 41, 60; Matadi to Kinshasa,

56–58, 64, 95, 140; postcolonial dilapi-
dation of, 233. *See also* colonial labor;
Congo Free State; diseases
RDC. *See* République Démocratique du
Congo
REGIDESO. *See* Régie des Eaux
Régie des Eaux (REGIDESO), 20, 112,
140, 142, 144, 218, 220
Republic of Congo (Brazzaville), xiv, 171,
235n7
République Democratique du Congo
(RDC). *See* Democratic Republic of the
Congo
respiratory infections, severe; 106, 223; as
principal disease, 77
rheumatism, 78
Richards, Audrey, 104
Riley, Genevieve, 237n6 (ch2)
Rosacker, Jennifer, 241n4 (ch7)
Rottenberg, Richard, 9, 162
Rusca, Maria, 8–9, 161

Sahlins, Marshall, 240n9 (ch6)
Salmonella Typhi, 82. *See also* typhoid fever
Sanderson, Jean-Paul, 44
SANRU. *See* Santé Rural du Congo
Santé Rural du Congo (SANRU), 112,
120–22, 133, 194, 217–18, 221, 224, 228,
231; as national NGO and broker for
fundraising and medical supplies, 122,
194, 217; origins and evolution of, 120–
22; research program of, 194. *See also*
Baer, Franklin; Église du Christ au
Congo
Sautter, Gilles, 41, 44
Schatzberg, Michael, 162–63
Schechter, Darrow, 160
schistosomiasis, 83, 135, 214, 216–17, 219,
222–23, 226, 231; as principal disease,
77–78. *See also* bilharzia
Schräpel, Norman, 235n2
Schwartz, Klaas, 8–9, 161
science, 29, 168, 213, 232; cultural construction of, 192; in evolutionary biology and
malaria, 195; and religion, 191–94; social,
162; and spirit, 200, 232; and technology

AFRICA AND THE DIASPORA:
HISTORY, POLITICS, CULTURE

Edited by Thomas Spear, Neil Kodesh,
Tejumola Olaniyan, Michael G. Schatzberg,
and James H. Sweet

www.ingramcontent.com/pod-product-compliance
Lightning Source LLC
Chambersburg PA
CBHW071016280326
41935CB00011B/1373